VETERINARY PUBLIC HEALTH :
NEW TRENDS

VETERINARY PUBLIC HEALTH: NEW TRENDS

Editors

H. RAHMAN

L.R. CHATLOD

Z.B. DUBAL

BIOTECH

2025

BIOTECH BOOKS

NEW DELHI

ISBN : 978-81-7622-230-3

Published by : **BIOTECH BOOKS**
4762-63/23, Ansari Road,
Darya Ganj, New Delhi - 110 002
Phone : 011-43003222
email : biotechbooks@yahoo.co.in

PRINTED IN INDIA

FOREWORD

I am happy to learn that the ICAR Research Complex for NEH Region, Sikkim Centre, Tadong, Gangtok is bringing out a publication entitled, "Veterinary Public Health New Trends" based on lead papers presented at National Symposium on "Transboundary Zoonotic Diseases: Challenges and Strategies" under aegis of Indian Association of Veterinary Public Health Specialists (IAVPHS). In view of the increasingly globalized world, threat of the transboundary diseases disrupting food supplies and posing serious human and animal health crisis is looming large. Sanitary and phytosanitary compliance under WTO/GATT regime is another dimension for agriculture and animal related international trade. To meet these challenges, professionals engaged in disease management, monitoring, surveillance and livestock related trade need to be exposed to recent advances in transboundary zoonotic diseases, food borne infections, molecular epidemiology and diagnostic tools for detection of pathogens and residue analysis of foods and feeds.

Perusal of the contents of "Veterinary Public Health New Trends" revealed that it covers wide ranging topics including trans-boundary diseases such as avian and swine flu, bacterial and parasitic zoonoses, food borne infections, environmental pollutants, etc. In view of the potential bioterrorism threats, it is national imperative to make the people aware of the bio-safety and biosecurity issues and the national and international regulations concerning these. Therefore, presenting information relevant to different aspects of veterinary public health, emerging and re-emerging zoonotic diseases, residue analysis, etc. is nationally relevant. In this perspective, I believe the information presented in "Veterinary Public Health New Trends" will be potentially useful to diverse group of people including veterinary professions, teachers, students, livestock and poultry farmers, policy makers, people dealing with animal and animal products related trade and common people interested in learning about public health in general.

I appreciate the efforts of Dr. H. Rahman and his associates for compiling the lectures in the form of a useful book.

KRISHI BHAVAN
NEW DELHI 110001

(K.M.L. Pathak)
Deputy Director General (AS)

PREFACE

The significant progress in the area of diagnosis and control of transmissible diseases particularly with advent of the advanced molecular techniques and increased public awareness about the safe food and environment are the important tools for the professionals, if they upkeep and use the knowledge wisely and judiciously. The documentation of the recent advances in the area of Veterinary Public Health including all the aspects related to hygiene and transboundry zoonotic diseases is a prime requisite to bring about an awareness amongst the vast majority of the veterinarians, medicos, researchers and environmentalists who are directly or indirectly involved in these activities.

One of the major responsibilities of the veterinary professionals is to provide health cover to the livestock population for production of safe food without degrading the environment. It encompasses the responsibilities to break the cycle of zoonotic infections and to minimize the animal husbandry related occupational and public health hazards. The present scenario under Sanitary and Phyto-sanitary regulations in the global trade of livestock products also call for development and use of appropriate technologies to overcome the WTO barriers in international trade.

This publication "Veterinary Public Health New Trends" is the outcome of lead lectures delivered by the experts during the VIIIth Conference of Indian Association of Veterinary Public Health Specialists (IAVPHS) and National Symposium on *"Transboundry Zoonotic diseases : Challenges and Strategies"* held at ICAR Research Complex for NEH Region, Sikkim Centre, Gangtok. We are deeply indebted to all the contributors for this lecture series as without their help, it could not have seen the light of the day.

The editors feel very much obliged to Dr. K.M.L. Pathak, Deputy Director General (Animal Sciences), Dr. S. V. Ngachan, Director, ICAR Research Complex for NEH Region and all those who have helped directly or indirectly in bringing out this publication.

Editors

CONTENTS

LIST OF CONTRIBUTORS

Dr. A.K. Bera
I.V.R.I., Eastern Regional Station
37, Belgachia Road, Kolkata–700 037

Dr. A. Deka
Division of Animal Health,
ICAR Research Complex for NEH Region,
Umiam, Meghalaya – 793 103

Dr. Ashwani Kumar
Department of Veterinary Public Health
CCS Haryana Agricultural University,
Hisar-125001, Haryana

Dr. A.M. Paturkar
Department of Veterinary Public Health
Bombay Veterinary College
Mumbai- 400 012

Dr. Ashok Kumar
Division of Veterinary Public Health
Indian Veterinary Research Institute,
Izatnagar-Bareilly 243 122

Dr. A.G. Karpe
Krantisinh Nana Patil College of Veterinary Science,
Shirwal, Dist-Satara, Maharashtra Animal and
Fishery Sciences University, Nagpur

Dr. Ahsan ul Haq
Department of Poultry Science
University of Agriculture, Faisalabad, Pakistan

Dr. B. Biswas
R.G. Kar Medical College and Hospital,
1, Belgachia Road, Kolkata

Dr. B.D.Sharma
Division of Livestock Products Technology
Indian Veterinary Research Institute,
Izatnagar - 243122, (U.P.)

Dr. B. Sharanagouda
Dairy Science College,
KVAFSU, Bangalore

Dr. B.M. Veeregowda
Dairy Science College,
KVAFSU, Bangalore

Dr. B.V. Venkateshaiah
Dairy Science College,
KVAFSU, Bangalore

Dr. D. Bhattacharya
I. V. R. I., Eastern Regional Station
37, Belgachia Road, Kolkata – 700 037

Dr. D.K. Sinha
Epidemiology section, CADRAD
Indian Veterinary Research Institute,
Izatnagar - 243122, (U.P.)

Dr. D.N.Garg
College of Veterinary Sciences,
& Ex-Addl. Director Research,
C.C.S. Haryana Agricultural University,
Hisar – 125004, Haryana

Dr. Fawwad Ahmad
Department of Poultry Science
University of Agriculture, Faisalabad, Pakistan

Dr. G.Leena
Dairy Science College,
KVAFSU, Bangalore

Dr. Gyanendra Gongal
Medical Officer (VPH)
WHO Regional Office for South-East Asia
New Delhi

Dr. H. Arunkumar
Dairy Science College,
KVAFSU, Bangalore

Dr. H.K. Sharma
Division of Veterinary Public Health & Hygiene
Faculty of Veterinary Sciences and Animal
Husbandry (SKUAST-Jammu)
R.S. Pura, Jammu - 181 102, J&K

Dr. H. Rahman
Project Director,
Project Directorate on Animal Disease Monitoring &
Surveillance,
Bangalore-560 024

Dr. H.V. Mohan
Division of Veterinary Public Health,
Indian Veterinary Research Institute,
Izatnagar-243 122, Bareilly,
Uttar Pradesh, India

Dr. I. Shakuntala
Division of Animal Health,
ICAR Research Complex for NEH Region,
Umiam, Meghalaya – 793 103

Dr. J. Deb
R. G. Kar Medical College and Hospital,
1, Belgachia Road, Kolkata - 700 004

Dr. J.K. Sharma
Department of Veterinary Public Health
Guru Angad Dev Veterinary and
Animal Sciences University,
Ludhiana-141 004

Dr. JPS Gill
Department of Veterinary Public Health
College of Veterinary Sciences
Guru Angad Dev Veterinary and
Animal Sciences University,
Ludhiana–141 004

Dr. K.N. Bhilegaonkar
Division of Veterinary Public Health
Indian Veterinary Research Institute,
Izatnagar, Bareilly-243 122, (U.P)

Dr. L.R. Chatlod
ICAR Research Complex for NEH Region
Sikkim Centre,
Tadong, Gangtok- 737102

Dr. Masood Akhtar
Department of Poultry Science
University of Agriculture, Faisalabad, Pakistan

Dr. Muhammad Ashraf
Department of Poultry Science
University of Agriculture, Faisalabad, Pakistan

Dr. M.Z. Siddiqui
Department of Poultry Science
University of Agriculture, Faisalabad, Pakistan

Dr. Nishi Pande
Division of Veterinary Public Health & Hygiene
Faculty of Veterinary Sciences & Animal
Husbandry (SKUAST-Jammu)
R.S. Pura 181 102, Jammu, J&K

Dr. N.N.Zade
Department of Veterinary Public Health
Nagpur Veterinary College
Seminary Hills, Nagpur (Maharashtra)

Dr. Papri Pal
ICAR Research Complex for NEH Region
Sikkim Centre,
Tadong, Gangtok- 737102

Dr. Rajesh Agrawal
Division of Veterinary Public Health & Hygiene
Faculty of Veterinary Sciences & Animal Husbandry
(SKUAST-Jammu)
R.S. Pura, Jammu-181 102, J&K

Dr. R.K. Agarwal
B & M Division
Indian Veterinary Research Institute,
Izatnagar, Bareilly - 243 122, (U.P.)

Dr. R.K. Joshi
Department of Veterinary Microbiology
College of Veterinary Science and A.H.
N.D. University of Agriculture and Technology
Kumarganj, Faizabad, U.P.

Dr. R.P. Kolhe
Krantisinh Nana Patil College of Veterinary Science,
Shirwal, Dist-Satara
Maharashtra Animal & Fishery Sciences University,
Nagpur-06

Dr. R.S. Rathore
Division of Veterinary Public Health,
Indian Veterinary Research Institute,
Izatnagar-243 122, (U.P.)

Dr. Rashmi Singh
College of Veterinary & Animal Sciences
G.B. Pant University of Agriculture & Technology
Pantnagar-263 145, Uttarakhand

Dr. R.J. Zende
Department of Veterinary Public Health
Bombay Veterinary College
Mumbai- 400 012

Dr. Samiran Bandyopadhyay
NRC on Yak,
Dirang, Arunachal Pradesh

Dr. Sandeep Ghatak
Department of Veterinary Public Health
Guru Angad Dev Veterinary and Animal
Sciences University, Ludhiana - 141 004

Dr. Sandeep P. Chaudhari
Department of Veterinary Public Health
Nagpur Veterinary College
Seminary Hills, Nagpur-06, Maharashtra

Dr. Sanjay Kumar
Division of Microbiology, Defence Research &
Development Establishment,
Jhansi Road, Gwalior-474 002, Madhya Pradesh

Dr. S.B. Barbuddhe
ICAR Research Complex for Goa,
Ela, Old Goa-403 402

Dr. S.K. Kotwal
Division of Veterinary Public Health & Hygiene
Faculty of Veterinary Sciences & A.H.
R.S. Pura, Jammu-181102, J&K

Dr. S.P. Singh
College of Veterinary & Animal Sciences
G.B. Pant University of Agriculture and Technology,
Pantnagar-263 145, Uttarakhand

Dr. S.R. Garg
Department of Veterinary Public Health,
College of Veterinary Sciences,
C.C.S. Haryana Agricultural University,
Hisar- 125 004, Haryana

Dr. Subhasish Bandyopadhyay
I. V. R. I., Eastern Regional Station
37, Belgachia Road, Kolkata – 700 037

Dr. S.V.S. Malik
Division of Veterinary Public Health
Indian Veterinary Research Institute,
Izatnagar - 243 122, (U.P.)

Dr. Shriya Rawat
Division of Veterinary Public Health
Indian Veterinary Research Institute,
Izatnagar, Bareilly - 243 122, (U.P)

Dr. Vijay J. Jadhav
Department of Veterinary Public Health
CCS Haryana Agricultural University,
Hisar-125001, Haryana

Dr. Y. Singh
Department of Veterinary Public Health
CCS Haryana Agricultural University,
Hisar–125 004, Haryana

Dr. Z.B. Dubal
Division of Animal Health,
ICAR Research Complex for NEH Region,
Umiam, Meghalaya – 793 103

SUBJECT INDEX

Hanta Virus
Japanese Encephalitis
Kyasanur Forest Disease
Rabies

Zoonotic Helminth Infection

Transmission
Zoonotic Cestode Infection
Zoonotic Nematode Infection
Zoonotic Trematode Infection

Zoonotic Mycoplasmoses

Classification
Conclusion
Definition
Detection
Obstacles and Proposals

THE EDITORS

Dr. H. Rahman did his M.V. Sc, from Punjab Agricultural University, Ludhiana, PhD from GB Pant Univ. Agril. Tech. Pantnagar and Post-Doc from Robert Koch Institute, Germany. He is currently holding the post of Joint Director of ICAR Research Complex, Sikkim Centre, Tadong. He has earlier worked at IVRI, Izatnagar and ICAR Research Complex for NEH Region, Umiam, Meghalaya as Head of Division and Associate Professor in Assam Agricultural University, Guwahati. Veterinary microbiology, public health, molecular biotechnology are major areas of his specialization. Dr. Rahman is a recipient of many awards and honors in the field of veterinary science. He has more than 150 publications including, books, research papers, bulletins, book chapters, manuals, souvenir, etc. in his credit. He is presently handling more than 10 externally funded projects on different field of agriculture and animal sciences. He has applied for patents on production of gamma irradiated Salmonella toxoid vaccine. He visited different countries like Germany, the Netherlands, Belgium, Italy, France, Bhutan and Nepal.

Dr. L.R. Chatlod did his M.V. Sc. and Ph.D. in Veterinary Public Health from Indian Veterinary Research Institute, Izatnagar, Bareilly. He joined Agricultural Research Service in 2003. Presently he is working as Scientist at ICAR Research Complex for NEH Region, Sikkim Centre, Gangtok. Food borne infection and intoxication and, molecular detection and characterization of enteric bacteria are major areas of his specialization. He has more than 40 publications including, research papers, book chapters, manuals, Conference papers, Popular Articles, Lead papers, Technical bulletins, souvenir and Extension folders etc. in his credit. He is presently associated with three externally funded projects and three institute project on different field of animal sciences.

Dr. Z.B. Dubal did his M.V. Sc. in Veterinary Public Health from Bombay Veterinary College, Konkan Krishi Vidyapeet, Maharashtra and Ph.D. from Indian Veterinary Research Institute, Izatnagar, Bareilly. After M.V. Sc., he was working as a SRF under the scheme of National Agricultural Technology Project and currently holding the post of Scientist, ICAR Research Complex for NEH Region, Umiam, Meghalaya. Food borne infection and intoxication and, molecular detection and characterization of enteric viruses are major areas of his specialization. He has more than 30 publications including, research papers, bulletins, book chapters, manuals, souvenir, abstracts etc. in his credit. He is presently handling one externally funded project and three institute project on different field of animal sciences.

1

SWINE FLUE (H_1N_1) - INDIAN SCENARIO

N.N. Zade and Sandeep P. Chaudhari

Swine flu (swine influenza) is a respiratory disease caused by viruses (influenza viruses) that infect the respiratory tract of pigs and result in nasal secretions, a barking-like cough, decreased appetite, and listless behaviour. Swine flu produces most of the same symptoms in pigs as human flu produces in people. Swine flu can last about one to two weeks in pigs that survive. Swine influenza virus was first isolated from pigs in 1930 in the U.S. and has been recognized by pork producers and veterinarians to cause infections in pigs worldwide. In a number of instances, people have developed the swine flu infection when they are closely associated with pigs (for example, farmers, pork processors), and likewise, pig populations have occasionally been infected with the human flu infection. In most instances, the cross-species infections (swine virus to man; human flu virus to pigs) have remained in local areas and have not caused national or worldwide infections in either pigs or humans. Unfortunately, this cross-species situation with influenza viruses has had the potential to change. Swine influenza (also called swine flu, hog flu, and pig flu) is an infection by any one of several types of swine influenza virus. Swine influenza virus (SIV) is any strain of the influenza family of viruses that is endemic in pigs. As of 2009, the known SIV strains include influenza C and the subtypes of influenza A known as H_1N_1, H_1N_2, H_3N_1, H_3N_2, and H_2N_3.

Influenza, A (H_1N_1) (earlier know as swine flu) is a new influenza virus causing illness in people. Investigators think the 2009 swine flu strain, first seen in Mexico, should be termed novel H_1N_1 flu since it is mainly found infecting people and exhibits two main surface antigens, H_1 (hemagglutinin type 1) and N_1 (neuraminidase type 1). Recent investigations show the eight RNA strands from novel H_1N_1 flu have one strand derived from human flu strains, two from avian (bird) strains, and five from swine strains.

H_1N_1 has included the Spanish Flu of 1918 to 1919, the Asian flu of 1957 to 1958 and the Hong Kong Flu of 1967 to 1968. India too was faced with the dilemma of whether it should call the latest pandemic threat 'swine flu' or 'Mexican flu'. The US embassy in Delhi informed the Union Health Ministry that Center for Disease Control and Prevention (CDC) in Atlanta had decided to abandon the term 'swine flu' and refer to the present outbreak as the 'H_1N_1 flu'. The two different diseases; swine flu (which is a disease in pigs) and human flu (associated with humans) need to have different names. The term "swine flu" for the ongoing H_1N_1 flu (in humans) was a factual error and has caused considerable and completely unnecessary damage to pork industry.

In Europe, the Paris-based World Organization for Animal Health, known by its French acronym, OIE, warned that the term 'swine flu' is a misnomer. Instead, the organization proposed the term 'North American Influenza' in keeping with a tradition of identifying outbreaks with the region of origin. The European Commission meanwhile had proposed changing the name of the virus to 'novel flu'. This incorrect nomenclature has lead many countries, in the beginning to impose unjustified ban and measures related to the import of pigs and pig products. It should be noted that the name of a disease always has heavy implications and has a very strong impact on the behaviour of consumers worldwide. As an example, it is easy to remember that at the beginning of the 'avian influenza crisis' in 2004 the consumption of poultry products decreased up to 50% in some countries and lead thousands of people to unemployment and economic distress, without any benefit for public and animal health. Also, because the disease was named 'swine flu' at the beginning, some countries decided to destroy all pig populations, without appropriate equipment, and again without any benefit for the animal or public health. Calling it swine flu had prompted countries like Russia and China to ban pork imports from Mexico and the US while Indonesia had expressed plans to destroy imported pork and other swine products. Health officials in Egypt ordered the slaughter of the estimated 300,000 pigs in that country because they thought H_1N_1 was spreading from swines to humans.

The World Health Organization announced on April 30, 2009 that it would stop using the term 'swine flu' to avoid confusing the public about the source and cause of the flu. The announcement was made after Egypt began slaughtering thousands of pigs in a misguided effort to prevent the spread of swine flu. WHO spokesperson Dick Thompson said that the agriculture industry and the UN food agency had expressed concerns that the term 'swine flu' was misleading consumers and needlessly causing countries to ban pork products and order the slaughter of pigs. Thus, "rather than calling this swine flu, we're going to stick with the technical scientific name H_1N_1 influenza A."

The term 'swine flu' is misleading, but the reason we're caught up in calling it 'swine' influenza is that the H_1N_1 was first found in pigs. Even though, the virus is a combination of genes from swine influenza, avian influenza and human influenza. It's a real combination of a lot of viruses which, is a common scenario in influenza viruses. The H_5N_1 was labeled 'avian' influenza because it was first found in birds. The novel H_1N_1 virus is derived originally from a strain that lived in pigs and this origin gave rise to the common name of 'swine flu', usually used by mass media.

Preliminary genetic characterization found that the hemagglutinin (HA) gene was similar to that of swine flu viruses present in U.S. pigs since 1999, but the neuraminidase (NA) and matrix protein (M) genes resembled versions present in European swine flu isolates. The six genes from American swine flu are themselves mixtures of swine flu, bird flu, and human flu viruses. While viruses with this genetic makeup had not previously been found to be circulating in humans or pigs, there is no formal national surveillance system to determine what viruses are circulating in pigs.

Influenza viruses can change its make-up in one of two ways : Antigenic drift is a series of mutations that cause the virus to gradually evolve over time. Antigenic shift is an abrupt change in the surface antigen proteins that suddenly creates a new subtype of the virus. In the history of influenza outbreaks, antigenic shift is the cause behind pandemics in 1918 (Spanish flu), 1957 (Asian flu) and 1968 (Hongkong flu) because the populations have not developed antibody protection against the virus.

Pigs are thought to be ideal 'mixing vessels' for the reassortment of human, swine and avian influenza A viruses. They probably play a crucial role in the emergence of new strains which can start a global pandemic. However, the reassortment could also occur in a human, infected with both human and animal influenza A viruses. Swine flu or the A/ H_1N_1 virus is a hybrid of the human influenza, avian influenza and swine influenza. It is an acute and highly contagious respiratory disease caused by the orthomyxovirus that caused the last influenza pandemic in 1917 that accounted for 20 million deaths worldwide.

The orthomyxoviruses are composed of one genus and three types, namely A, B and C. The diseases caused by these viruses are acute respiratory with prominent systemic symptoms. The type A is associated with worldwide epidemics. The B and C types are not as severe as the A type and there is no animal reservoir associated with these types. The orthomyxoviruses contain a single stranded negative RNA genome divided into 8 segments. The virus is surrounded by a lipid bilayer with surface glycoproteins, namely hemagglutinin (H) and neuraminidase (N). The H and N antigens are variable. There are 13 different H antigens and 9 different N antigens found in birds. This translates into 117 different combinations that can occur and affect humans. Viral attachment is mediated by hemagglutinin. At a cellular level, the virus enters the cell through pinocytosis and the viral RNA fuses with the host vacuole membrane thereby capping the viral RNA and is transported to the nucleus where replication starts. Viral particles are released into the blood via budding from infected cells. These infected cells then die via a mechanism of programmed cell death or apoptosis. The segmented genome of the influenza virus allows the possibility of rearrangement of genetic material to occur and this may account for the appearance of new variants in simultaneously infected cells.

Swine influenza virus is common throughout pig populations worldwide. Transmission of the virus from pigs to humans is not common and does not always lead to human influenza, often resulting only in the production of antibodies in the blood. If transmission does cause human influenza, it is called zoonotic swine flu. People with regular exposure to pigs are at increased risk of swine flu infection. The meat of an infected animal poses no risk of infection when properly cooked.

The H_1N_1 virus has adapted itself to humans and is highly contagious. By contrast, the H_5N_1 'bird flu' was (and is) spreading between birds, only occasionally spreading from a bird to a human, and even more rarely spreading from one human to a second (and maybe a third) and then stopping. So the new H_1N_1 isn't behaving like a swine flu virus in the sense that H_5N_1 is behaving like a bird flu virus, even though by the conventions of virology it is still classified as a swine flu virus.

WHO has begun probing the claim that H_1N_1 may have evolved while growing virus in labs for making vaccines. The swine flu causing H_1N_1 virus that is threatening to wreak havoc in the world through unleashing a pandemic may have been created in a lab as a result of a human error. H_1N_1 virus could have accidentally evolved in eggs scientists use to grow viruses and drug makers while making vaccines, as suspected by Adrian Gibbs, an Australian researcher.

Swine flu became the media's and publics favourite topic and thus made a troubling impact on swine producers and pork processors in the country. The swine industry suffered a lot of damage and it will take time for the industry to recover from this. Even after WHO urged the use of the virus' technical name, A(H_1N_1), while referring to it. Still radio, television and print media continue to use the term 'swine flu'. Though there is no formal or state policy banning the use of 'swine flu', a term 'A (H_1N_1)' may be used when referring to this type of flu.

ORIGIN OF CURRENT INFLUENZA H_1N_1 VIRUS

Influenza viruses of two subtypes, H_1N_1 and H_3N_2, have been causing respiratory infections in humans since 1977. Before that, it was believed that only one human subtype circulated each flu season.

Major changes in the surface glycoproteins of influenza virus called antigenic shift, lead to worldwide epidemics of influenza known as pandemics. There have been six instances of antigenic shift since 1889. In that year, H_2N_2 viruses circulated, followed by H_3N_8 in 1900, H_1N_1 in 1918, H_2N_2 in 1957, H_3N_2 in 1968, and H_1N_1 in 1977. Each pandemic strain carries HA and NA proteins that have been absent in humans for many years, and therefore immunity is either very low or nonexistent.

Influenza viruses of the H_3N_2 subtype were still circulating in humans in May of 1977 when H_1N_1 viruses were isolated in China and then Russia. In the winter of 1977-78 the H_1N_1 viruses caused epidemic infection throughout the Northern Hemisphere. The results of serological tests indicated that the HA and NA glycoproteins of the 1977 H_1N_1 viruses were very similar to those from viruses of the same subtype which circulated in 1950. It is possible that the 1950 H_1N_1 influenza virus was truly frozen in nature or elsewhere and that such a strain was only recently introduced into man. The suggestion is clear; the virus was frozen in a laboratory freezer since 1950, and was released, either on intent or accident, in 1977.

The close genetic identity between the 1950 and 1977 H_1N_1 strains was revealed by oligonucleotide mapping. In this technique, purified viral RNA is cleaved with an enzyme,

RNAse T_1 that cuts the RNA after every G base. The oligonucleotides are labeled at the 52-end with 32P, separated by two-dimensional gel electrophoresis, and detected by exposing the gel to X-ray film. The oligonucleotides form a pattern ('fingerprint', pictured) that can reveal genetic differences between virus isolates. This technique is more sensitive than serologic assays, but only provides information on about 10-15% of the viral RNA. However, the larger oligonucleotides are a representative sample of the entire genome. There was a minimum of 8 bases changes among the large oligonucleotides of the RNAs of the 1950 and 1977 H_1N_1 viruses. In contrast, the RNA of the 1977 H_1N_1 isolate had 38 base changes compared with a 1947 H_1N_1 isolate (Racaniello, 2009).

VIRUS CHARACTERISTICS

The virus is a novel strain of influenza. It was also determined that the strain contained genes from five different flu viruses: North American swine influenza, North American avian influenza, human influenza, and two swine influenza viruses typically found in Asia and Europe. Further analysis showed that several of the proteins of the virus are most similar to strains that cause mild symptoms in humans (Wilkinson, 2009).

CONTAGIOUSNESS

The virus is contagious and is believed to spread from human to human in much the same way as seasonal flu. The most common mechanisms by which it spreads are by droplets from coughs and sneezes of infected people, and touching a surface or the hand of a person contaminated with virus, and then touching one's mouth or nose (UK HPA, 2009). The US CDC had recommended that people should wait at least a day after their fever subsides (usually 3-4 days after the onset of symptoms) before resuming normal activities, but it has been found that they can continue to shed virus for several days after that (ABC News, 2009). The contagiousness of the virus may change as it mutates.

EVOLUTION POTENTIAL

Experts are of concern that the new virus strain could mutate over the coming period, as new H_1N_1 influenza virus has been described as 'very unstable', meaning it could mix and swap genetic material when exposed to other viruses. Both H_1N_1 and H_5N_1 are unstable so the chances of them exchanging genetic material are higher, whereas a stable (seasonal flu) virus is less likely to take on genetic material. The H_5N_1 virus is mostly limited to birds, but in rare cases when it infects humans it has a mortality rate of 60% to 70% (Reuters, 2009). Experts worry about the emergence of a hybrid of the more virulent Asian-lineage HPAI (highly pathogenic avian influenza) A/H_5N_1 strain (media labeled 'bird flu') with more human-transmissible Influenza A strains such as this novel 2009 swine-origin A/ H_1N_1 strain (media labeled 'swine flu'), especially since the H_5N_1 strain is and has been for years endemic in birds in countries like China, Indonesia, Vietnam and Egypt (FAO, 2008; Reuters 2009).

TRANSMISSION

Transmission Between Pigs

Influenza is quite common in pigs and antibodies to the virus are also common in pigs. The main route of transmission is through direct contact between infected and uninfected animals. These close contacts are particularly common during animal transport. Intensive farming may also increase the risk of transmission, as the pigs are raised in very close proximity to each other (Saenz *et al.*, 2006; Gilchrist *et al.*, 2007). The direct transfer of the virus probably occurs either by pigs touching noses, or through dried mucus. Airborne transmissions through the aerosols produced by pigs coughing or sneezing are also an important means of infection .The virus usually spreads quickly through a herd, infecting all the pigs within just a few days. Transmission may also occur through wild animals, such as wild boar, which can spread the disease between farms (Saenz *et. al.*, 2006).

Transmission to Humans

People who work with poultry and swine, especially people with intense exposures, are at increased risk of infection with influenza virus endemic in these animals, and constitute a population of human hosts in which zoonosis and reassortment can co-occur (Gray and Kayali, 2009). Other professions at particular risk of infection are veterinarians and meat processing workers, although the risk of infection for both of these groups is lower than that of farm workers (Myers *et. al.*, 2006).

SPECIES AFFECTED

Swine

Before being transmitted to humans, the viruses circulated in swine which has allowed for the undetected persistence and evolution of this potentially pandemic strain for many years. Pigs are known to have been infected by humans. Pigs are susceptible to influenza viruses that can also infect both humans and birds, so they may act as a "mixing vessel" in which reassortment can occur between flu viruses of several species.

Humans

Humans have been affected since early 2009.

Birds

In Chile it has been discovered that the human H_1N_1/09 virus had jumped, unmutated, to birds. The infected turkeys suffered only mild effects. The turkey meat remains safe to eat.

Swine influenza virus is common throughout pig populations worldwide. Transmission of the virus from pigs to humans is not common and does not always lead to human influenza, often resulting only in the production of antibodies in the blood. If transmission does cause human influenza, it is called zoonotic swine flu. People with regular exposure to pigs are at increased risk of swine flu infection. The meat of an infected animal poses no risk of infection when properly cooked.

SIGNS AND SYMPTOMS

In Swine

In pig's influenza infection produces fever, lethargy, sneezing, coughing, difficulty in breathing and decreased appetite. In some cases the infection can cause abortion. Although mortality is usually low (around 1–4%), the virus can produce weight loss and poor growth, causing economic loss to farmers. Infected pigs can lose up to 12 pounds of body weight over a 3 to 4 week period.

In Humans

Direct transmission of a swine flu virus from pigs to humans is occasionally possible (called zoonotic swine flu). According to the Center for Disease Control and Prevention (CDC), in humans the symptoms of the 2009 "swine flu" H_1N_1 virus are similar to those of influenza and of influenza-like illness in general. Symptoms include fever, cough, sore throat, body aches, headache, chills and fatigue. The 2009 outbreak has shown an increased percentage of patients reporting diarrhea and vomiting (CDC, 2009). The 2009 H_1N_1 virus is not zoonotic swine flu, as it is not transmitted from pigs to humans, but from person to person. The most common cause of death is respiratory failure. Other causes of death are pneumonia (leading to sepsis), high fever (leading to neurological problems), dehydration (from excessive vomiting and diarrhea) and electrolyte imbalance. Fatalities are more likely in young children and the elderly.

DIAGNOSIS

The two major tests that are being used are the nasopharyngeal (or back of the throat) swab for viral culture, the gold standard, and the indirect evidence test by detection of antibodies to novel H_1N_1 with PCR studies.

PREVENTION

Prevention of swine influenza has three components: prevention in swine, prevention of transmission to humans, and prevention of its spread among humans.

In Swine

Methods of preventing the spread of influenza among swine include facility management, herd management and vaccination. Because much of the illness and death associated with swine flu involves secondary infection by other pathogens, control strategies that rely on vaccination may be insufficient. Control of swine influenza by vaccination has become more difficult in recent decades, as the evolution of the virus has resulted in inconsistent responses to traditional vaccines.

Facility management includes using disinfectants and ambient temperature to control virus in the environment. The virus is unlikely to survive outside living cells for more than two weeks, except in cold (but above freezing) conditions and it is readily inactivated by disinfectants. Herd management includes not adding pigs carrying influenza to herds that have not been exposed to the virus. The virus survives in healthy carrier pigs for up to 3 months and can be recovered from them between outbreaks. Carrier pigs are usually responsible for the introduction of SIV into previously uninfected herds and countries, so new animals should be quarantined (CFSPH, 2009). After an outbreak, as immunity in exposed pigs wanes, new outbreaks of the same strain can occur.

In Humans

Prevention of Pig to Human Transmission : Swine can be infected by both avian and human influenza strains and therefore are host where the antigenic shifts can occur that create new influenza strains. The transmission from swine to human is believed to occur mainly in swine farms where farmers are in close contact with live pigs. Although strains of swine influenza are usually not able to infect humans this may occasionally happen, so farmers and veterinarians are encouraged to use a face mask when dealing with infected animals. The use of vaccines on swine to prevent their infection is a major method of limiting swine to human transmission. Risk factors that may contribute to swine-to-human transmission include smoking and not wearing gloves when working with sick animals (Ramirez *et. al.*, 2006).

Prevention of Human to Human Transmission : Influenza spreads among humans through coughing or sneezing and people touching infected surface and then touching their own nose or mouth. Consumption of pork products does not spread swine flu, since the virus is not transmitted through food (CDC, 2009). The swine flu in humans is most contagious during the first five days of the illness. Although some people, most commonly children, can remain contagious for up to ten days. Diagnosis can be made by sending a specimen, collected during the first five days for analysis (CDC, 2009b).

Recommendations to prevent spread of the virus among humans include using standard infection control against influenza. This includes frequent washing of hands with soap and water or with alcohol-based hand sanitizers, especially after being out in public. Chances of transmission are also reduced by disinfecting household surfaces, which can be done effectively with a diluted chlorine bleach solution (WQHC, 2009). Influenza can spread via cough or sneezes, but an increasing body of evidence shows small droplets containing the virus can linger on tabletops, telephones and other surfaces and be transferred via the fingers to the mouth, nose or eyes. Alcohol-based gel or foam hand sanitizers work well to destroy viruses and bacteria. Anyone with flu-like symptoms such as a sudden fever, cough or muscle aches should stay away from work or public transportation and should contact a doctor for advice.

Social distancing is another tactic. It means staying away from other people who might be infected and can include avoiding large gatherings, spreading out a little at work, or perhaps staying home and lying low if an infection is spreading in a community. Public health and other responsible authorities have action plans which may request or require social distancing actions depending on the severity of the outbreak.

VACCINATION

Vaccines are available for different kinds of swine flu. Although the current trivalent influenza vaccine is unlikely to provide protection against the new 2009 H_1N_1 strain CDC (2009c). Vaccines against the new strain are being developed and could be ready as early as November 2009 (Petty, 2009).

TREATMENT

In Swine

As swine influenza is rarely fatal to pigs, little treatment beyond rest and supportive care is required (CFSPH, 2009). Vaccination and animal management techniques are most important in these efforts. Antibiotics are also used to treat this disease, which although they have no effect against the influenza virus, do help prevent bacterial pneumonia and other secondary infections in influenza-weakened herds (CFSPH, 2009).

In Humans

If a person becomes sick with swine flu, antiviral drugs can make the illness milder and make the patient feel better faster. They may also prevent serious flu complications. For treatment, antiviral drugs work best if started soon after getting sick (within 2 days of symptoms). Beside antivirals, supportive care at home or in hospital, focuses on controlling fevers, relieving pain and maintaining fluid balance, as well as identifying and treating any secondary infections or other medical problems. The U.S. Centers for Disease Control and Prevention recommends the use of Tamiflu (oseltamivir) or Relenza (zanamivir) for the treatment and/or prevention of infection with swine influenza viruses; however, the majority of people infected with the virus make a full recovery without requiring medical attention or antiviral drugs.

INDIAN SCENARIO

The number of Swine Flu infected people rose to more than 1000 for the first time. The hardest hit state is Maharashtra with its two mega-cities, Mumbai and Pune on the top of the list of the victims.

Total Confirmed Cases in India	4885**
Total Deaths in India	134***
Total Confirmed Cases Worldwide	Over 2094378*
Total Deaths Worldwide	2185*
Last Updated September, 2009	

Sources : **PIB *WHO

India's battle with the H_1N_1 virus has been aided by relatively high summertime temperatures and by the sheer fact that the virus has been more prevalent in the country's urban centres and amongst the middle to upper class. An internal government report estimates that 3-5 million people will require vaccination after a full-fledged pandemic hits the country, with the WHO estimating that approximately 33% of India's population will be infected. As all viruses, H_1N_1 will mutate and is likely to pose a major challenge to the socio-economic stability of the country. Thus, the health professionals (including the veterinary and medical) should be properly equipped to combat the situation (Honawar, 2009).

Cases of the virus have been largely limited to the country's urban centres. However, with a population density of approximately 345 people per square kilometer, it could be only a matter of time before the number of confirmed cases surge. By comparison, Australia, the UK and the US have population densities of 2.84, 246 and 31 respectively, yet they comprise some of the worst hit countries. An outbreak of H_1N_1 amongst India's rural population or slum dwellers is likely to go by relatively unnoticed, as the common man remains oblivious to the symptoms which are deceivingly similar to the common flu (Honawar, 2009).

EFFECT OF SWINE FLU ON INDIAN INDUSTRY/ ECONOMY

1. Tourism Industries

Tourism Industry which has already been hit by the global economic slowdown is now scared that if the swine flu is not controlled by the time of tourism peak season, it will take a toll on the tourism industry.

2. Airline

As the swine flu is likely to slow down the movement of people across the country and within the country, it is likely to bring down the occupancy rate of the airlines thereby, hitting the top line and bottom line.

3. Bollywood Industry

The flu has also disrupted the business of Bollywood. Shootings were cancelled and cinema halls were shut down in some cities as the toll from the H_1N_1 pandemic rose to eight. More than 850 have so far tested positive from the virus.

4. Media

Community and people have a propensity to gaze at more news in times of scourge. Media companies will gain more advertisements in times of crisis and also due to festival season.

5. Multiplexes and Retail

Just when multiplexes thought business was reverse on trail, the virus has punched movie theaters. Peoples started avoiding going to multiplexes and malls thus, impacting the sales of shops and multiplexes.

Pandemics typically diminish GDP growth rates by 0.5-2% according to viciousness. Swine Flu and monsoons will affect GDP adversely and it is approximated to be lower by 1%. Thus, GDP growth rate and Indian GDP growth rate will be relegated to 5.8-6.2% (Gupta, 2009).

The global spread of the virus indicates that cooler temperatures are more conducive to the survival and commutability of the disease, with countries in the southern hemisphere bearing the brunt of H_1N_1 to date. Chile, Argentina, Australia, and the UK have been hit the hardest, with England recording over 30,000 confirmed cases in a week. The World Health Organization (WHO) reports that close to 1800 people have died globally and more than 182,000 have been infected, a number that is expected to increase as the more heavily populated northern hemisphere slips into winter season. Of increasing concern however, is that as the influenza survives within societies for longer period of time, a more virulent strain of the virus could become increasingly dominant and durable within clusters of society, even during the summer months. H_1N_1 virus could infect more than two billion people globally within the next two years, an aspect which is particularly worrying given that this strain has never been witnessed and everyone on the planet is immunologically vulnerable (Honawar, 2009).

REFERENCES

ABC News (2009). Swine Flu Might Be Even More Contagious, 16 September, 2009. www.google.com.

CDC (2009). Swine Flu and You. http://www.cdc.gov/swineflu/swineflu_you.htm.

CDC (2009a). Q & A : Key facts about swine influenza (swine flu) – Spread of Swine Flu. http://www.cdc.gov/swineflu/key_facts.htm

CDC (2009b). Q & A : Key facts about swine influenza (swine flu) – Diagnosis. http://www.cdc.gov/swineflu/key_facts.htm.

CDC (2009c). Q & A : Key facts about swine influenza (swine flu) – Virus Strains. http://www.cdc.gov/swineflu/key_facts.htm

CFSPH (2009). Influenza Factsheet. Iowa State University. http://www.cfsph.iastate.edu/Factsheets/pdfs/influenza.pdf.

FAO (2008). Avian Influenza Disease Emergency Situation Update http://www.fao.org/docs/eims/upload//246457/aj097e00.

Gilchrist, M.J., Greko, C., Wallinga, D.B., Beran, G.W., Riley, D.G. and Thorne, P.S. (2007). The potential role of concentrated animal feeding operations in infectious disease epidemics and antibiotic resistance. *Environ. Hlth. Perspect.* **115** : 313–6.

Gray, G.C. and Kayali, G. (2009). Facing pandemic influenza threats: the importance of including poultry and swine workers in preparedness plans. *Poultry Sci.* **88** : 880–4.

Gupta, V.P. (2009). Impact of Swine Flu on India and its Economy. Indian MBA.com

Honawar, R. (2009). Swine Flu and India–Are we panicking unnecessarily? Strategic fortnight group. www.google.com

Myers, K.P., Olsen, C.W., Setterquist, S.F. (2006). Are swine workers in the United States at increased risk of infection with zoonotic influenza virus? *Clin. Infect. Dis.* **42** : 14–20.

Petty, L. (2009). Swine Flu Vaccine Could Be Ready in 6 Weeks. NBC Connecticut. http://www.nbcconnecticut.com/news/local/CT-Company-Making-Swine-Flu-Vaccine.html

Racaniello, V. (2009). Origin of current influenza H1N1 virus. Virology blog, about viruses and viral disease.

Ramirez, A., Capuano, A.W., Wellman, D.A., Lesher, K.A., Setterquist, S.F and Gray, G.C. (2006). Preventing zoonotic influenza virus infection. *Emerg. Infect. Dis.* **12** : 996–1000.

Reuters (2009). New virus very unstable, more changes seen-expert http://www.reuters.com/article/asiaCrisis/idUSHKG147261.

Saenz, R.A., Hethcote, H.W. and Gray, G.C. (2006). Confined animal feeding operations as amplifiers of influenza. *Vector Borne Zoonotic Dis*. **6** : 338–46.

UK HPA (2009) Public information on swine flu. www.google.com

Wilkinson, E. (2009), "What scientists know about swine flu"? BBC News. http://news.bbc.co.uk/2/hi/health/8028371.stm

WQHC (2009). Chlorine Bleach: Helping to Manage the Flu Risk. Water Quality & Health Council.

http://www.waterandhealth.org/newsletter/new/winter_2005/chlorine_bleach.html.

2

BIRD FLU-ZOONOSIS THREAT AND PREVENTIVE STRATEGIES

Ahsan ul Haq, Masood Akhtar, M.Z. Siddiqui, Fawwad Ahmad and Muhammad Ashraf

Zoonosis is the communication of infectious animal diseases to human. It may be due to parasitic, bacterial, fungal or viral agents. The infectious diseases could spread by various routes *e.g.* respiratory, through vectors, feco-oral route, and contaminated hands or through direct contact. Toxoplasmosis, Brucellosis, Mad Cow, Rabies, Trichomoniosis, Anthrax, Babesiosis are some major zoonotic diseases in large animals. While Newcastle disease, Fowl Pox, Salmonellosis, Colibacillosis, Chlamydiosis and Avian Influenza are the major zoonotic problems in birds.

Bird flu (H_5N_1) is still prevalent in many countries including China, Pakistan, Bangladesh, India, Nepal, Thailand and Vietnam. Data analysis shows that in Pakistan, 29 out breaks of bird flu were recorded in 2006, 59 in 2007 and 8 in 2008. During 2007 three humans became sick and one of them died due to H_5N_1 infection.

Types of Avian Influenza Viruses

Type A, B and C, type A virus can attack on birds and mammals while type B and C can attack on human. Viruses consist of 13H and 9N surface proteins and can attack in following manners.

H_1N_1 and H_3N_2 can attack on pigs.

H_1N_1 and H_2N_2 and H_3N_2 can attack on humans.

H_3N_8 and H_7N_7 can attack on horses.

While 117 of H and N surface viruses can attack the birds.

Mostly bird flu is caused by H_5N_1, H_7N_1 and H_9N_1 influenza virus. Composition of influenza virus is reported as 0.0–1.1% RNA, 70–75% protein, 20–24% lipid and 5–8% carbohydrate. Virus that can transfer from bird to human is H_5N_1.

SIGN AND SYMPTOMS IN BIRDS

The symptoms like cough, fever, sore throat, muscle aches, decreased activity, decreased feed consumption and emaciation, decreased egg production, huddling, oedema of head and face, nervous disorders and diarrhea are generally found in birds infected with the influenza virus. Whereas, acute respiratory distress, coughing, fever, sore throat and sneezing are the major symptoms found in humans caused by bird flu virus. Deaths due to bird flu are mainly because of viral pneumonia and acute respiratory distress.

TRANSMISSION OF DISEASE FROM BIRD TO HUMAN

Most of the avian viruses cannot affect the human. During 1990, bird flu cases in human were found in many areas like Hong Kong, Europe, Middle East and Asia.

1. Transmission directly from infected bird to the human.
2. Droppings, saliva and nasal secretion of the wild or infected migratory birds.
3. Some domestic birds may be infected through contaminated feed, water and soil, while the human may be infected from domestic birds, cages, equipments and infected air etc.
4. Unhygienic open-air markets of poultry eggs and birds.

Table 2.1 : Status of Human Cases and Deaths in the Regional Countries

Sr. No.	Country	2003		2004		2005		2006		2007		2008		Total	
		C	D	C	D	C	D	C	D	C	D	C	D	C	D
1.	Azerbaijan	0	0	0	0	0	0	8	5	0	0	0	0	8	5
2.	Cambodia	0	0	0	0	4	4	2	2	1	1	0	0	7	7
3.	China	1	1	0	0	8	5	13	8	5	3	0	0	27	17
4.	Djibouti	0	0	0	0	0	0	1	0	0	0	0	0	1	0
5.	Egypt	0	0	0	0	0	0	18	10	25	9	0	0	43	19
6.	Indonesia	0	0	0	0	20	13	55	45	42	37	10	8	127	103
7.	Iraq	0	0	0	0	0	0	3	2	0	0	0	0	3	2
8.	Lao PDR	0	0	0	0	0	0	0	0	2	2	0	0	2	2
9.	Nigeria	0	0	0	0	0	0	0	0	1	1	0	0	1	0
10.	Thailand	0	0	17	12	5	2	3	3	0	0	0	0	25	17
11.	Turkey	0	0	0	0	0	0	12	4	0	0	0	0	12	4
12.	Vietnam	3	3	29	20	61	19	0	0	8	5	2	2	103	49
13.	Pakistan	0	0	0	0	0	0	0	0	1	1	0	0	1	1
14.	Myanmar	0	0	0	0	0	0	0	0	1	0	0	0	1	0
TOTAL		4	4	46	32	98	43	115	79	86	59	12	10	361	227

Source : World Health Organization. C : Case, D : Death.

VACCINE

Killed vaccine of bird flu is recommended at the age of 30-32 days. This vaccine is injected intramuscular, when the titer of vaccine decreases, there is a need to repeat this vaccine. Normally it is repeated after 4-5 months.

PREVENTION AND ERADICATION

To reduce the risk of transfer of infectious diseases from animals/birds to human, research findings indicated that following measures should be adopted.

1. Hygienic measures during working with animals / birds.

2. Wearing of gloves, masks and gum boots.
3. Special care in laboratory.
4. Stopping of eating and drinking while working with birds/animals or in laboratory, elimination of the carrier birds from flocks.
5. Burning or proper disposal of contaminated litter/ manure and proper disinfections of the cages/nests are the best preventive measures, which can reduce the chance of zoonosis.
6. Wild birds are main source of disease spreading; prohibit the entry of wild bird in the farm.
7. Separation of healthy birds from the infected birds.
8. Cleaning of footwear, clothing, vehicles, insemination equipment, feed and water etc.
9. Stopping the spread of virus carried by fecal matter.
10. Carefully wash the utensils used for slaughtering and preparing chicken meat. After and before handling of poultry we should wash our hands thoroughly.
11. Proper medicine has not been prepared for the treatment of bird flu but as a primary treatment a flu drug Oseltamivir (Tamiflu) is recommended.
12. High temperature during cooking can reduce chances of bird flu virus. So we should cook the chicken until the juices remain as minimum as possible.

CONTROL STRATEGIES

1. There must be national programme for the control and prevention of avian influenza in each country so that transboundary chances can be reduced.
2. There is a need to strengthen disease control, to increase awareness among the farmers/consumers.
3. Research based proper vaccine development is required.

4. Vaccine evaluation and quality assurance system needs strengthening.

5. Surveillance for detection of various influenza sub types infecting commercial and backyard poultry is required/ improvement.

6. There is a need of establishing regional surveillance units/laboratories across the countries.

7. National capacity building in each country can improve the condition.

8. Payment of compensation against depopulation of H_5N_1 affected poultry flocks requires quick action.

9. National reference laboratory for poultry must be established in each country.

10. Proper checking of poultry and its products also reduce the chances.

11. Information exchange system must be active and up dated among the countries affected.

With the help of above mentioned preventive measures and strategies the transfer of bird flu to human can be controlled. Currently, Pakistan is free from clinical avian influenza at the moment and OIE has confirmed Pakistan Poultry free from avian influenza.

3

IMPACT OF ZOONOTIC DISEASES ON HUMAN HEALTH AND ECONOMY

H. Rahman, L.R. Chatlod and Papri Pal

The word Zoonosis (Pleural: Zoonoses) was introduced by Rudolf Virchow in 1880 to include collectively the diseases shared in nature by man and animals. Later WHO in 1959 defined that Zoonoses are "those diseases and infections which are naturally transmitted between vertebrate animals and man." Zoonoses include only those infections where there is either a proof or a strong circumstantial evidence for transmission between animals and man. Zoonoses (zoonotic diseases) are a heterogeneous group of diseases with a variety of causative agents. More than 300 such diseases of diverse etiology have been recognized.

EMERGING ZOONOSES

Contrary to "lingering" zoonoses, public awareness of "emerging" zoonoses is very high. WHO/FAO/OIE joint consultation on emerging zoonotic diseases held in Geneva, 3-5 May 2004, defined an emerging zoonosis as "a zoonosis that is newly recognized or newly evolved, or that has occurred previously but shows an increase in incidence or expansion in geographical, host or vector range".

Emerging zoonotic diseases have potentially serious human health and economic impacts and their current upwards trends are likely to continue. Examples are avian influenza, severe acute respiratory syndrome (SARS), Bovine Spongiform

Encephalitis (BSE) and the Nipah virus. Some of the "lingering" zoonoses are re-emerging in some regions, although they seem to attract less public awareness. Brucellosis, dog rabies and parasitic diseases such as cysticercosis/taeniasis and echinococcosis/hydatidosis are few examples.

CLASSIFICATION

With the advanced laboratory techniques and increased awareness among medical and veterinary scientists, ecologists and biologists, more than 300 zoonoses of diverse etiology are now recognized. Thus, a very large number of zoonoses call for classification especially for easy understanding. It can be classified in many ways.

A. According to the Mechanism of Transmission

1. **Anthropozoonoses :** Infections transmitted to man from lower vertebrates (ex: rabies, toxoplasmosis).
2. **Zooanthropozoonoses :** Infections transmitted from man to animals (ex: diphteria, amebiosis).
3. **Amphixenoses :** Infections maintained in both man and lower vertebrates, and may be naturally transmitted in either direction (*e.g.* : *Staphylococcus*, Mycobacterium).

B. According to the Life Cycle

1. **Direct Zoonoses :** Transmitted from infected vertebrate host to a susceptible vertebrate host by direct contact or by a mechanical vector. No developmental change or propagation of the organism occurs during the transmission (*ex.:* Rabies, trichinosis, and brucellosis).
2. **Cyclozoonoses :** Requires more than one vertebrate host, but no invertebrate host. (*Ex.:* Echinococcosis, human taeniasis and Pentastoma infections).
3. **Metazoonoses :** Agent multiplies, develops, or both in an invertebrate host before transmission to a vertebrate host is possible. (This means that a definite prepatent

or incubation period must be completed before transmission.) (*Ex.*: Arboviruses, plague, and schistosomiasis).

4. **Saprozoonoses** : To transmit these infections a non-animal development site or reservoir is required, such as food plants, soil, or other organic material. (*Ex:* larva migrans and some of the mycotic diseases).

C. According to the Etiology (Mostly Used)

1. Bacterial zoonoses *e.g.*, anthrax, brucellosis, plague, salmonellosis, etc.
2. Viral zoonoses *e.g.*, Rabies, influenza, Japanese encephalitis, yellow fever etc.
3. Rikettsial zoonoses *e.g.*, Q-fever, typhus fever, etc.
4. Fungal zoonoses *e.g.*, cryptococcosis, candidiasis, ringworms, etc.
5. Protozoal zoonoses *e.g.*, toxoplasmosis, leishmaniasis, trypanosomiasis, etc.
6. Helminthic zoonoses *e.g.*, echinococcosis (hydatid disease), taeniasis, guineaworm infection, etc.
7. Ectoparasitic zoonoses *e.g.*, scabies, myiasis, etc.
8. Zoonoses caused by unconventional agents (Prions) *e.g.*, transmissible spongiform encephalopathies, bovine spongiform encephalopathy (TSE, Mad cow disease), etc.

D. According to the Mode of Transmission

Zoonoses can be transmitted in many ways. On this they are classified as :

1. Contact borne.
2. Food and Water borne.
3. Air borne.
4. Vector-borne.

E. According to Occupation

Specialized professional activities provide opportunities for intimate contact between man and animals. The activities promote exposure to the pathogen and may act as risk factors for the transmission of select zoonoses.

1. ***Agriculture :*** Anthrax, Brucellosis, Leptospirosis, Japanese Encephalitis, Rabies.
2. ***Animal Product Manufacture :*** Anthrax, Brucellosis, Salmonellosis, Tuberculosis.
3. ***Sylvan and Camp Dwellers :*** Brucellosis, Vibriosis, Leptospirosis, Plague, Tuberculosis, Japanese encephalitis.
4. ***Recreational :*** Salmonellosis, Leptospirosis, Glanders, plague, Rabies, Ornithosis.
5. ***Laboratory :*** Anthrax, Brucellosis, Leptospirosis, Salmonellosis, Marburg, Ebola.
6. ***Epidemiological :*** Salmonellosis, Campylobacteriosis, Ornithosis, JE, Rabies.
7. ***Emergency :*** Plague, Rabies.

TRANSFER WAYS OF ANIMAL DISEASES TO HUMAN

1. Human Consumption of Raw or Undercooked Meat, Poultry, or Seafood. For example, if meat contains harmful bacteria, and it is not thoroughly cooked to kill the bacteria, food borne illness/disease may result once the food is eaten.
2. Human being bitten or stung by an insect or animal. For example, dog bites may seriously injure tissues and can also transmit bacterial infections and rabies, a disease of viral origin. The bite of a diseased rat may transmit any of several diseases to man, including plague, salmonellosis, leptospirosis, and rat-bite fevers; the bites of venomous snakes and fish can lead to human discomfort and death.

3. Human Contact with the Flesh of an Animal. The flesh of various types of fish is toxic to man. For example, Japanese puffers contain the poisonous chemical compound tetrodotoxin; scombroid fish harbor *Proteus morganii,* which causes gastrointestinal diseases; and mullet and surmullet can cause nervous disturbances.

FACTORS THAT INFLUENCE THE EMERGENCE OR REEMERGENCE OF ZOONOSES

Microbiologic infections acquired from animals, known as zoonoses, pose a risk to public health. An estimated 60% of emerging human pathogens are zoonotic. Of these pathogens, >71% have wildlife origins. These pathogens can switch hosts by acquiring new genetic combinations that have altered pathogenic potential or by changes in behavior or socio-economic, environmental, or ecologic characteristics of the hosts.

1. Recreational Zoonoses

Sporting activities can expose humans to zoonotic infections. Hunting wildlife has been associated with infections such as brucellosis and tularemia. Less obvious routes arise from activities such as water sports. *Leptospira* spp.–infected animals excrete viable organisms in their urine, which can persist in aquatic environments for prolonged periods. After a triathlon event in 1998, a total of 52 of 474 athletes tested were diagnosed with leptospirosis.

2. Role of Companion Animals

Companion animals have many forms of contact and opportunities to transmit multiple zoonoses. The sexual stage of the life cycle of *Toxoplasma* spp. occurs in cats, thus exposing humans to infection in situations in which hygienic measures have not been observed. Cats also serve as reservoir for *Bartonella henselae,* the etiologic agent of cat-scratch fever. Animal bites can result in zoonotic infections, typified by infection with *Pasteurella multocida*. Dogs are the most likely source when humans become infected with rabies virus and are potential sources of *Toxocara* spp. This emerging threat is becoming apparent with importation of rescued dogs and global movement of dogs with their owners, which has resulted in several cases of leishmaniasis in the absence of sand fly vectors.

Table 3.1 : Examples of Pathogenic Microbes and the Diseases they Cause, Identified Since 1973

Year	*Microbe*	*Type*	*Disease*
1973	Rotavirus	Virus	Infantile diarrhea
1977	Ebola virus	Virus	Acute hemorrhagic fever
1977	*Legionella pneumophila*	Bacterium	Legionnaires' disease
1982	*Escherichia coli O157:H7*	Bacterium	Hemorrhagic colitis; hemolytic uremic syndrome
1982	*Borrelia burgdorferi*	Bacterium	Lyme disease
1983	Human Immunode-ficiencyVirus (HIV)	Virus	Acquired Immuno-Deficiency Syndrome (AIDS)
1989	Hepatitis C	Virus	Parentally transmitted non-A, non-B liver infection
1992	*Vibrio cholerae O139*	Bacterium	New strain associated with epidemic cholera
1993	Hantavirus	Virus	Adult respiratory distress syndrome
1994	Cryptosporidium	Protozoa	Enteric disease
1995	Ehrlichiosis	Bacterium	Severe arthritis?
1996	nvCJD	Prion	New variant Creutzfeldt-Jakob disease
1997	H_1N_1	Virus	Influenza
1999	Nipah	Virus	Severe encephalitis

Source : US Institute of Medicine, 1997; WHO, 1999.

3. Bush Meat

Zoonotic diseases associated with hunting and eating wildlife is of increasing global concern. Bush meat is considered a delicacy by many and has resulted in its growth as a commercial enterprise. Tracking, capturing, handling, butchering in the field, and transporting of carcasses involve risks of cross-species transmission. Zoonotic pathogens from wildlife may infect humans with little or no human-to-human transmission (*e.g.*, Avian influenza virus and Hendra virus). Alternatively, increased travel or migration and increased between-person contacts have facilitated emergence of simian immunodeficiency virus/HIV/AIDS in Africa.

4. Globalization and Livestock Movement

Large-scale movement of persons, livestock, food, or goods is now commonplace and provides increasing opportunities for rapid spread of pathogens. Trichinellae in horsemeat have been transported across the Pacific Ocean and infected consumers in other parts of the world. Discarded tires provide new habitats for mosquitoes in addition to their usual ecologic niches. Transport of animals can result in mingling of different species in crowded and stressful conditions. This mingling can suppress immune responses to persistent infections and increase pathogen shedding. Under such circumstances, susceptible species can readily become infected.

5. Tourism

Tourism has exponentially increased in recent years. This finding has resulted in increasing numbers of imported zoonoses, such as a variety of rickettsial spotted fevers, brucellosis, melioidosis, genotype I hepatitis E, tick-borne encephalitis, and schistosomiasis. An estimated >1 million international journeys are made each day, and a staggering 700 million tourists travel on an annual basis.

6. Changed Land Use and Urbanization

Deforestation and development of natural habitats have been seen on a global scale to accommodate intensification of agriculture and living areas for humans. As a result, ecologic habitats have been disrupted, reservoir abundance has changed, and transmission dynamics have been altered. Reduced host abundance may force vectors to seek alternative hosts, increasing opportunities for disease transmission.

Development of forests to provide rubber plantations in Malaysia has been correlated with increases in schistosomiasis. Wildlife may modify feeding practices as a consequence of changing land use, bringing them closer to humans and livestock. This modification was suggested to have been instrumental in the Nipah virus outbreak that affected pigs and humans in Malaysia in 1999. Nipah virus persists as a serious problem in many rural areas of Bangladesh and India, where infected bats living near human dwellings, urinate in date palm sap, which is later consumed raw by humans.

Close contact between humans and animals in the context of farming will increase the incidence of zoonotic diseases—those transmitted from animals to humans. Water management efforts, such as dam building, will encourage the spread of water-breeding vectors such as mosquitoes and snails that have contributed to outbreaks of Rift Valley fever and schistosomiasis in Africa.

7. Human Demographics and Behavior

Population growth and urbanization, particularly in the developing world, will continue to facilitate the transfer of pathogens among people and regions. Frequent and often sudden population movements within and across borders caused by ethnic conflict, civil war, and famine will continue to spread diseases rapidly in affected areas, particularly among refugees. As of 1999, there were some 24 major humanitarian emergencies worldwide involving at least 35 million refugees and internally displaced people. Refugee camps facilitate the spread of TB, HIV, cholera, dysentery, and malaria. Behavioral patterns, such as unprotected sex with multiple partners and intravenous drug use, will remain key factors in the spread of HIV/AIDS.

8. Technology, Medicine, and Industry

Although technological breakthroughs will greatly facilitate the detection, diagnosis, and control of certain infectious and noninfectious illnesses, they also will introduce new dangers, especially in the developed world where they are used extensively. The globalization of the food supply means that non hygienic food production, preparation, and handling practices in originating countries can introduce pathogens endangering foreign as well as local populations. Disease outbreaks due to *Cyclospora* spp., *Escherichia coli*, and *Salmonella* spp. in several countries, result from such food practices.

9. International Travel and Commerce

The increase in international air travel, trade, and tourism will dramatically increase the prospects that infectious disease pathogens such as influenza—and vectors such as mosquitoes and rodents—will spread quickly around the globe, often in less time than the incubation period of most diseases. The cross-border movement of some 2 million people each day, including 1 million between developed and developing countries each week, and surging global trade ensure that travel and commerce will remain key factors in the spread of infectious diseases.

10. Breakdown in Public Health Care

Alone or in combination, war and natural disasters, economic collapse, and human complacency are causing a breakdown in health care delivery and facilitating the emergence or reemergence of zoonotic diseases.

11. Climate Change

Climatic shifts are likely to enable some diseases and associated vectors—particularly mosquito-borne diseases such as malaria, yellow fever, and dengue—to spread to new areas. Warmer temperatures and increased rainfall already have expanded the geographic range of malaria to some highland areas in Sub-Saharan Africa and Latin America and could add several million more cases in developing country regions over the next two decades.

Table 3.2 : Factors Contributing to Zoonotic Disease Reemergence and Associated / Diseases

Contributing factor(s)	*Associated Infectious Diseases*
Human demographics and behavior	Dengue/dengue hemorrhagic fever, AIDS, giardiasis.
Technology and industry	Nosocomial (hospital-acquired) infections, hemorrhagic colitis/ hemolytic uremic syndrome.
Economic development and land use	Lyme disease, plague, rabies, yellow fever, Rift Valley fever, schistosomiasis.
International travel and commerce	Malaria, cholera.
Microbial adaptation and change	Influenza, HIV/AIDS, malaria, *Staphylococcus aureus* infections.
Breakdown of public health measures.	Rabies, tuberculosis, cholera
Climate change	Malaria, dengue, cholera, yellow fever.

Source : Adapted from US Institute of Medicine, 1997.

ZOONOSES : A SOCIAL AND ECONOMIC BURDEN

People have always depended on animals as sources of food, transport, labour and companionship. However, these animals are also sources of viral, bacterial and parasitic diseases transmitted in many ways, including direct contact or water contamination by them. For many years and in many countries these diseases, with their reservoirs in domestic and wild animals, have imposed and are still imposing a very heavy burden, especially among the people who are living and working in rural areas.

The significance of zoonotic and parasitic diseases and related food borne diseases, is growing continuously and their health and socioeconomic impacts are increasingly being felt by many countries and most particularly, although not exclusively, by developing countries. Apart from causing human suffering, morbidity and mortality, they hamper agricultural production, decrease availability of food, and create barriers to international trade. The persistent zoonotic disease burden is likely to aggravate and, in extreme cases, may even provoke social fragmentation, economic decay, and political polarization in the hardest hit countries in the developing world.

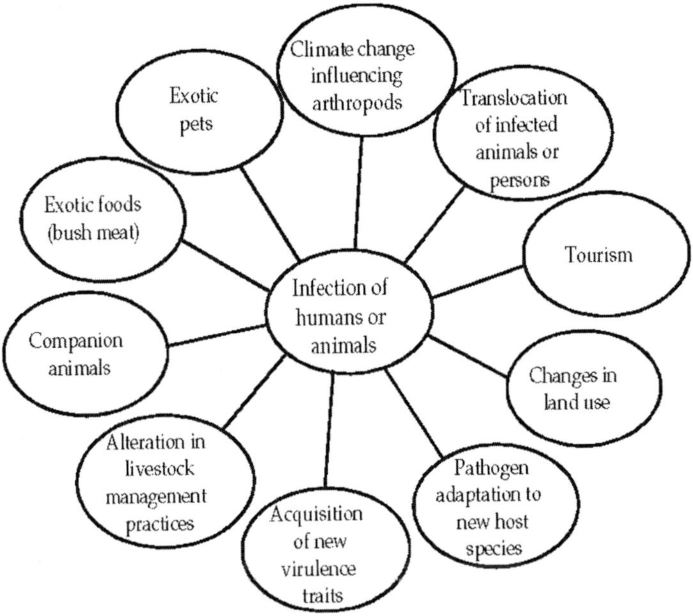

Fig. 3.1 : Factors influencing new and reemerging zoonoses.

The Broad-Based Economic Impact of Zoonotic Disease in Humans and in Animals

Independent of its origin, zoonotic disease has many costs related to prevention and response. There is also significant and likely greater cost associated with failing to develop and implement prevention and response capabilities.

Even when plans and capabilities exist, the more insidious costs of failure to follow known prevention methods may be incurred in research facilities, food production and processing, and health care facilities. The former increases the likelihood of contamination from handling, storing, and transporting high-risk pathogens. The latter manifests as Hospital Acquired Infection (HAI). Across all of these industries, the potential impact on operational, financial, and reputational integrity can be extremely severe. In addition, negligence in high-containment laboratory settings can compromise public confidence, potentially delaying development of the therapeutic interventions and countermeasures needed to prevent or mitigate the effects of severe epidemics or pandemics.

Animals removed from the food supply through infection or suspected infection can significantly damage the global economy. The recent Foot and Mouth Disease (FMD), Bovine Spongiform Encephalopathy (BSE) and avian influenza outbreaks are striking examples of the cost of these outbreaks. These diseases have generated billions of dollars in losses globally in the past decade.

The Economic Impact of Zoonotic Disease can be Extensive : Reaching from the local farmers' market to global trade agreements. Understanding these impacts is the first step in designing plans for preventing the spread of zoonoses as well as the resumption of trade and the continued operation of services after an outbreak.

While exposure to naturally occurring, highly transmissible zoonoses poses a global risk, certain industries have higher susceptibility to zoonoses exposure and therefore may be more vigilant about planning to mitigate the social and economic outcomes. On the front line are life sciences, food and agriculture, and health care. Certain other industries may indirectly suffer severe economic losses due to a decrease in public gatherings, travel, and tourism. These industries include retail, wholesale, consumer packaged goods, aviation, hospitality, gaming, sports, media, entertainment, financial institutions, professional services, transportation, and logistics.

Impact on Employment : Zoonoses can affect global employment in several ways. Companies may experience reduced attendance due to infection, fear of infection, or absenteeism of workers caring for their families. Broader economic problems caused by reduced workforces may then initiate economic downturn and further unemployment.

Impact on Economy and Global Trade : Disease outbreaks among livestock are a major risk for the farming sector. Previous crises or fear associated with perceived contamination of the food supply have reduced consumer confidence, causing sudden and drastic cuts in consumption of the affected products and reductions in its price. In addition, losses can result from culling of infected livestock, reduced animal value due to control measures such as compulsory emergency vaccination, and business interruption costs. The loss of access to regional and international markets tends to have much more important economic implications than local production losses alone. The extent of the economic damage is contingent upon the volume of exports from the affected area. Naturally, the impact can be severe for those areas that had an important and established export market before the outbreak.

Impact on Transport, Travel, Tourism, and Social Gatherings : With modern communications, news of even a small outbreak in a country can spread rapidly throughout the global community. Travelers intending to visit that country may perceive a threat and have concern for their personal safety. Economies in the affected countries can be severely impacted as commuters and vacationers cancel trips or immediately leave the affected country. Social gatherings such as symposia or conventions may be cancelled for public health reasons.

Impact on Delivery of Health Care : Concern continues to mount that a pandemic, or serious epidemic like SARS, will have an enormous and potentially incapacitating impact on the health care industry. Quality of health care might further be compromised as employees on the front line of infectious exposure must deal with large numbers of patients and uninfected people seeking medical reassurance. These same workers must also bear the mental burden as they may pose in spreading the disease to their families.

These planning and response considerations raise a host of ethical, legal, commercial, and policy questions as to how to balance the duty of care with the occupational health and safety of employees and the financial needs of facilities. If unanswered prior to the occurrence of zoonoses, the social and economic impacts could be catastrophic.

Disruptive Social Impact : At least some of the hardest-hit countries, initially in Sub-Saharan Africa and later in other regions, will face a demographic catastrophe as zoonotic diseases reduce human life expectancy dramatically.

ECONOMIC IMPACT OF ZOONOTIC DISEASE IN SOUTH EAST ASIA

1. Plague in India

The 1994 plague outbreak in Surat, India and resulting panic brought about a sudden exodus of 0.5 million people from the region and led to abrupt shutdowns of entire industries, including aviation and tourism. Several countries froze trade, banned travel from India, and sent some Indian migrants home. The WHO estimated the outbreak cost India some $2 billion.

2. Bird Flu in India

India has suffered the incidence of bird flu thrice since 2006. In early 2006, bird flu in poultry occurred in western parts of the country. In July 2007 bird flu occurred in Manipur and in the early part of 2008 in West Bengal, Tripura and other states of north-eastern part of the country. In 2006, the poultry industry suffered an estimated loss of Rs 30,000 million, while in 2007 it was Rs 6,700 million. In 2006, when bird flu hit Maharashtra and Gujarat, more than 12 countries had imposed a ban on Indian poultry products resulting in a loss of Rs. 10,500 crores.

3. Avian Flu in Hong Kong

The avian influenza outbreak in 1997 cost hundreds of millions of dollars in lost poultry production, commerce, and tourism. Airport arrivals in November of that year alone were down by 22 per cent from the preceding year.

4. Nipah in Malaysia

In 1999, the Nipahvirus caused the shutdown of over half of the country's pig farms and an embargo against pork exports.

ECONOMIC IMPACT OF ZOONOTIC DISEASE IN THE AMERICAS

1. Cholera in Peru

The outbreak of cholera in 1991 cost the Peruvian fishing industry an estimated $775 million in lost tourism and trade because of a temporary ban on seafood exports.

2. Pandemic Flu in the US (Projected)

The estimated economic impact of Pandemic Influenza would be US$71.3 to $166.5 billion, excluding disruptions to commerce and society.

3. SARS in Canada

Research suggests a loss in national economic activity in 2003 of roughly $1.5 billion, representing 0.15 per cent of Canada's real GDP. Real GDP in the City of Toronto itself was lowered by $950 million, or 0.5 per cent, with about $570 million of this total concentrated in the travel and tourism sector.

ECONOMIC IMPACT OF RECENT EPIDEMICS

1. The Impact of Severe Acute Respiratory Syndrome (SARS)

In 2002 and 2003, SARS—a novel virus that causes acute respiratory disorder—is believed to have emerged in China where it is assumed to have made a zoonotic leap. Within months, this communicable disease spread around the world, from Asia to North and South America and Europe. Before it was finally contained, SARS infected 8,098 people, nearly 800 of them died.

Many more around the world felt the deep financial impact of SARS. It measurably lowered the GDP of Asian countries and Canada. The total worldwide impact of $50 billion in losses was largely from industries such as tourism, retail, and trade, as people cancelled trips and business deals due to the fear and uncertainty about transmissibility of this previously unknown pathogen. Health care also suffered immense panic and concern about a disease that had no known cure. A significant number of those infected were health care workers, causing high levels of distress amongst hospital staff, a situation that raises legal and ethical issues about the obligation of health care workers to perform their duties and the protection they are provided during such an event.

2. The Projected Impact of Pandemic Influenza

No other anticipated global zoonotic scenario is causing as much concern as pandemic influenza. In 1918, pandemic influenza was responsible for an estimated 50 million deaths worldwide.

A new influenza pandemic is expected when the virus mutates to a form that is readily transmitted among humans. The projected losses to global economies could top $1.25 trillion, and the pandemic could kill as many as 150 million people worldwide. To date, current strains of avian influenza, the anticipated source of pandemic influenza have killed tens of millions of domestic birds (poultry) and wild birds worldwide. This has amounted to billions of dollars in losses for economies in Asia, which have been hit the hardest. As avian flu spreads throughout the world's poultry food supply, it is causing import/export bans as it did in France in 2006 and in the U.S. in 2008.

Once the virus becomes capable of efficient human-to-human transmission, the potential disruption to industry, services, and government is anticipated to be enormous. Stockpiling of vaccines and antiviral medication is happening on a global basis and massive planning efforts are underway to mitigate the effects of the pandemic.

3. Bovine Spongiform Encephalopathy (BSE)

BSE, a zoonotic neurodegenerative disease found in cattle also known as "mad cow disease", can be transmitted to humans through the consumption of infected cattle products. In humans, it is known as "Variant Creutzfeldt-Jakob disease" (VCJD), a long incubation disease that is fatal and has killed 204 people.

By far, the greatest impact of BSE has been economic. In the UK, more than 4.4 million head of cattle were destroyed to stop the spread of a BSE outbreak. The combined effects of a fall in consumer confidence throughout the UK and Europe, and the subsequent bans and restrictions on beef trade caused the British cattle and beef market to collapse, costing nearly $6 billion. In Canada, a single cow infected with BSE led to the ban of Canadian beef imports in the United States, costing an estimated $5 billion.

CONCLUSION

Diseases transmitted from animals have assumed substantial public health importance. Avian influenza, severe acute respiratory syndrome, and Nipah virus infection are a few examples of growing number of diseases that humans can contract from animals. These diseases can cause huge economic losses in addition to mortality and morbidity.

Prevention and control of major zoonoses depend on the firm decision of national authorities to face these diseases and on their capabilities to mobilize resources in different sectors, to establish coordination of activities, promote much needed intersectoral cooperation, especially between national veterinary and public health services in association with public health education campaigns and community involvement. Only comprehensive national approaches supported by inter national technical collaboration will alleviate or eliminate the public health and economic impact of zoonotic diseases.

REFERENCES

Meslin, FX., Stöhr, K., Heymann, D. (2000). Public Health Implications of Emerging Zoonoses. *Rev. Sci. Tech.* **19** : 310-7.

Meslin, FX. (2008). Public health impact of zoonoses and international approaches for their detection and containment. *Vet. Ital.* **44** : 583-90.

Murphy, FA. (2008) Emerging Zoonoses: The Challenge for Public Health and Biodefense. *Prev. Ve.t Med.* **86** : 216-23.

Morse, S.S. (1995). Factors in the Emergence of Infectious Diseases. *Emerg. Infect. Dis.* **1**.

Morse, S.S. (2004). Factors and Determinants of Disease Emergence. *Rev. Sci. Tech. Off. Int. Epiz.* **23** : 443-451.

Sally J. Cutler, Anthony R. Fooks, and Wim H. M. van der Poel (2010). Public Health Threat of New, Reemerging, and Neglected Zoonoses in the Industrialized World. *Emerg. Infect. Dis.* **16** : 1–7.

Seimenis, A. (1998). Zoonoses: A Social and Economic Burden. Eastern Mediterranean *Hlth. J.* **4** : 220-222.

4

EMERGENCE OF ZOONOTIC MYCOPLASMOSES

D.N. Garg

About 30,000 people die of zoonotic diseases every year in the world and there are about 300 zoonotic diseases prevalent in the world. Out of 1461 diseases (now recognized in human) approximately, 62% are caused by multiple-host pathogens characterized by their movement across species lines. Given the rate of population growth, changes in climatic conditions and rapid urban development, the infectious diseases are here to stay over a large part of 21st century. Over the past 3 decades approximately, 75% of new emerging human infections have been zoonotic. Mycoplasmoses, as of public health importance, has not been accepted in any part of the world. Though mycoplasmas, acholeplasmas and ureaplasmas are widely distributed in animal hosts but whether they are significant colonizers of human is still not certain. The importance of mycoplasmas in human and animal infections has accentuated with recent reporting of instances of human infections with animal mycoplasmas and *vice-versa* leading to recognition of zoonotic mycoplasmoses. The slow reporting of zoonotic mycoplasmoses can be attributed mainly to difficulty in measuring zoonotic potential of mycoplasmoses as in some complex diseases *viz.* multiple sclerosis, rheumatoid arthritis, leukemia, atherosclerosis, chronic fatigue syndrome, CJD, Crohn's colitis *etc.* This chapter provides the current status of possible zoonotic mycoplasmas and recorded instances of zoonotic mycoplasmoses.

DEFINITION

Zoonotic mycoplasmoses may best be defined as sharing of mycoplasmal infections, which are naturally transmitted between vertebrate animals and man. This kind of sharing occurs under natural conditions permitting bidirectional movement of mycoplasmas and is not based on experimental evidence of occurrence.

In case, if man acts as a reservoir for mycoplasmosis in animals, the zoonosis is called zooanthroponotic mycoplasmosis; animals acting as reservoir for human mycoplasmosis lead to anthropozoonotic mycoplasmosis. Transmitted between man and animals, mycoplasmosis is called amphizoonotic.

ZOONOTIC MYCOPLASMAS (GARG, 2009)

The concept of zoonotic mycoplasmoses is new and only some mycoplasmas and acholeplasmas belonging to *Mycoplasmatales* and *Achopleplasmatales* show existence of zoonotic mycoplasmoses. So far, eight species in the genus *Mycoplasma* of family *Mycoplasmataceae* and two species of genus *Acholeplasma* of family *Acholeplasmataceae* can be claimed as zoonotic. No other mollicute including ureaplasma, aneroplasma and asteroplasma has yet been recorded as zoonotic. The zoonotic mycoplasmas, thus far recorded, are classified (Table-4.1) on the basis whether man or animals acts as reservoir of the mycoplasmas.

Table 4.1 : Classification of Recorded Zoonotic Mycoplasmas/ Acholeplasmas

Zooanthropozoonotic	*Anthropozoonotic*	*Amphizoonotic*
M. pneumoniae	*M. arthritidis*	*A. laidlawii*
M. salivarium	*M. arginin*	*A. oculi*
	M. bovis	
	M. canis	
	M. edwardii	
	M. sp. (Str. M.7806)	

ZOOANTHROPOZOONOTIC MYCOPLASMOSES

In humans, mycoplasmas, acholeplasmas and ureaplasmas are mucosally associated, residing predominantly in the respiratory and urogenital tract. Till now, 13 species in the genus *Mycoplasma*, 2 in the genus *Acholeplasma* and 1 in the genus *Ureaplasma* have been isolated from humans. Out of these, only 2 *Mycoplasma* species viz. *M. pneumoniae, M salivarium* have been recorded as zooanthropozoonotic.

1. *Mycoplasma pneumoniae*

Mycoplasma pneumoniae was first identified and described in the early 1960s. Primary site of colonization of *M. pneumoniae* is oropharynx and is pathogenic to humans. The pneumonia is designated 'primary atypical' to distinguish it from 'typical' pneumonia due to *Streptococcus pneumoniae*, the pneumococcus. A detailed definition of epidemiology of *M. pneumoniae* disease has emerged (Lind and Bentzon, 1988). Attack rate is low and disease spreads slowly in communities with close contact among their members. Transmissions by droplets require a rather high inoculum unless the host is immunocompromised. A zoonotic outbreak of *M. pneumoniae* infection in a class of a Budapest secondary school has been reported (Mikola *et al.*, 1997). Thirty students became feverish and upper respiratory tract catarrh. When 2 were hospitalized with pneumonia, a mycoplasma infection was confirmed by cold agglutination test. Their classroom contained a terrarium with hamsters, from which *M. pneumoniae* was isolated.

2. *Mycoplasma salivarium*

Mycoplasma salivarium exists as commensal organisms in the oropharynx of human and nonhuman primates. Pathogenicity of *M. salivarium* is not known. However, isolation of the organism with a significantly higher incidence from the gingival sulci of individuals with periodental disease (87%) than in persons with healthy periodentium (32%) has stimulated interest in its possible role in periodental pathoplogy (Engel and Kenny, 1970; Forest, 1979). Also, it is the predominant mycoplasmal species in dental plaques. Likewise, this organism has been identified as a causative agent of septic arthritis in hypogammaglobulnaemia (So *et al.*, 1983). *M. salivarium*, usually confined to humans or other primates, was repeatedly isolated from nasal and pharyngeal secretions of swine (Erickson *et al.*, 1988). It has also been isolated from the tonsils of 3 horses (Poland and Lemcke, 1978). *Mycoplasma salivarium* is neither a true equine nor porcine mycoplasma and thus might have been acquired by them from their environmental companion. No further report came on this account.

Comments

Mycoplasma pneumoniae organisms are usually confined to humans, which is the only natural host of *M. pneumoniae. Mycoplasma salivarium* is a common parasitic inhabitant of the oropharynx of human and nonhuman primates. The isolation reports of *M. pneumoniae* from hamsters in the reported zoonotic outbreak (Mikola *et al.*, 1997) and *M. salivarium* from horses (Poland and Lemcke, 1978) and swine (Erickson *et al.*, 1988) were preliminary. Whether these were zooanthroponotic has not proved conclusively.

ANTHROPOZOONOTIC MYCOPLASMOSES

Numerous mycoplasmas are known to exist as animal pathogen (Ross, 1993), opportunist and as non pathogen. However, only a few, as described briefly below has taken a zoonotic route.

1. *Mycoplasma arthritidis*

Mycoplasma arthritidis is a common pathogen of laboratory and wild rats causing purulent polyarthritis, sometimes occurring as localized outbreaks in stocks of laboratory rats. Also, isolated repeatedly from apparently healthy rats. Between 1948 and 1965, several mycoplasma strains were isolated from human urogenital tract and synovial tissues in laboratories at widely diverse geographical locations. These organisms did not relate to other known human mycoplasmas but were designated as *M. hominis* type 2. Later these strains were reclassified as *M. arthritidis* (Lemcke, 1965). The justification of this reclassification was subsequently confirmed by nucleic acid homology, by enzyme analysis and by examination of electrophoretic patterns of the cell proteins of these strains. No subsequent isolates of the organism from human tissues have been reported and no adequate role in human disease has been documented.

Comments

Mycoplasma arthritidis is causative agent of chronic proliferative arthritis of rodents and possess superantigen called MAM (*M. arthritidis* mitogen). It is the only mycoplasma species which has been demonstrated to induce differentiation of mouse lymphocytes into cytotoxic/suppressor effector cells. Arthritogenic potential of some mycoplasmas led to speculations concerning their role in human rheumatoid arthritis. Besides, the earlier isolations of *M. arthritidis* from synovial tissues, numerous other investigations over the past 4 decades have either failed to isolate mycoplasmas or have resulted in inconsistent findings.

2. *Mycoplasma canis*

Mycoplasma canis is found as a common parasitic inhabitant of the mucous membrane of upper respiratory tract, conjunctivae and genitals of dogs. It has also been isolated occasionally from nonhuman primates. Several strains of *M. canis* were isolated from the oropharynx of members of a family at the time when their dog had an acute respiratory disease infection. (Armstrong *et. al.*, 1971). Although one member of the family was taking immunosuppressant, the pathogenic role of *M. canis* in human disease was neither established nor the dynamics of zoonotic transfer of *M. canis* studied.

Comments

Pathogenicity of *M. canis* is not known under natural and experimental conditions. Experimentally, a strain isolated from the pericardium of a dog did not produce any lesion in dogs and small rodents. Thus, the zoonotic transfer of *M. canis* may be regarded as of no public health significance.

3. Mycoplasma bovis

Mycoplasma bovis is a potential bovine pathogen causing mastitis, pneumonia, arthritis and genital disorders (Pfutzner and Sachse, 1996). Once established in a herd, the organism persists and may become endemic; producing mastitis in dairy herd. Madoff *et al.* (1979) have reported the isolation of *M. bovis* from sputum of a woman with lobar pneumonia.

Comments

The significance of frequent isolations of *M. bovis* from respiratory tract of cattle with respiratory disease is yet to be resolved though the incidence of pneumonia due to *M. bovis* can be as high as 100 % (Pfutzner, 1990). *Mycoplasma bovis* infection may spread by aerosol, which may be a logic way of its transmission to human in the case reported by Madoff *et al.* (1979). The possibility of transfer of *M. bovis via* consumption of infected bovine-milk is another possibility as this organism appears more invasive and may cause septicaemia.

4. *Mycoplasma arginini*

Mycoplasma arginini is a mammalian parasite with an apparently wide host range. It is found with a high frequency in the respiratory tract and less frequently in the conjunctivae and genital tract of sheep, goats and cattle. Occasionally, isolations have also been reported from pigs, horses, dogs, domestic and wild cats. It is also frequently isolated from bovine serum used in tissue culture. A septicaemic infection caused by *M. arginini* in a patient with advanced Hodgkin's disease and marked immunodeficiency emphasizes the potentially heightened risk to immunocompromised hosts with mollicutes of both human and nonhuman organisms (Yechouron *et. al.*, 1992). This organism was repeatedly isolated from the blood and bronchial washings of a patient during the course of the disease. *M. arginini*, commonly found in a variety of species of large animals, was thought to have been acquired by the patient during his work as a slaughter-house employee. Prayson *et al.* (2008) have recently reported isolation of *M. arginini* from an unusual case of deep infection of open femur fracture in a 56-year hunter; organisms identified at CDC, Georgia after extensive DNA testing. The hunter had an attack of African lion causing crushing bite leading to open femur fracture and after some time bone culture was found positive for *M. arginini.* Authors put the theory that the lion had fed on goat prior to the attack on hunter resulting in deep tissue inoculation of *M. arginini*. Quirk *et al.* (2001) detected mycoplasma DNA in 6 (13.0%) of the 46 tumor-DNA samples. Nucleotide sequence similarity searches of nested PCR products revealed that 1 *M. salivarium* and 5 *M. arginini* DNA sequences were amplified from the ovarian tissues.

Comments

Evidence that *M. arginini* is pathogenic for animals and man is yet to be presented. However, the circumstantial evidence in the cases reported so far (Yechouron *et al.* 1992; Prayson *et. al.*, 2008; Quirk *et al.*, 2001) suggests the zoonotic transfer and pathogenic role of *M. arginini.*

5. *Mycoplasma felis*

Mycoplasma felis is a common parasitic inhabitant of the upper respiratory and lower genital tract of asymptomatic and diseased cats. Strains related to *M. felis* have also been isolated frequently from tonsils and other regions of respiratory tract of healthy and diseased horses. *Mycoplasma felis* is associated with conjunctivitis in cats, being isolated significantly more frequently from the conjunctivae of diseased cats than in the convalescent or healthy cats. Bonilla *et al.* (1997) described first documented case of *M. felis* infection in a woman who had common variable immune deficiency and who presented with septic arthritis of the left hip and right knee. *Mycoplasma felis* was isolated from both the joints. She has been exposed to cat before the diagnosis of *M. felis* septic arthritis was made.

Comments

Evidences so far that the *M. felis* is pathogenic are inconclusive though conjunctivitis can be experimentally induced in cats. Prevalence of *M. felis* in Oligoathritis patients exposed to cats, the possible role of *M. felis* as arthritogenic agent and the routes as well as risk of transmission is under investigation.

6. *Mycoplasma edwardii*

M. edwardii is frequently found in the upper respiratory and urogenital tracts of male and female dogs. It has also been isolated from shrews. *M. edwardii* has recently been reported from septicaemic infection in a patient with advanced acquired immuno-deficiency syndrome (AIDS). This has been reported by Baseman and Tully (1997) as a personal communication to them by M.K. York.

Comments

Its pathogenicity is not known although occasionally isolated from pneumonic lungs of dogs, and recently has been reported from an advanced case of AIDS.

7. *Mycoplasma* sp. (Strain M 7806)

McCabe *et al.* (1987) described a mycoplasmal infection in the hands of a veterinarian acquired through a cat - bite. The infection resulted in severe soft tissue cellulitis with tissue destruction sufficient to require a tendon graft. The organism (Strain M 7806) was identified as an unclassified, glucose-fermenting *Mycoplasma* species and resolved after vibramycin was administered. Although other serologically related strains were later isolated from the oropharynx of feline, the organism remained unclassified.

Comments

This unclassified strain of *Mycoplasma* has never been isolated subsequently either from human or animals. Therefore, no comment can be offered about its pathogenic, epidemiologic and zoonotic potential.

AMPHIZOONOTIC ACHOLEPLASMOSES

Currently, 13 species of *Acholeplasma* exist in nature, which are apparent parasites of vertebrate hosts. Only two species *viz.* *A. laidlawii* and *A. oculi*, are commonly isolated from diseased sites of various animals and humans. These are described briefly.

1. *Acholeplasma laidlawii*

Acholeplasma laidlawii was originally isolated from sewage, manure, humus and soil but its designation as true saprophyte was challenged later by its occurrence in mammals and birds. It is frequently recovered from oral cavity, respiratory and genital tract secretions, eye, lymphnodes, semen and serum. Its pathogenicity has not been well established, although some strains are lethal for chicken embryos. A limited number of *A. laidlawii* strains have been isolated from oral cavity (Razin *et al.*, 1964) and from flora of human burns (Markham and Markham, 1969).

2. *Acholeplasma oculi*

Acholeplasma oculi has been isolated from conjunctivae of goats with keratoconjuntivitis, nasal secretions of porcines, nasopharynx, lungs, spinal fluid, joints, and semen of equines and external genitals of guinea pigs. Experimentally, it has been shown to produce conjunctivitis, pneumonia and death in goats. A single isolate of *A. oculi* was cultured from amniotic fluid at 19 weeks of gestation (Waites *et al.*, 1987). Its identification by direct immunofluorescence appeared to preclude contamination. The remainder of pregnancy in question was unremarkable and a full term infant was delivered without any complication.

Comments

As *A. laidlawii* is abundantly isolated from a wide variety of syndrome in man and animals, it looks like a perfect example of amphizoonosis; being freely transmitted between man and animals. A fresh look to *A. laidlawii* is required for its possible potential role when it is found associated with diseased hosts. Pathogenicity of *A. oculi* can not be ignored. However, in absence of any record of prooven virulence, it is not wise to draw any conclusion as to its zoonotic potential.

CURRENT STATUS OF ZOONOTIC MYCOPLASMOSES IN INDIA

There are no recorded evidence of any episode of zoonotic mycoplasmoses, whether zooanthropozoonotic or anthropozoonotic or amphizoonotic, in India till date.

DETECTION OF ZOONOTIC MYCOPLASMAS

Details of media, cultural conditions and other requirements for isolation and identification of mollicutes are available in the literature (Razin and Tully, 1995; Tully and Razin, 1995). The current biotechnological approach to laboratory diagnosis of mollicutes infection has also been described earlier by Garg (1993).

Differential characteristics of zoonotic species of genus *Mycoplasma* and *Acholeplasma* so far recorded are given in the Table 4.2. Final identification, however, depends on determination of serological relatedness, for which commonly used methods *viz.* growth inhibition, direct or indirect immunofluorescence and/are metabolic inhibition tests are available. Rapid detection for quick diagnosis of zoonotic mycoplasmas and to prevent severe consequences in affected humans and animals seems essential. Although culture is well adapted to most but not all species of zoonotic mycoplasmas listed in this chapter. Thus, many methods for direct (DNA probes, rDNA) and amplified detection of mycoplasmas (PCR) of possible zoonotic significance are used currently. Reviews on use of diagnostic DNA probes and PCR for mycoplasma are available (Razin *et al.*, 1987; Johansson, 1993; Razin, 1994).

Table 4.2 : Differential Characteristics of Zoonotic Species of *Mycoplasma* and *Acholeplasma*

Mollicutes Organism	*Gl*	*Ma*	*Arg*	*Phos*	*Film, Spot*	*Tet A/an*	*Gel*	*SD*	*CD*	*H*	*G+C Mol%*
Mycoplasma											
M. arginini	–	–	+	–	–	–/+		–		–	27.6-28.6
M. arthritidis	–	–	+	–	–/–	+	–	–		–	30.03-2.6
M. bovis	–	–	–	+	D	+/+	–	–	X		27.8-32.9
M. canis	+	–	–	–	–	–/+	D	–	–	+	28.4-29.1
M. felis	+	–	–	+	+	–/+	–	–	–	–	25.2
M. edwardii	+	–	–	–	+	–/+	–	–	–	–	29.2
M .pneumoniae	+	+	–	–	–	+/+	–	–	–	+	38.6-40.8
M. salivarium	–	–	+	–	+	–/w	–	–	–	–	27.3-31.4
M.sp. (Str.M 7806)	+										
Acholeplasma *A. laidlawii*	+	–	–		w/+	D		–	–	–	31.0-36.0
A. oculi	+	–			+/+						26.0-27.0

+= 90 % or more strains are positive , – = 90 % or more strains are negative, d = 11 to 90% strains are positive, x= not definitely setteled, Gl=glucose catabolization, Ma=mannose, Arg= arginine deimination, Phos= phosphatase, Tet=tetrazolium reduction, A/An=aerobic/anerobic, Gel=gelatin hydrolysis, SD=coagulated serum digestion, CD=casein digestion, H= haemadsorption, the test performed with RBC from species from which mycoplasma originated plus guinea pig (sometimes with a variety RBC). (Gonalez *et al.*, 1995), an immunoenzyme assay using MOAb and streptavidin-biotin detection for *M. arginini, M. salivarium, A. laidlawii* (BRL, Maryland, USA).

Rapid detection of *M. pneumoniae* antigen (total antigen, P1 adhesin or glycolipids) includes direct immunofluorescence; counter-immuno-electrophoresis, immunoblotting and antigen capture enzyme immunoassay (EIA). Detection of *M. pneumoniae* by probing for specific nucleotide sequence by primers of P1 or cytoadhesin gene with product identified by dot-blot-hybridization (DBH) following PCR amplification (P1-PCR-DBH-Assay).

Amongst other zoonotic mycoplasmas, available rapid detection systems are : a PCR diagnosis for *M. arthritidis* (Van Kupperveld *et al.*, 1992); an antigen capture ELISA using monoclonal antibodies (Heller *et al.*, 1993); a DNA probe (Hotzel *et al.*, 1993) and PCR system based on amplification of 16S rRNA gene for *M. bovis* (Chavez *et al.*, 1995).

DNA probes to detect either mycoplasmal DNA or mycoplasmal rRNA and 16S rRNA based PCR for *M. arginini, M. salivarium, A. laidlawii* (Gobel and Stanbridge, 1984. Razin *et al.* 1984, Mattson and Johansson, 1993; Teysson *et al.*, 1993). An oligonucleotide array has also been recently developed to detect and genotype mollicutes based on internal transcribed spacer (ITS) (*Jang et al.*, 2009). This method proposed oligonucleotide array effective for 23 mycoplasmas including many zoonotic mycoplasmas, in a single hybridization. Whereas 16S rDNA identity of mycoplasma ranges from 62.7 to 98.8%, the ITS sequence identity of mycoplasma ranges from 32.0 to 99.0%. Thus, it is more rapid and accurate detection method for species specific identification using sequence based molecular technique. However, such fast detection methods are neither available for *M. canis* nor for *A. oculi* providing scope for research on this account.

ZOONOTIC MYCOPLASMOSES : OBSTACLES AND PROPOSALS

Is zoonotic mycoplasmoses emerging? Should microbiological examination of foods of animal origin *viz.* meat, milk and their product include their screening for mycoplasmas? Answer to such question has been provided reasonably by Garg and Singh (2009) in a recent paper. Though the available reports on zoonotic mycoplasmoses are limited but it appears that it is just waiting to happen at the verge of emergence.

Obstacles in the way of recognition of zoonotic mycoplasmoses include: (i) absence of specific or distinguishable clinical sign in the affected individuals (s) or difficulty in diagnosing healthy or convalescent carriers capable of transmitting zoonotic mycoplasmas, and (ii) lack of training to recognize the pathogenic mycoplasmas. Presently, zoonotic aspects are beginning to surface at the hands of those expertising in mycoplasma work. Our human or veterinary clinical or diagnostic laboratories are not yet ready to diagnose mycoplasmal infections, either in man or in animals. Thus, laboratory training in mycoplasma work increasing the competency of medical and veterinary diagnosticians will flip the reporting of zoonotic occurrence of mycoplasmas. Fastidious nature of mollicutes is reflected in slow cultivation, identification and diagnostic procedures.

Recently developed molecular methods *viz.* nucleic acid probes/ PCR, 16S rRNA sequence analysis, molecular based ELISA has certainly obviated the need to cultivate and identify mollicutes organisms. These sophisticated and fast methods, however, are usually applied in research laboratories and remain limited there, unless these methods are routinely used by diagnosticians, slow reporting of zoonotic mycoplasmoses will continue. Development of diagnostic kit and their commercial availability will go a long way; leading to mounted occurrence of zoonotic mycoplasmas helping to understand the epidemiological linkages *viz.* transmission path, geographic locations of zoonotic mycoplasmoses.

It is assumed that mycoplasma, being Gram-negative, in large numbers in foods of animal origin could lead to some sporadics or outbreaks of food-borne gastroenteritis, which remains undiagnosed etiologically. As mycoplasmas do not grow on conventional SPC plating media and limulus amoebocyte lysate (LAL) as screen test for endotoxin or mycoplasmological examination is not used routinely, it will be a wise step to introduce such tests in food analysis/public health laboratories so as to define the possible association of mycoplasma with contaminated foods.

CONCLUSIONS

Emerging zoonotic mycoplasmoses is a direct challenge to veterinary and medical profession. So far episodes of zoonotic mycoplasmoses has occurred in the form of an out break and a few sporadic incidences only; all being occupational zoonoses and involvement of a veterinarian in the life cycle of mycoplasma is incidental or accidental as dead end host. Zoonotic mycoplasmas and acholeplasmas recorded so far include; *M. pneumoniae, M. salivarium, M. arthritidis, M. canis, M. bovis, M. arginini, M. felis, M. edwardii, A. laidlawii* and *A. oculi*. This list of zoonotic mycoplasmas may possibly extend in future. The recorded reports support the apparent transmission of animal mollicutes to human and *vice-versa*. Immediate concern is where serious clinical infections in human have occurred with a fatal outcome from apparently animal derived mollicute. The slow reporting of zoonotic mycoplasmoses is possible to circumvent if only diagnostic mycoplasma antigen and antisera as well as rapid molecular tests (nucleic acid probes/PCR, 16S rRNA sequence analysis, MOAb-ELISA) as kits are made available commercially. Till now, a few reports on zoonotic mycoplasmas provide only incomplete and inconclusive information. Generation of competent human resource capable to work with mycoplasma-biotechnology is a prerequisite to increase the capability of diagnostic laboratories for diagnosis of mycoplasmoses. Aim to diagnose zoonotic mycoplasmoses should always be directed to gather information on involved transmission vehicles and routes, ecological parameters as well as on spatial and temporal distribution. All this will provide better understanding of hidden aspects of zoonotic mycoplasmas/zoonotic mycoplasmoses.

ZOONOTIC HEMOTROPHIC MYCOPLASMA

Hemotrophic mycoplasma infection is a neglected zoonotic disease, which poses a threat to public health and the animal industry, especially in China (Hu *et al.*, 2009). So far, 6 hemotrophic *Mycoplasma* species have been identified in rodents and mammals (Yang *et al.*, 2000).

REFERENCES

Armstrong, D., Yu, B.H., Yagoda, A. and Kagnoff, M.F. (1971). Colonization of humans by *Mycoplasma canis*. *J. Infect. Dis.* **124** : 607-609.

Baseman, J.B. and Tully, J.G. (1997). Mycoplasmas: Sophisticated, reemerging and burdened by their notoriety. *Emer. Infect. Dis.* **3** : 21-32.

Bonilla, H.F., Chenoweth, C.E., Tully, J.G., Blythe, L.K., Robertson, J.A. and Kauffman, C.A. (1997). *Mycoplasma felis* septic arthritis in a patient with hypogammaglobulinemia. *Clin. Infect. Dis.* **24** : 222-225.

Chavez Gonzalez, Y.R., Bascunana, C.R., Bolske, G., Mattsson, J.G., Molina, C.F. and Johansson, K-E. (1995). *In-vitro* amplification of the 16S rRNA genes from *Mycoplasma bovis* and *Mycoplasma agalactiae* by PCR. *Vet. Microbiol.* **47** : 183-190.

Engel, L.D. and Kenny, G.E. (1970). *Mycoplasma salivarium* in human gingival sulci. *J. Periodon. Res.* **5** : 1- 9.

Erickson, B. Z., Ross, R.F. and Bove, J.M. (1988). Isolation of *Mycoplasma salivarium* from swine. *Vet. Micrbiol.* **16** : 385-390.

Forest, N. (1979). Caracterisation de *Mycoplasma salivarium* dans les parodontopathies. *J. Biol. Buccale.* **7** : 321-330.

Garg, D.N. (1993). Current biotechnological approaches to laboratory diagnosis of mollicutes infection. In: Srivastava, Prasad, Kalra, Gupta (Eds.) *Ani. Hlth, Bio l.* 164-174.

Garg, D.N. (2009). Mycoplasmas of zoonotic signifinace.CME-Emerging Trends in mycoplasmas. Himachal Institute of Public Administration (HIPA), Shimla, Himachal Pradesh, India. 26 March, 2009.

Garg, D. N. and Singh, Y. (2009). Zoonotic mycoplasmoses: Waiting to happen. *In*: Singh, Funk, Tripathi, Joshi (Eds.) Food Safety Quality Assurance and Global Trade: Concerns and Strategies (Int. Book Dist. Coy., Lucknow, India). pp. 167-172.

Gobel, U. B. and Stanbridge, E. J. (1984). Cloned mycoplasma ribosomal RNA genes for detection of mycoplasma contamination in tissue cultures. *Science* **226** : 1211-1213.

Heller, M., Berthold, E., Pfutzner, H., Leirer, R. and Sachse, K. (1993). Antigens capture ELISA using a monoclonal antibody for detection of *Mycoplasma bovis* in milk. *Vet. Microbiol.* **37** : 127-133.

Hotzel, H., Dermuth, B., Sachse, K., Pflitsch, A. and Pfutzner, H. (1993). Detection of *Mycoplasma bovis* using *in-vitro* deoxyribonucleic acid amplification. *Rev. Sci. Tech. Off. Int. Epiz.* **12** : 581- 591.

Hu, Z., Yin, J., Shen, K., Kang, W. and Chen, Q. (2009). Outbreaks of Hemotrophic *Mycoplasma* infections in China. *Emer. Infect Dis.* **15** : 1139-1140.

Jang, H., Kim, H., Kang, B., Kim, C., and Park, H. (2009). Oligonucleotide array-based detection and genotyping of mollicutes (*Acholeplasma, Mycoplasma* and *Ureaplasma*). *J. Micrbiol. Biotechnol.* **19** : 265-270.

Johansson, K.E. (1993). Detection and identification of mycoplasmas with diagnostic DNA probes complimentary to ribosomal RNA. In: Khane, Adoni (Eds.). Rapid Diagnosis of Mycoplasmas. (Plenum Press, New York). pp. 139-154.

Lemcke, R. M. (1965). A serological comparison of various species of *Mycoplasma* by an agar gel double-diffusion technique. *J. Gen. Micrbiol.* **38** : 91-100.

Lind, K. and Bentzon, M.W. (1988). Changes in the epidemiological pattern of *Mycoplasma pneumoniae* infections in Denmark: a 30 years survey. *Epidemiol Infect.* **101** : 377-386.

Madoff, S., Pixley, B.Q., Del Guidice, R.A. and Modellering, Jr. (1979). Isolation of *Mycoplasma bovis* from a patient with systemic illness. *J. Clin. Micrbiol.* **9** : 709-711.

Markham, J.G. and Markham, N.P. (1969). *Mycoplasma laidlawii* in human burns. *J. Bacteriol.* **98** : 827-828.

Mattson, J.G. and Johnasson, K-E. (1993). Oligonucleotide probes complimentary to 16S rRNA for rapid detection of mycoplasma contamination in cell cultures. FEMS *Microbiol. Lett.* **107** : 139-144.

McCabe, S.J., Murray, J.F., Ruhnke, H.L. and Rachlis, A. (1987). *Mycoplasma* infection of the hand acquired from a cat. *J. Hand. Surg.* **12A** : 1085-1088.

Mikola, I., Balogh, G., Nagg, A., Matyas, M., Rady, M., Glavits, R. and Stipkovits, L. (1997). Zoonotic outbreak of *Mycoplasma pneumoniae* infection. *Magyar allatorvosok Lapja.* **119** : 403-405.

Pfutzner, H. (1990). Epizootiology of *Mycoplasma bovis* infection in cattle. Zbl. Bakt. *(suppl)*: **20** : 394-399.

Pfutzner, H. and Sachse, K. (1996). *Mycoplasma bovis* as an agent of mastitis, pneumonia, arthritis and genital disorders in cattle. *Rev. Sci. Tech. Off. Int. Epiz.* **15** : 1477-1494.

Poland, J. and Lemcke, R. (1978). Mycoplasmas of the respiratory tract of horses and their significance in upper respiratory tract disease. Proc. 4th Int. Cong. On Equine Infect. Dis. Lyon. *J. Equine Med. Surg. (Suppl.)* **1** : 437-446.

Prayson, M.J., Venkatarryappa, I., Srivastava, M., Northern, I. and Burdette, S.D. (2008). Deep infection with *Mycoplasma arginini* in an open femur fracture secondary to an African lion bite: A case report. *Injury Extra.* **39** : 243-246.

Quirk, J.T., Kupinski, J.M. and DiCioccio, R.A. (2001). Detection of Mycoplasma ribosomal DNA sequences in ovarian tumors by nested PCR. *Gynecologic Oncol.* **83** : 560-562.

Razin, S. (1994). DNA probes and PCR in diagnosis of mycoplasma infections. *Mol. Cell. Probes.* **8** : 497-511.

Razin, S. and Tully, J.G. (1995). Molecular and Diagnostic Procedures in Mycoplasmology.Vol. I. Molecular characterization (Acdemic Press, New York).

Razin, S. Gross, M., Wormser, M. Pollack, Y. and Glaser, G. (1984). Detection of mycoplasmas infecting cell cultures by DNA hybridization. *In Vitro.* **20** : 404-408.

Razin, S., Hyman, H. C., Nur, I and Yogev, D. (1987). DNA probes for detection and identification of mycoplasmas. *Isr. J. Med. Sci.* **23** : 735-741.

Razin, S., Michmann, J. and Shimshoni, Z. (1964). The occurrence of mycoplasma pleuropneumonia like organisms, (PPLO) in the oral cavity of dentulous and edentulous subjects. *J. Dent. Res.* **43** : 402-405.

Ross, R.F. (1993). Mycoplasmas: Animal pathogens. In: Khane, Adoni (Eds.). Rapid Diagnosis of Mycoplasmas. (Plenum Press, New York). pp. 69-109.

So, A.K.L., Furr, P.M., Taylor-Robinson, D. and Webster, A.D.B. (1983). Arthritis caused by *Mycoplasma salivarium* in hypogammaglobulinaemia. *Brit. Med. J.* **286** : 762-763.

Teysson, R., Poutiers, F., Saillard, C., Grau, O., Laigret, F., Bove, J. M. and Bebear, C. (1993). Detection of mollicute contamination in cell cultures by 16S rRNA amplification. *Mol. Cell.* Probes. **7** : 209-216.

Tully, J.G. and Razin, S. (1995). Molecular and Diagnostic Procedures in Mycoplasmology. Vol. II. Diagnostic Procedures. (Academic Press, New York). Van Kupperveld, F.J.M., van der Logt, J.T.M., Angulo, A.F., van Zoest, M.J., Quint, W.G.V., Neisters, H.G.M., Galama, J.M.D. and Melchers, W.J.G. (1992). Genus and species specific identification of mycoplasmas by 16S rRNA amplification. *Appl. Environ. Micrbiol.* **58** : 2006-2615.

Waites, K.B., Tully, J.G., Rose, D.L, Marriot, P.A., Davis, R.O. and Casell, G.H. (1987). Isolation of *Acholeplasma oculi* from human amniotic fluid in early pregnancy. *Curr. Microbiol.* **15** : 325-327.

Yang, D. Tai, X. Quin, and Yun, S.Y. (2000). Prevalence of *Eperythrozoon* spp. Infection and congenital eperthrozoonosis in humans in Inner Mangolia. *Clin. Epidemiol. Infect.* **125** : 421-426.

Yechouron, A., Lefebvre, J., Robson, H.G., Rose, D.L. and Tully, J.G. (1992). Fatal septicemia with *Mycoplasma arginini*: A new human zoonosis. *Clin. Infect. Dis.* **15** : 434-438.

5

CHANGING PATTERN OF VIRAL ZOONOSES : INDIAN PERSPECTIVE

R.K. Joshi

Zoonotic infections are defined as those transmissible, directly or indirectly, between vertebrate animals and humans. Zoonoses account for many of the recently emerging infectious diseases with high potential for public health and socio-economic impact. In recent years, changing patterns of infectious diseases has caught the attention of scientific community. The factors that lead to increase in the rates of these so-called 'emerging infectious diseases' (EIDs) have primarily involved the role of human activities such as population growth, increased association of populations and wild animal reservoirs, change in the land use system and the degradation of health care resources. Increase in international trade and travel, migration of people from rural to urban, deforestation, industrialization, urbanization, encroachment in animal habitat and changing agricultural practices are the major contributory factors in the changing pattern of transmission. It is estimated that the majority of these emerging diseases are derived from animals. These zoonoses come out of their natural reservoirs either through direct contact or indirectly through close contact with domestic animals and subsequently into human populations. The most important key factor in emergence of a new disease is genetic changes in the pathogen that establish them in a new host species, made them to productively infect new individuals and create local, regional or world wide health threats. Many of these key factors significantly increase the potential of transmission.

In India, the zoonotic viruses have always been a cause of concern as they are responsible for large scale involvement of human population. They usually reach to an epidemic proportion in a particular season. There are well established tracts of these infections in India and cause substantial human deaths every year. Some of the important viral zoonoses are as follows :

JAPANESE ENCEPHALITIS (JE)

Japanese Encephalitis (JE) is a mosquito borne viral zoonotic disease of Public health importance because of its epidemic potential and high case mortality rate. The virus infects mainly animals through migrating birds. Pig is the amplifier host. Man is affected incidentally. JE is primarily a disease of rural, semi urban, agricultural areas where vector mosquitoes proliferate in close association with pigs and other animal reservoirs. Man-to-man transmission is not possible.

JE occurs chiefly in three areas: (1) China and Korea (2) the Indian sub-continent consisting of India, parts of Bangladesh, southern Nepal, and Sri Lanka (3) the Southeast Asian countries of Burma, Thailand, Cambodia, Laos, Vietnam, Malaysia, Indonesia and the Philippines. JE may also occur with a lower frequency in Japan, Taiwan, Singapore, Hong Kong, and eastern Russia. The virus was isolated for the first time in the world from a post-mortem human brain in Japan in 1933. JE was clinically diagnosed for the first time in India in 1955 at Vellore, erstwhile North Arcot district of Tamil Nadu. Since, than the disease has been reported from 24 states / Union Territories so far. Frequently affected states include Andhra Pradesh, Assam, Bihar, Goa, Haryana, Karnataka, Manipur, Tamil Nadu, Uttar Pradesh and West Bengal. There was a rise of JE incidence in 1980s and has dropped significantly and maintained till 1995. Later the disease spread to new areas probably due to agricultural development and intensive rice cultivation supported by irrigation schemes that lead to an increase in mosquito population. It is a seasonal disease. Epidemics coincide with the heavy rainfall and or floods during monsoon and post monsoon period (August to December), agricultural practices, due to high density of the mosquito vector (because of stagnant water), and presence of reservoir host (pigs). Northern India, including North-eastern India, receives summer monsoons and as such the transmission season begins from May, with incidence reaching peak in August-October depending on the advancement of monsoon. With onset of winter, JE outbreaks subside. However, in endemic areas, sporadic cases may occur throughout the year due to congenial climatic conditions throughout the year (*e.g.*, Southern India).

Pigs are the most important reservoirs. Though they do not manifest the disease, they develop very high titers of virus and infect mosquitoes. Thus, pigs are the amplifying hosts. Susceptible children are infected by infected mosquito bites. Frogs, snakes, egrets, bats and most domestic animals like cattle also are infected by the virus.

Man is an incidental and dead-end host. Man-to-man transmission does not occur in nature. Cattle also act as dead-end host in the transmission cycle. From Ardeid birds, JE infection is transmitted by mosquitoes to pigs/ducklings. The pigs/ducklings serve as amplifying hosts since the virus multiplies in them. Man or cattle get infected either from birds or pigs/ducklings through mosquito bite. Ardeid bird–mosquito–Ardeid bird and pig/duckling–mosquito–pig/duckling cycle exist in nature.

The longest and most severe epidemic of JE in 3 decades occurred from July through November 2005 in Gorakhpur, Uttar Pradesh, India. Overall, 5,737 persons were affected in 7 districts of eastern Uttar Pradesh, and 1,344 persons died (WHO, 2005). Japanese encephalitis virus (JEV) is the most common cause of childhood viral encephalitis in the world; it causes an estimated 50,000 cases and 10,000 deaths annually (Monath and Heinz, 1996; Solomon *et al.*, 2003). JEV is endemic in the Gorakhpur and Basti divisions of eastern Uttar Pradesh. The geographic features of this region are conducive for the spread of JEV; an abundance of rice fields and a bowl-shaped landscape allow water to collect in pools. Heavy rains saturated the ground in 2005, which caused ideal breeding conditions for mosquitoes that transmit the virus from pigs to humans. In addition, high temperature and relative humidity provided a suitable environment for JEV transmission.

CHIKUNGUNYA VIRUS

Chikungunya fever is a viral illness that is transmitted by mosquito bite. The disease resembles dengue fever, and is characterized by severe, sometimes persistent, joint pain (arthritis), as well as fever and rash. It is rarely life-threatening. Epidemics of fever, rash and arthritis, resembling Chikungunya fever have been recorded as early as 1824 in India and elsewhere. However, Chikungunya virus (CHIKV) was first isolated in 1952 from humans, and *Aedes aegypti* and *Culex pipiens* mosquitoes during an epidemic of a non-fatal dengue-like illness on and near the Makonde plateau in south-eastern Tanzania (McCrae *et al.*, 1971). This Alphavirus (Family Togaviridae) is considered to be transmitted principally by various members of the mosquito genus *Aedes* (Diallo *et al.*, 1999) in a cycle between mosquitoes and various wildlife species. Sporadic spillover to humans has been characterized by mostly small, localized outbreaks.

Until recently it has been primarily restricted to countries surrounding or near the Indian Ocean, (McCrae *et al.*, 1971). Beginning in 2004 in East Africa, and continuing across many islands in the Indian Ocean and the Indian subcontinent in 2005–2006 an epidemic thought to affect more than 1.5 million people has occurred (Sourisseau *et al.*, 2007). Of special significance are hundreds of cases in holiday and business travelers from Europe and North America who returned to their homes under incubation (Lanciotti *et al.*, 2007, Taubitz *et al.*, 2007). Virus might have become established in southern Europe following the arrival of an incubating human visitor and was transmitted in 2007 by a previously introduced *Aedes* (*A. albopictus*) mosquito species in the region, potentially creating a new endemic (Rezza *et al.*, 2007).

In South East Asia, frequent outbreaks were reported from the 1960s through to 2003 in India, Malaysia, Indonesia, Cambodia, Vietnam, Myanmar, Pakistan and Thailand (Chastel, 1963; Jadhav *et al.*, 1965; Myers *et al.*, 1965; Munasinghe *et al.*, 1966; Halstead *et al.*, 1969a, b, c, d; Nimmannitya *et al.*, 1969; Thaung *et al.*, 1975; Thein *et al.*, 1992; Thaikruea *et al.*, 1997; Mourya *et al.*, 2001; Kit, 2002; Laras *et al.*, 2005; Parola *et al.*, 2006). Numerous large cities in South East Asia particularly Calcutta and Bangkok have been identified as active sites of transmission of disease (Pavri, 1964; Sarkar *et al.*, 1965b; Halstead *et al.*, 1969d; Burke *et al.*, 1985).

Chikungunya fever has an interesting epidemiology. It shows cyclical pattern of appearance and disappearance, of which major epidemics occur at an interval of 7-8 years and sometimes as long as 20 years between two episodes. Between 1960 and 1982, outbreaks of Chikungunya fever were reported from Africa and Asia. In Asian subcontinant, virus strains were first isolated in Bangkok in 1960s; then from various parts of India such as Vellore, Calcutta and Maharastha in 1964; from Sri Lanka in 1969; Vietnam in 1975; Myanmar in 1975 and Indonesia in 1982. After an interval of more than 20 years, Chikungunya fever reappeared in several countries including India, Indonesia, Maldives, Thailand and various Indian Ocean islands *viz.* Comoros, Mauritius, Reunion and Seychelles. Till 10th October 2006, 151 districts of eight states/provinces of India have been affected by chikungunya fever. The affected states are Andhra Pradesh, Andaman & Nicobar Islands, Tamil Nadu, Karnataka, Maharashtra, Gujarat, Madhya Pradesh, Kerala and Delhi. More than 1.25 million cases have been reported from the country with 7,52,245 cases from Karnataka and 2,58,998 from Maharashtra provinces (Chhabra *et al.*, 2008).

RABIES

Rabies is highly fatal zoonotic viral encephalitis that infects almost all warm-blooded animals including those living in wild and human beings. The disease is most commonly seen in carnivores from which it is transmitted to herbivores and other hosts. Both sylvatic and urban cycles of rabies perpetuate in

India since ancient times. Rabies is present throughout the country, except in the islands of Lakshadweep, Andaman and Nicobar (Sudarshan, 2004). India has the highest incidence of human rabies in the world. There is no organized system of surveillance of rabies cases, and hence there is a lack of reliable data. From 1985, India reported about 25,000 to 30,000 human deaths with rabies every year, which accounted to about 60% of the global report of 50,000 (WHO, 2005). The Indian Association for the Prevention and Control of Rabies estimates that about 8,000,000 people receive treatment for dog bites every year. Some even postulated that the true incidence of human rabies could be even ten times more than those officially reported. Once symptoms of rabies develop, it is almost invariably fatal. The problem with dog rabies in India is that dogs are asymptomatic carriers and they are freely available in every human establishment. Large geographical areas of the country did not report animal rabies in the last 10 years. The dog population was estimated to be about 25 million, most of which are ownerless and not immunized against rabies. The estimated animal bite load per year was 2.28 million. Thus, the current statistics of animal bites, rabies in animal population are scanty, unreliable and controversial due to poor surveillance/reporting system (Sudarshan, 2004).

India has the highest incidence of rabies world-wide. About 35,000 people die annually in our country and this is when the first successful vaccine was discovered on July 6, 1885 by Louis Pasteur. About one million people receive postexposure vaccination. Newspapers carry stories of deaths due to rabies and of valiant efforts by animal activists. Rabies is not a notifiable disease in India and our surveillance mechanisms are poor. A study carried out in four cities of India has reported the annual incidence of animal bites to be 2.1 per 1000 population. The number of animal bites in our capital city of Delhi had increased from 23852 in 1995 to 29905 in 1998 of which over 95% were dog bites (Bansal, 2004). Children constitute 30 to 50% of those receiving post-exposure vaccination or from dying from the disease. The nuisance of stray dogs seems to have assumed epidemic proportions everywhere.

Municipal bodies across India avoid catching these stray dogs due to animal rights activists, for instance the number of stray dogs culled in Delhi had decreased from 50,000 to 2500 a year (Bansal, 2004).

KYASANUR FOREST DISEASE (KFD)

Kyasanur Forest Disease (KFD), a tick-borne flavivirus infection was first described by Telford Work and Harold Trapido in a small forested region of Shimoga district of Karnataka in India in 1955 (Work and Trapido, 1957). The virus came to light when scientists heard that, monkeys were dying in large numbers in the area, and a number of local villagers also developed a mysterious illness comprising of severe headache, chills and a high fever. The human mortality rate was about ten percent (Work and Trapido, 1957). Initially, the disease was localized within a small area of Sagar Sorab taluka of Shimoga district. Then the disease moved to adjoining areas as a result of deforestation, increased human/ animal activity in the forest area. KFD is mainly seasonal and most cases appear during inter monsoon period i.e. December to June when man enters the forest for collecting wood and plants for fuel purposes and bitten by infected ticks. During this period, larval and nymphal stages of ticks also become very active.

Following the discovery of KFD, small but consistent numbers of cases continued to be reported annually. But in 1983 there was a large scale epidemic of KFD involving 1500 human cases and 150 deaths. The outbreak coincided with the clearing of large tracts of the forest to build cashew nut plantations and for the grazing of cattle (Varma, 2000). This has had a two-fold effect on KFD biology and epidemiology. First, clearing of natural patch of forest and farming the former forest has led to a significant increase in human presence in the area, which has in turn increased human exposure to the agent and its vectors (ticks). Second, the addition of cattle to the region has led to a relative shift host for these adult ticks as *Haemaphysalis spinigera* prefer to feed on large animals, including humans (Varma, 2000, Chomel *et al.*, 2007).

As a result up to three hundred cases of KFD are now reported annually, with a mortality rate of about ten percent. An understanding of the disease has enabled control measures to be introduced including the use of insecticides to control tick populations, public information (since the majority of infections occur during the dry pre-Monsoon months January to May), and the development of a killed vaccine that can protect about seventy percent of recipients. However, none of these strategies tackles the root of the problem, which is raising human population and the pressure that this applies to the local environment.

BUFFALOPOX VIRUS (BPV)

Buffalopox is a zoonotic and contagious viral disease, which mostly affects buffaloes, but rarely cows and human beings. Buffalopox is caused by buffalopox virus (BPV), classified in *Orthopoxvirus* genus of *Poxviridae* family. Occurrence of outbreaks is accompanied with 80% morbidity and significant productivity losses. The disease is being reported from all the buffalo rearing states of India, including Uttar Pradesh, Rajasthan, Andhra Pradesh, Gujarat and Karnataka.

NIPAH VIRUS

Nipah Virus Infection (NiV) is an emerging infectious disease of public health importance in the South-East Asia Region. The virus is named after the Malaysian village where it was first discovered. This virus along with Hendra virus comprises a new genus designated Henipavirus in the subfamily *Paramyxovirinae*. Fruit bats of the genus *Pteropus* have been identified as natural reservoirs of NiV. A seroepidemiologic study in Malaysia implicated four fruit bat species, *Pteropus hypomelanus, P. vampyrus, Cynopterus brachyotis, Eonycteris spelaea,* and an insectivorous bat, *Scotophilus kuhlii.* Nipah virus has been isolated from the brain and spinal fluid of victims in Malaysia. Infective virus has also been isolated from environmental samples of bat urine and partially-eaten fruit in Malaysia.

There were focal outbreaks of NiV in Bangladesh and India in 2001 during winter. Drinking of fresh date palm sap, possibly contaminated by fruit bats (*P. giganteus*) during the winter season, may have been responsible for indirect transmission of Nipah virus to humans (Luby *et al.*, 2006). There is circumstantial evidence of human-to-human transmission in India in 2001. During the outbreak in Siliguri, 33 health workers and hospital visitors became ill after exposure to patients hospitalized with Nipah virus illness, suggesting nosocomial infections (Chadha *et al.*, 2006). Antibodies to a Nipah-like virus have been found in sera from fruit bats collected in India, Indonesia and Timor-Leste (Heymann, 2008).

HANTA VIRUS

Hanta virus infections are currently underestimated or not recognised by the medical and public health authorities in many countries, largely because diagnostics are not available. Hanta virus infections are widely distributed in Europe with the exception of the far north and the Mediterranean regions. The underlying causes of varying epidemiological patterns differ among regions: in western and central Europe epidemics caused by hanta virus infections follow years with increased seed production by oak and beech trees followed by increased rodent reproduction. In the northern regions, hanta virus infections in three to four year cycles and are thought to be driven by prey – predator interactions. Hanta virus infections and HFRS seem to be on the increase in Europe, partly because of better diagnostics, partly perhaps due to environmental changes.

REFERENCES

Bansal, R.K. (2004). Making India a rabies-free country. JAPI **52** : 2-3.

Burke, D. S., Nisalak, A. & Nimmannitya, S. (1985). Disappearance of Chikungunya virus from Bangkok. *Trans R Soc Trop Med Hyg* **79** : 419–420.

Chadha, M.S., Comer, J.A., Lowe, L., Rota, P.A., Rollin, P.E., Bellini, W.J (2006). Nipah virus-associated encephalitis outbreak, Siliguri, India. *Emerg. Infect. Dis.* **6** : 235-40.

Chastel, C. (1963). Human infections in Cambodia by the chikungunya virus or an apparently closely related agent. I. Clinical aspects. Isolations and identification of the viruses. Serology. *Bull Soc Pathol Exot Filiales* **56** : 892–915 (in French).

Chhabra, M., Mittal, V., Bhattacharya, D., Rana, U., and Lal. S. (2008). Chikungunya fever: A re-emerging viral infection. *Indian J Med Microbiol* **26** : 5-12.

Chomel, B.B., Belotto, A. and Meslin. F. (2007). *Emerg. Infect. Dis.* **13** : 6-11.

Diallo, M., Thonnon, J., Traore-Lamizana, M. and Fontenille, D. (1999). Vectors of Chikungunya virus in a Senegal: Current data and transmission cycles. *American Society Tropical Medicine Hygiene.* **60** : 281–286.

Halstead, S. B., Nimmannitya, S. & Margiotta, M. R. (1969a). Dengue and chikungunya virus infection in man in Thailand, 1962–1964. II. Observations on disease in outpatients. *Am J Trop Med Hyg* **18** : 972–983.

Halstead, S.B., Scanlon, J.E., Umpaivit, P. and Udomsakdi, S. (1969d). Dengue and chikungunya virus infection in man in Thailand, 1962–1964. IV. Epidemiologic studies in the Bangkok metropolitan area. *Am J Trop Med Hyg* **18** : 997–1021.

Halstead, S.B., Udomsakdi, S., Scanlon, J.E. & Rohitayodhin, S. (1969c). Dengue and chikungunya virus infection in man in Thailand, 1962–1964. V. Epidemiologic observations outside Bangkok. *Am J Trop Med Hyg* **18** : 1022–1033.

Halstead, S.B., Udomsakdi, S., Singharaj, P. & Nisalak, A. (1969b). Dengue chikungunya virus infection in man in Thailand, 1962–1964. 3. Clinical, epidemiologic, and virologic observations on disease in non-indigenous white persons. *Am J Trop Med Hyg* **18** : 984–996.

Heymann, D.L. (2008). Henipavirus: Hendra and Nipah viral diseases. *Ctrl. of Comm. Dis.* **19** : 275-278.

Jadhav, M., Namboodripad, M., Carman, R.H., Carey, D.E. & Myers, R.M. (1965). Chikungunya disease in infants and children in Vellore: a report of clinical and haematological features of virologically proved cases. *Indian J Med Res* **53** : 764–776.

Kit, L. S. (2002). Emerging and re-emerging diseases in Malaysia. *Asia Pac J Public Hlth.* **14** : 6–8.

Lanciotti Robert, S., Kosoy Olga, L., Laven Janeen, J., Panella Amanda, J., Velez Jason, O., Lambert Amy, J. and Campbell Grant, L. (2007). Chikungunya virus in US travelers returning from India, 2006. *Emerg. Infect. Dis.* **13** : 764–767.

Laras, K., Sukri, N.C., Larasati, R.P., Bangs, M.J., Kosim, R., Djauzi, Wandra, T., Master, J., Kosasih, H. (2005). Tracking the re-emergence of epidemic chikungunya virus in Indonesia. *Trans R Soc Trop Med Hyg* **99** : 128–141.

Luby, S.P., Rahman, M., Hossain, M.J., Blum, L.S (2006) Foodborne transmission of Nipah virus, Bangladesh. *Emerg. Infect. Dis*. **12** : 1888-1894.

McCrae, A.W.R., Henderson, B.E., Kirya, B.G. and Sempala, S.D.K. (1971). Chikungunya virus in the Entebbe area of Uganda: Isolations and epidemiology. *Trans R Soc Trop Med Hyg*. **65** : 152–168.

Monath, T.P. and Heinz, F.X. (1996). *Flaviviridae*. In: Fields BN, Knipe DM, Howley PM, editors. *Fields virology*. **3** : 961–1034.

Mourya, D.T., Thakare, J.R., Gokhale, M.D., Powers, A.M., Hundekar, S.L., Jayakumar, P.C., Bondre, V.P., Shouche, Y.S. and Padbidri, V.S. (2001). Isolation of chikungunya virus from Aedes aegypti mosquitoes collected in the town of Yawat, Pune District, Maharashtra State, India. *Acta Virol* **45** : 305–309.

Munasinghe, D.R., Amarasekera, P.J. and Fernando, C.F. (1966). An epidemic of dengue-like fever in Ceylon (chikungunya)–a clinical and haematological study. *Ceylon Med J* **11** : 129–142.

Myers, R.M., Carey, D.E., Reuben, R., Jesudass, E.S., De Ranitz, C. and Jadhav, M. (1965). The 1964 epidemic of dengue-like fever in South India: isolation of chikungunya virus from human sera and from mosquitoes. *Indian J Med Res* **53** : 694–701.

Nimmannitya, S., Halstead, S.B., Cohen, S.N. and Margiotta, M.R. (1969). Dengue and chikungunya virus infection in man in Thailand, 1962–1964. I. Observations on hospitalized patients with hemorrhagic fever. *Am J Trop Med Hyg* **18** : 954–971.

Parola, P., de Lamballerie, X., Jourdan, J., Rovery, C., Vaillant, V., Minodier, P., Brouqui, P., Flahault, A., Raoult, D. and Charrel, R.N. (2006). Novel chikungunya virus variant in travellers returning from Indian Ocean islands. *Emerg. Infect. Dis.* **12** : 1493–1499.

Pavri, K. M. (1964). Presence of chikungunya antibodies in human sera collected from Calcutta and Jamshedpur before 1963. *Indian J. Med. Res.* **52** : 698–702.

Rezza, G., Nicolettim L., Angelinim R., Romi, R., Finarelli, A.C., Panning, M., Cordioli, P., Fortuna, C (2007). Infection with chikungunya virus in Italy: an outbreak in a temperate region. *Lancet.* **370** : 1840–1846.

Sarkar, J.K., Chatterjee, S.N., Chakravarty, S.K. and Mitra, A.C. (1965b). The causative agent of Calcutta haemorrhagic fever: chikungunya or dengue. *Bull Calcutta Sch. Trop. Med.* **13** : 53–54.

Solomon, T., Ni, H., Beasley, D.W.C., Ekkelenkamp, M., Cardosa, M.J. and Barret, A.D. (2003) Origin and evolution of Japanese encephalitis virus in Southeast Asia. *J. Virol.* **77** : 3091–8.

Sourisseau, M., Schilte, C., Casartelli,. N., Trouillet, C., Guivel-Benhassine, F (2007) Characterization of reemerging Chikungunya virus. *PLOS Pathogens.* **3** : 804–817.

Sudarshan, M.K. (2004) Assessing burden of rabies in India.WHO sponsored national multi-centric rabies survey. *Assoc Prev Control Rabies India J* **6** : 44-5.

Taubitz Winfried, Cramer Jakob P, Kapaun Anette, Pfeffer Martin, Drosten Christian, Dobler Gerhard, Burchard Gerd D, Loschen Thomas.(2007) Chikungunya fever in travelers: Clinical presentation and course. *Clin. Infect. Dis.*. **45** : e1–e4.

Thaikruea, L., Charearnsook, O., Reanphumkarnkit, S., Dissomboon, P., Phonjan, R., Ratchbud, S., Kounsang, Y. and Buranapiyawong, D. (1997). Chikungunya in Thailand: a re-emerging disease? *Southeast Asian J. Trop. Med. Publ. Hlth.* **28** : 359–364.

Thaung, U., Ming, C. K., Swe, T. and Thein, S. (1975). Epidemiological features of dengue and chikungunya infections in Burma. *Southeast Asian J. Trop. Med. Publ. Hlth.* **6** : 276–283.

Thein, S., La Linn, M., Aaskov, J., Aung, M.M., Aye, M., Zaw, A. and Myint, A. (1992). Development of a simple indirect enzyme-linked immunosorbent assay for the detection of immunoglobulin M antibody in serum from patients following an outbreak of chikungunya virus infection in Yangon, Myanmar. *Trans R Soc. Trop. Med. Hyg.* **86** : 438–442.

Varma MGR. (2000). The encyclopedia of arthropod-transmitted infections. New York : *CABI Pub.*, **200** : 254-60

WHO (2005). Outbreak encephalitis 2005: cases of Japanese encephalitis in Gorakhpur, Uttar Pradesh, India. 2005. Core Programme Clusters. Communicable Diseases and Disease Surveillance. 2005 Oct 21 [cited 2006 Jul 11].

Work T. and Trapido H., (1957). Proceedings of the Ninth Pacific Science Congress **17** : 80-84.

6

TRANSBOUNDARY ANIMAL DISEASES AND ZOONOSES - NEED OF HOLISTIC APPROACH

Gyanendra Gongal

Transboundary Animal Diseases (TADs) may be defined as those epidemic diseases which are highly contagious or transmissible and have potential for very rapid spread, irrespective of national borders, causing serious socio-economic consequences and possibly disruption of international trade in animals and animal products. The importance of TADs is increasing in the context of commercialization of livestock sector, globalization of livestock trade and informal nature of live animal movement and transport of livestock products, livestock production materials in cross border areas. The outbreak of highly pathogenic avian influenza, foot-and-mouth disease (FMD), Peste des petits ruminants (PPR) are classical examples of TADs in South Asia Region.

Zoonoses are those infections and diseases which are naturally "transmissible from vertebrate animals to man". Over 30 new human pathogens have been detected in the last three decades, 75% of which have originated from animals. New pathogens from animals, particularly viruses, remain unpredictable, continue to emerge and spread across countries and many of them have profoundly affected countries in Asia. The emerging diseases of epidemic potential in Asia are SARS, avian influenza (AI) and the Nipah virus infection. The major endemic zoonotic diseases are rabies, leptospirosis, Japanese encephalitis, anthrax and brucellosis.

The economic and public health costs of highly pathogenic, emerging and re-emerging diseases are so great globally that, preventive strategies are not only cost-effective, but imperative. Regional cooperation is a prerequisite for control and eradication of TADs and zoonoses. In the contest of the global and regional effort for the prevention, control and eradication of TADs and zoonoses, Food and Agriculture Organization, World Organization for Animal Health (OIE) and World Health Organization (WHO) are working together to promote holistic approach through implementation of Regional Cooperation Project in coordination with ASEAN and SAARC Secretariats. The project emphasizes the enhancement of surveillance and response capacity and improvement of laboratory diagnostic capacity for highly pathogenic and emerging and re-emerging diseases which involves training and capacity building activities.

The spread of infectious diseases emerge from the interfaces between animals and humans and the ecosystems in which they live. It is clear that no one discipline or sector of society has enough knowledge and resources to prevent the emergence or resurgence of diseases in todays globalized world. The need of "One World One Health" approach was originated from New Delhi Ministerial Conference on Avian Influenza in December 2007. The One World One Health (OWOH) concept proposes an international, interdisciplinary, cross-sectoral approach to surveillance, monitoring, prevention, control and mitigation of emerging diseases, as well as to environmental conservation. The OWOH concept provides a framework for preventing emerging infectious diseases of animal origin, instead of simply responding to them once they have occurred.

The risk factors associated with persistence and emergence of TADs and zoonoses have been elaborated. Various activities have been discussed in details for effective management of TADs and zoonoses in the context of regional and international frameworks.

7

TRANSBOUNDARY ANIMAL DISEASES : AN OVERVIEW

S.K. Kotwal, Rajesh Agrawal, Nishi Pande and H.K. Sharma

Transboundary animal diseases (TADs) are defined as those epidemic diseases which are highly contagious or transmissible and have the potential for very rapid spread, irrespective of national borders, causing serious socio-economic and possibly public health consequences. TADs cause a high morbidity and mortality in susceptible animal populations and thus constitute a constant threat to the livelihood of livestock farmers and detrimental effect on national economies. TADs have the potential to threaten food security, increase poverty levels in livestock depending poor communities, major production losses for livestock products such as meat, milk, wool, fibres, skins and hides, thereby reducing farm incomes. They may also limit upgrading the production trait of local livestock population by making it difficult to utilize exotic high producing breeds which tend to be very susceptible to the transboundary diseases. It also increases the cost of livestock production through costly disease control measures; inhibit national/international trade in livestock and livestock products besides public health (i.e. zoonoses) and environmental consequences. Another characteristic being the rapidity with which they can spread in susceptible livestock populations. This renders individual farmers and veterinary services relatively powerless to take effective action to avoid or overcome outbreaks of these diseases.

Basic Conditions that Influence the Establishment, Spread in Region, Countries or Zones within Countries Are :

- Climate
- Geographical isolation
- Livestock production system
- Prevalent host and vectors
- Control methods

Factors Contributing to the Dynamic Nature of Transboundary Animal Diseases Are :

Transboundary animal diseases show dynamism as new diseases emerge, and old diseases re-emerge, sudden and unexpected spread to new regions over great distances. These trends are likely to continue and even speed up in the future. In last 30 years many new infectious diseases emerged in human like AIDS, Lassa fever, Ebola, Influenza etc. The same has occurred with animal diseases, with the appearance of BSE, porcine reproductive and respiratory syndrome (PRRS) and equine morbilli virus disease. Not only do new infections emerge, but also new biotypes or antigenic types of existing infectious diseases. There are a number of factors contributing to the dynamic nature of transboundary animal diseases :

- ***Globalization :*** Globalization facilitates the sea, land, air transport and marketing opportunities (livestock and products) and increase the movement of animals and human thus favouring spread of such diseases. Nomadism and the movement of human and their animals away from wars and civil disturbances also help in the spread of infectious animal diseases creating immense pressure on countries in maintaining effective quarantine barriers at airports, seaports and along international borders.
- ***Livestock Production Systems :*** Intensification and commercialization of livestock production has increased

the concentration of animals with greater opportunity for transboundary animal diseases to spread and cause greater economic losses.

- ***Government Veterinary Services :*** Funding of veterinary services is poor and even declining in many countries, resulting in uncontrolled livestock movements, poor diagnostic capacity and the inability to handle quickly and effectively to disease outbreaks. Farmers fear for disease losses and thus often tend to sell still healthy-looking livestock to reduce their financial losses when a disease problem is occurring on their farm. As a proportion of these apparently healthy animals may be in early stages of infection where clinical signs are not yet apparent, this behavior of farmers may significantly contribute to the spread of disease.
- ***Biological and Ecological Factors :*** In some regions of the world, tropical rain forests and other wilderness areas are being converted to livestock farming. This exposes human communities and farm animals to a completely new range of infectious diseases which may have previously only circulated in wild life reservoirs and had remained unknown. Some of these diseases may be transmissible to susceptible humans and/or livestock. Global warming trends, may change rainfall and weather patterns in a number of regions, affecting particularly the global distribution of insect vectors, *e.g.* mosquitoes and *Culicoides* midges and the important viral and protozoal transboundary animal diseases that they transmit.

Fight Against Transboundary Animal Diseases

An effective national animal quarantine system should always be the first line of defence against the entry and establishment of transboundary animal diseases. However, even the most sophisticated quarantine service cannot provide an absolute barrier. Countries therefore need a second line of defence, which is the development of contingency plans and capabilities to respond quickly to high threat diseases should they enter. If an introduced transboundary animal disease can be recognised early whilst it is localised and then a disease control programme be quickly implimented, the prospects for eradication of the disease with minimal production losses and other costs are markedly enhanced. Conversely, if the disease is allowed to become well established in the country, eradication may be very costly and difficult or even impractical (particularly if the disease becomes established in wildlife). Thus, the two key principles in combating transboundary animal diseases are :

(a) Early Warning System : This is to rapidly detect the introduction or sudden increase in the incidence of any disease of livestock which has the potential of developing to epidemic proportions and/or causing serious socio-economic consequences or public health concerns. It embraces all initiatives, mainly based on disease surveillance, reporting and epidemiological analysis that would lead to improved awareness and knowledge of the distribution and behaviour of disease outbreaks (and of infection) which allow forecasting of the source and evolution of the disease outbreaks and the monitoring of the effectiveness of disease control campaigns.

(b) Early Reaction System : This is to carry out without delay the disease control activities needed to contain the outbreak and then to eliminate the disease and infection in the shortest possible time frame and in the most cost-effective way, or at least to return to the status-quo that existed previously and to provide scientific evidence that one of these objectives has been achieved.

Use of new technology in the fight against transboundary animal diseases.

The last two decades or so have seen exceedingly rapid strides in scientific knowledge in the fields of genetic engineering and computer science. Such new technology can now be applied to combat transboundary animal diseases. The areas in which technical advances to combat these diseases have been most pronounced are :

- Disease surveillance and animal health information systems (like GLEWS, EMPRES).
- Other methods for studying the epidemiology of disease outbreaks.
- Disease diagnosis and methods for the characterization of etiological agents.
- Better vaccines for disease control and eradication programmes.
- Sanitary measures for management of such diseases (see table).

Some major transboundary animal diseases and their current geographical distribution :

1. *Foot-and-Mouth Disease (FMD)* is the most contagious disease in animals, affecting mainly cattle, sheep and pigs with high morbidity and production losses, and is a major hurdle to international trade in livestock and livestock products. The disease has been absent from south Eastern Europe and rest of Europe. Considerable progress has been made towards eradication in South America, with the southern countries of Chile, Argentina, Paraguay, and Uruguay not having recorded outbreaks for two years or longer and the southern states of Santa Catarina and Rio Grande do Sul have been declared 'FMD free with vaccination'. FMD is still endemic in many parts of Africa, the Middle East and Asia, but a regional control programme is in place in South-East Asia.

2. *Rinderpest (RP)* is a viral disease affecting mainly cattle and buffaloes. It usually causes a very high mortality, although less virulent virus strains circulating in East Africa have complicated eradication there. RP has been progressively eliminated in West Africa, but here are still three endemic foci in East Africa. Great progress has been made towards RP eradication in India, but the disease is endemic in Pakistan and has spread to

Afghanistan. There are endemic foci in the Middle east. Sporadic outbreaks, the origins of which are unknown, have occurred in Eastern Russia and Mongolia in recent years.

3. *Peste des Petits Ruminants (PPR)* is a rinderpest-like disease of sheep and goats. In recent years there has been serious spread of this disease from Africa, to the Middle East and in Asia as far east as India.

4. *Rift Valley Fever (RVF)* is a serious mosquito-borne virus disease of sheep, cattle and goats which causes very high mortality rates in young animals and abortion of pregnant animals. It is also transmitted to humans causing a potentially fatal disease. Major epidemics have occurred at irregular intervals of 10-30 years in the eastern half of Africa, from South Africa to Egypt.

5. *Lumpy Skin Disease (LSD)* is a disease of cattle which may cause serious production losses, through prolonged debility and loss of hides. LSD is mainly confined to Africa, where it has caused periodic, major epidemics in many countries.

6. *Classical Swine Fever (CSF)* is a generalised virus disease of pigs which may cause high mortalities. It is endemic in much of South and South-East Asia, where it is a constraint to the development of the pig industry. It is the most significant transboundary animal disease in Europe, where it caused 611 outbreaks in the European Community in 1997. These occurred in the Netherlands, Germany, Spain and Italy and are estimated to have cost these countries more than $7 billion. Recent outbreaks have also occurred in Latin America.

7. *African Swine Fever (ASF)* is another generalized virus disease of pigs which is endemic in much of sub-Saharan Africa. There have been very serious outbreaks over the last few years in previously free areas of West Africa. ASF has shown great propensity for inter-continental spread. Outbreaks have occurred at different times in parts of Europe and Latin America.

Table 7.1 : Sanitary Measures for Managing Animal Diseases (Quinlan, 2000)

Sequence of Control Measures	*Reduce Risk of Entry*	*Verification of Compliance*	*Control or Mitigation*	*Adaptation or Acceptance*
When to take Measures	• Request to import new commodity, or from new country • Surveillance indicates change in pathway risk or epidemiology • Policy review on existing pathways or disease status	• Entry and distribution points for commodities and live animals	• Outbreak or incursion detected and control options exist • Natural pathway led to introduction and control deemed appropriate	• Impact found to be less than predicted • Improved ability to adapt • Ineffective control ended • Disease not controllable with existing technology • Cost of control exceeds benefits
Examples of Measures Aimed at Preventing Introduction of Diseases	• Training, technical assistance, and surveys in control of origin • Network with officials and experts areas of risk • Review of interception lists • Development of restricted lists in accordance with SPS guidelines • Inspection in country of origin	• Inspection • Visual • Random sampling • Targeted by risk • Detector dogs • Review of permits zoo sanitary certificates, bills of landing • Isolation for observation period • Treatment, re-export or destruction in response to interception	• Detection and delineation of infected zone • Monitoring of surrounding zone • Suppression, containment or eradication using • Quarantine stations • Stamping-out • Vaccines • Pesticide applications • Sterile insect relase • Systems approach using a combination of measures	• Research new control options for producers • Registration of new vaccine that is effective in control options for producers • Registration of new vaccine that is effective in control • Create disease-free stock supply and certification • Control programme keeps disease at tolerable level

Contd....

Sequence of Control Measures	*Reduce Risk of Entry*	*Verification of Compliance*	*Control or Mitigation*	*Adaptation or Acceptance*
	• Restrict imports to a designated free area in a country with disease • Require advance treatment for high-risk commodities • Analysis to find pathways for preventive action • Identify potential range of organism and survival parameters	• Limited ports of entry according to type of cargo and/or risk • Limited market destination • Containerisation for transit through vulnerable zone • Public education	• Treatment of animals leaving the area to avoid spread • Emergency reporting systems to inform of movement to new areas (leads back to risk reduction measures)	• Addition of water treatment for water-borne diseases.
Reasons for failure of control measures *Note* : All measures may fail with inadequate funding or political will to carry them out	• Information non-existent or misleading • Treatment options limited • Pathway not yet recognised • Host not yet recognized • Inadequate data	• Inspection fails due to volume of entry, poor sampling, etc. • Cryptic life stage at time of entry or difficult to identiry or diagnose • Natural pathway not regulated • Smuggling of high-risk items • Transhipment obscures country of origin	• Detection techniques not successful (*i.e.* disease not detected) • Insufficient monitoring • Vaccines not available	• Control methods used by some producers but not by all • Disease agent may become resistant to the control measures • New populations or strains cause outbreaks of non-indigenous disease

Contd....

Sequence of Control Measures	*Reduce Risk of Entry*	*Verification of Compliance*	*Control or Mitigation*	*Adaptation or Acceptance*
Problems from relying on Above Measures	• Requirements to reduce risk become onerous • Trade dispute results from imbalance between risk reduction and free trade values • Consumers in importing country lose benefit of new supply.	• Delays in release of cargo and passenger delays • Civil rights could be violated • Smuggling may increase	• More severe environmental impact from control versus prevention • Repeated introductions lead to high costs when the original pathway is not closed	• Secondary impacts from the disease may not be recognized initially • Existence of disease is accepted, ending control efforts.

8. *Newcastle Disease (ND)* is perhaps the most lethal disease of poultry, outbreaks of which have occurred in most parts of the world, including two major pandemics during this century. It is a major constraint to the development of village chicken industries, particularly in Asia and Africa.

9. *Highly Pathogenic Avian Influenza (HPAI)* this is another serious poultry disease, which may produce high mortalities. There is some concern about the potential for the appearance of avian influenza virus strains transmittable to humans. Wild water birds constitute the major reservoir for avian influenza viruses and HPAI outbreaks in domestic poultry may occur suddenly anywhere in the world. There have been a number of outbreaks in recent years in North America, Asia and Australia. Same is true about swine influenza which is creating public health crisis affecting human health across the globe.

10. *Contagious Bovine Pleuropneumonia (CBPP)* Although this is an insidious disease in areas where it is well established, it causes serious epidemics with high mortality rates in cattle when it moves into new areas. Major CBPP epidemics have been experienced in Eastern, Southern and West Africa over the last few years. The disease is also endemic in some parts of Asia.

CONCLUSION

The livestock sector plays a vital role in the economies of many developing countries. The diseases of animals adversely affect the human populations by reducing the quantity and quality of food, livestock products like hides, skins, fibers, wool and animal draught power *i.e.* traction, transport etc. Transboundary animal diseases are a permanent threat for health of livestock and man with most serious consequences. Such diseases are no respecters of national or administrative borders. The control efforts of individual countries (with contiguous borders) against these diseases may be continually frustrated by the fact that neighboring countries are not taking equivalent action. Such diseases therefore need to be tackled on a regional basis, with cooperation between countries and harmonization of their prevention and response programmes. An international approach should take advantage of natural geographical barriers and broader epidemiological patterns of the diseases.

8

STRATEGIES FOR CONTROL OF RABIES WITH SPECIAL REFERENCE TO HILLY STATES

S.K. Kotwal

Rabies is one of the oldest documented and most feared maladies in medical history. Despite significant progress in Lyssa virus research *viz.* pathogenesis, prophylaxis, molecular virology, control and epidemiology, the rabies remains a neglected and poorly controlled disease throughout much of the developing countries. The global mortality from rabies is substantial compared to many other human diseases. However, the reported cases of rabies represent only the 'tip of iceberg' from a public health point of view, as per one estimate, for each reported death, ten or more may go unreported. An estimated 2.7 billion people live in developing countries where canine rabies is endemic; the mortality can be estimated to 30,000 to 35,000 cases per year (Meslin *et al.,* 1994). In every country where rabies is a public health problem, its elimination is justified in terms of its public health and economic significance. If animal rabies is eliminated most of the mortality and related expenses associated with public health activities can be diverted for other public health priorities. In many developing countries rabies is not a notifiable disease in animals or humans and remains the most neglected zoonosis inspite of the fact that rabies kills more people than Dengue, JE, Yellow fever combined. In India with serious canine rabies problem, the economic burden justifies elimination of the disease. If the disease is not eliminated the expenses related to prevention and control of disease in both man and animals are likely to increase dramatically.

EXTENT OF THE PROBLEM

Exact extent of the rabies problem in the developing countries is not known and whatever estimates available are extrapolated from the informations such as human rabies Post Exposure Therapy (PET), post vaccinal complications and the animal rabies and occasionally vaccination failures reports. Hilly states with unique topography and interspersed wild life which often overlaps with domestic animals and pets require special attention.

RABIES IN HUMANS

Approximately 98% of estimated deaths due to rabies were reported from developing countries as per world Rabies Survey (WHO, 1992). The disease is mainly contacted through bites or licks of a rabid dog and occasionally the wild animals. More than 70% of the population of two most populated countries in the world, India and China reside in canine rabies infested areas of the world. In India, an estimated 25,000 to 30,000 persons (20,565 per annum as per APCRI- 2003) die of rabies annually, thus it continues to be a major Public Health problem. Estimates of the actual number of rabies deaths / morbidity that occur annually can be derived from the mortality figures for rabies from those developing countries where rabies surveillance is adequate. In such areas rates of the human rabies vary from one to more than 10 cases per million inhabitants.

POST EXPOSURE TREATMENT (PET)

In India an estimated 3-3.5 million persons are reported to receive PET annually requiring more than 40,000 liters of antirabic vaccine (sheep brain) each year. In China about 2 million persons receive PET (Lin *et al.*, 1990). Data from 30 countries with dog rabies revealed a mean rate of 867 rabies PET per million inhabitants (Meslin *et al*, 1994). Globally an estimated 10 million people require post exposure treatments annually (WHO, 1999). Annual bite incidence in India as reported by ARCRI, 2003 is 17.4/1000 population.

POST VACCINATION COMPLICATIONS

Vaccination failure and rates of neurological complication following rabies vaccines of nerve tissue origin must be considered as an indirect burden of the disease warranting concern. Reactions occur in about 1.5 persons per thousand vaccines (range 0.1 – 5 per 1000) and up to 25% of these patients die or suffer permanent disability, these complications or deaths could have been avoided.

ANIMAL RABIES

Dogs are responsible for vast majority of human rabies deaths; in India this figure approaches 98 – 99%. Thus canine rabies requires most attentioning programmes for rabies elimination. Completeness of Animal Rabies Surveillance varies from country-to-country and from species-to-species. For every one human death there are four cases in dogs (WHO, 1992 a). In Thailand, with a well developed network of regional rabies laboratories, an estimated 8422 dog rabies cases were recorded during the year 1987. It was roughly about 1 case for every 961 dogs (estimated owned dog population is 7 million). Rabies cases in food and draught animals are grossly under reported due to several reasons like difficult and inaccessible terrain, lack of laboratories, infrastructure etc. The economic losses in livestock on account of rabies are substantial. As per one survey (in Punjab) spanning over a decade (Singh, 2007) dog bite alone accounted for 61.4% rabies deaths in cattle, 48.7% in goats, 48.4% in dogs, 45% in horses and 22% in cats.

RABIES SURVEILLANCE

The main aim of rabies surveillance lies in estimating the public health burden of the disease but there are a number of difficulties in establishing and conducting appropriate surveillance before elimination programmes are launched. In most developing countries generally only those animals that bite man (*e.g.* dog) are included in surveillance programmes for rabies testing. Investigation of every suspect animal rabies case is important since a single case of rabies indicates that elimination is not complete. The elimination programmes and rabies surveillance activities should go side by side as they provide a deep insight on the magnitude of the problem. The surveillance aspects are incomplete in India in spite of the developments of a number of techniques for diagnosis, sampling, shipping brain material etc.

The cost of rabies surveillance represents only a small proportion of total cost of rabies control programme. Citing an example for Philippines, it represents only one percent of the total cost (Fishbein *et al.*, 1991). The logistical difficulties and cost of establishing comprehensive surveillance of animal rabies in developing countries are some impediments. In such developing regions where rabies is known to exist and the resources are scanty, it may be technically more practical to rely on indirect estimates for example vaccination coverage data to assess the success of prevention activities in the dog population.

RATIONAL FOR ELIMINATING RABIES

In spite of the fact that the rabies is public health problem in most developing countries including India yet it is the most neglected disease. The high case fatality rate (1% of total morbidity due to infectious diseases) and the uncertainty associated with the treatment make it most feared disease. Rabies elimination programmes in the country can be justified on these grounds :

(*i*) Reduction of mortality.

(*ii*) Reduction of morbidity and associated expenses.

(*iii*) Economic benefits by discontinuing animal vaccination.

Surge in economic burden recently seen in developing countries is due to a rising trend in PET together with quality improvement of the vaccines (cell culture vaccines) which is likely to further increase the expenses. In Thailand the cost of PET (1989) was estimated at US $ 2700,000 (51% of total annual cost of rabies prevention in the country). Whereas, the dog immunization and removal accounted for only 18% and 28% of these costs respectively. The remaining 3% represented the surveillance related expenses. If the 80% of Thailands' dog population (72,000,000) is to be vaccinated than expenses would be approximately 3500,000 US $ an amount 25% more than spent on human vaccines (Meslin, 1989). Thus, the elimination of rabies is justified as it can halt mortality, morbidity and psychological suffering besides other economic benefits. The reduction in mortality and morbidity is justified on humanitarian and economic grounds.

ECONOMIC AND HEALTH BURDEN OF RABIES IN INDIA

Based on the results of the rabies survey, 2003 by APCRI revised annual incidence of rabies is at around 20,565. The principal animal reservoir is dog (96.3%), frequency of human rabies deaths is at approximately 1 per 30 minutes. The pet dog: man ratio reported was 1 : 36, pet, owned, household dog population is at 28 million and the annual bite frequency of 17.4/1000 population. The annual man days lost from animal bites is reported to be 38 million man days with annual medical expenses around 2 billion rupees. The most common reservoir of rabies were dogs, cattle, goats, cats, pigs and among the wild animals were mongoose, jackals and monkeys.

STRATEGIES FOR RABIES PREVENTION

The disease has been eliminated from number of countries for example, UK – 1922, Japan – 1957, Malaysia – 1957. Recently, only a hand full of countries have eliminated this disease, these include Taiwan – 1961, Portugal – 1961, Uruguay – 1983. Different strategies have been adapted to control/eliminate rabies broadly *viz.*; those directed at humans (PET/pre exposure treatment) and those directed at the main animal host species (population control, parentral or oral vaccination). These strategies may be used alone or in combination. In order to eliminate canine rabies in the northern hilly states of India and elsewhere, there are at least five pre-requisites *viz.*, availability of a potent cell culture vaccine (both for animal and human use), Medical and veterinary professional interactions, effective methods of control and prevention with sound backing of diagnosis, an increased awareness in public, implementation of dog control strategies, political and financial backing and other intersectoral cooperation etc.

CANINE RABIES ELIMINATION

Studies on Dog Behaviour

This requires knowledge of certain characteristics of dog *e.g.* ecology, population dynamics, human animal bond because it is the most important species in developing countries. The programmes based on combination of dog elimination and vaccination campaigns have been carried out under WHO regime. Dog population studies in most countries with different socio-economical and religious background had certain major characteristics in common (WHO, 1988).

Common Characteristics of Dog Population

1. Animals aged 1 year or less represented 21-42% of population.
2. Majority of the dogs were mostly owned by an individual, by a family or community.
3. Only small proportion (7-12%) was owner less.
4. 85% of dog population was accessible to parentral vaccination.

Dog Population and Turn Over

The WHO coordinated projects had demonstrated that dogs have huge population turn over (25-30% of the dogs are replaced by new individuals within a year). Thus biannual vaccination can not in most areas maintain immunization coverage compatible with elimination of the disease.

Dog Population Management

The four different approaches to dog population management are :

(*a*) Dog movement restriction.

(*b*) Reproduction control.

(*c*) Habitat control

(*d*) Dog removal.

The dog removal has been extensively applied in past. The other three approaches having been recently implemented and are still being assessed (WHO, 1990, 1993). Removal is believed to disrupt the naturally established social organization of dog population and is reported to increase the contact rate between dogs, who take over the space formally occupied by another individual. Thus the recent studies have concluded that dog elimination is least efficient (manpower, cost and opposition to dog rabies control).

Parentral Vaccines

Success of vaccination can achieve the desired coverage if significant proportion of dogs are covered by parentral vaccination (for example, dogs aged under 2 – 3 months, owner less dogs, owned dogs found in or near the household, un-catchable, free roaming etc). These categories together represent about 15–25% of total dog population. Besides this the annual 25% new additions may also interfere in desired vaccine coverage.

Public Cooperation

The sensitization of the public for the success of the programme is a pre-requisite. In Sri Lanka a two step strategy *i.e.* extensive information campaigns on the days before actual vaccination and high density of vaccination centers in the area involved (1 centre for every 250–500 meters) led to the satisfactory vaccination coverage.

Planning Strategies

Both at the national and regional levels, we need to establish task forces with sound organizational setup duly empowered with financial and administrative powers. In this connection Animal Welfare Board of India (AWBI) could coordinate the various states in this endeavour. At the regional level, where actually control programmes are to be executed we require Programme Implementation Committees as well as implementation teams. These constituent committees should be familiar with the regional as well as local requirements for implementation of rabies control programmes.

Area Under Rabies Control

We must choose such an area in the beginning for this programme that is actually facing the problem of rabies both in man and animals. In this regard the habits and habitats of principal animal species (Dog) need to be exploited. In this area immunization of dogs as well as birth control may be carried out before moving to another area and return only for annual booster. Strategically the approach should be from the periphery towards the center of the adopted area. Systematic and effective implementation of the programme requires thorough details of the area for the sake of convenience. An Inter-sectoral collaboration in the adopted area has to be ensured amongst health, veterinary, municipality, environment, police, NGOs, media, urban/rural developments and wild life experts (if required). Once the urban cycle is broken the disease can be pushed back into its sylvatic habitat wherefrom it can be eliminated by other efforts.

Training of Personals/Volunteers

This can be achieved by proper trainings/practical demonstration (dog catching, oral bait feeding of community/ stray dogs, immunization, maintenance of records etc) of those involved in these programmes.

IS ORAL VACCINATION OF DOGS A KEY TO RABIES ELIMINATION?

This technique is still under study and no large scale field experiment seems to have been conducted with respect to canine rabies. The few baiting trials using placebo baits however, have been carried out in Mexico (Frontini *et al.*, 1992), Tunisia (Kharmachi *et al.*, 1992), Zimbabwe (Perry *et al.*, 1988) and Nepal (Suchowiecki *et al.*, 1992). Result of few trials on the efficacy of orally administered vaccines in dogs have shown promising results and vaccinated dog's withstood virulent challenge (WHO, 1988, 1991). Two types of vaccines, one the rabies recombinant (Vaccinia vectored) and the SAG-2 vaccines were found to protect dogs for over one year after oral immunization (WHO, 1993). At present baits for delivering vaccines orally are available for foxes and Raccoons. Oral vaccine can be used alone or in association with parentral vaccination. There are three delivery systems which can be adopted for use in dogs :

(*a*) Distribution of baits through owners.

(*b*) Placement of baits at strategic spots where they can be picked up by stray and free roaming dogs (wild life immunization model).

(*c*) The distribution of baits to dogs encountered in the streets (hand–out model).

The first technique is, if owners could be motivated that could lead to a high percentage of coverage of owned dogs (approx-90%). Deposition of the baits at strategic spots would target mainly free roaming ownerless or owned dogs. The efficacy being dependent up on the dog population parameters etc. (WHO, 1993). This technique is thought to be more effective in rural areas with higher proportion of free roaming dogs and could lead up to 85% of coverage. The last delivery technique that is hand out model was experimented in Tunisia but resulted only up to 30 % coverage of dog population in the experimental area (WHO, 1992). The oral vaccination technique may play a complementary role to parentral vaccination especially in areas where a large number of unrestrainable owned dogs, free roaming dogs are abundant. This technique with little improvement could replace parentral vaccination in future.

Another problem in the hilly states is the chances of exposure of dogs and other domestic animals to rabies in such areas as mosaics/interfaces of forests and habitations. These areas are frequented by wild animal vectors *e.g.*, jackals, foxes, mongooses (some could be rabid) etc. Sending animals to such areas for grazing requires careful monitoring.

CONCLUSION

The success of rabies elimination in a number of countries suggests that elimination is feasible and should be considered in developing countries where the only reservoir of rabies is dog. Some studies carried out during the past decade have provided information on strategies which may be adopted to eliminate the disease. Rabies control programmes must be designed for sustainability from the planning stage with sound technical, political and administrative support which should be assured and the flow of information should be from bottom to top (WHO, 1992). Vaccine availability, merging/sharing of personals and equipments and other resources is desired but requires strong political backing and will.

9

STATUS AND STRATEGIES FOR CONTROL OF BRUCELLOSIS IN INDIA

D.K. Sinha

Brucellosis is an acute or chronic contagious disease of domestic animals. It is one of the most ancient and world's major zoonoses accounting for enormous economic losses and significant human morbidity in endemic areas. It is caused by intracellular, Gram's negative, coccobacilli, 0.6 to 1.5 micron in size of genus *Brucella*, which infect macrophages with principal involvement of liver, spleen and bone marrow. There are six species of *Brucella* namely, *B. abortus* (cattle), *B. melitensis* (sheep and goat), *B. suis* (pigs), *B. ovis* (rams), *B. canis* (dogs) and *B. neotomae* (wood rats). Two new species, provisionally called *B. pinnipediae* and *B. cetaceae*, have been isolated from marine hosts in recent years (Ewalt *et al.* 1994, Ross *et al.* 1996). Their zoonotic potential has been demonstrated by reports of human infection (Brew *et al.* 1999, Sohn *et al.* 2003, McDonald *et al.* 2006).

Brucellae are fairly hardy, organisms have been recovered from fetal and manure samples that remained in a cool environment for longer than 2 months. However, exposure to sunlight kills the organism within a few hours (Waring 2005) and the organism is susceptible to many common disinfectants, including 1% sodium hypochlorite (Anon 2008).

The classical species *viz. B. abortus, B. melitensis,* and *B. suis* have been identified as Category B bioterrorism agents

(Rotz *et al.* 2002, CDC 2005) because they are easily capable of causing considerable morbidity with low mortality if used in a mass event.

OCCURRENCE AND TRANSMISSION

Animal brucellosis is worldwide in distribution and bovine brucellosis, caused by *B. abortus*, remains the most widespread form in animals (Corbel 1997). Brucellosis causes considerable economic losses through reduced productivity, abortions and weak off springs of livestock which is a major stumbling block for trade and export. Among animals, the predominant route of exposure is through ingestion or inhalation of organisms that are present in fetal fluids or other birth products; herds are typically exposed following the introduction of an infected animal that subsequently gives birth or aborts a fetus, whereupon pasture or water become contaminated by these excretions. Transient disease (*e.g.* abortions) can also develop following administration of a live *Brucella* vaccine, particularly the *B. abortus* vaccine strain (Paulsen *et al.* 2002). Among sheep, transmission is more common via the venereal route. Among dogs, the urine of males and vaginal secretions of females are the main sources of infection via the venereal, oral, nasal, or conjunctival routes (Wanke 2004, Hollew 2006).

Human brucellosis is a severely debilitating disease manifesting a lot of complications that requires prolonged treatment with a combination of antibiotics ensuing considerable medical expenses in addition to loss of income due to loss of working hours. Human brucellosis is mainly caused by four species – *B. melitensis, B. abortus, B. suis and B. canis.* However, till date no *B. ovis* infection has been reported in humans. *B. canis* infection in humanbeing is of decreased severity and frequency, compared with illness caused by the classical strains of *Brucella* spp. It has been estimated that as many as 1% of human brucellosis cases are attributable to *B. canis* (Scheftel 2003).

B. melitensis remains the principal cause of human brucellosis worldwide and may account for upto 90% of all brucellosis cases with *B. melitensis* type 1 predominating in India (Mantur *et al.* 2006). The infective dose of *B. melitensis* is very low (10 organisms). Estimated 5 lakh human infections per year still occur worldwide. The reported incidence in endemic areas varies from <1 / lakh population in UK, USA and Australia, to >20-30/ lakh in southern European countries such as Greece and Spain and upto >70/ lakh in Middle Eastern countries like Kuwait and Saudi Arabia (Cutler *et al.* 2005).

Consumption of unpasteurized milk and their products especially soft cheese, yoghurts and ice-cream (Eckman 1975), undercooked traditional delicacies such as liver and spleen are mainly responsible for human brucellosis (Malik 1997). Though rare, occasionally human-to-human transmission takes place through tissue transplantation or sexual contact (Mantur *et al.* 1996). Also contact with vaginal discharge, urine, feces and blood of infected animals through broken skin and mucous membrane of conjunctiva and inhalation of the organism can cause the disease. The disease is an occupational hazard for livestock owners, abattoir workers, dairy workers, shepherds, farmers, veterinarians and laboratory workers. Brucellosis has been shown to be one of the most common laboratory acquired infections (Noviello *et al.* 2004). With the increase in global tourism, brucellosis is emerging as a common imported disease in the developed world (Memish and Balkhy, 2004).

PREVALENCE

In India, the presence of brucellosis was first established early in the previous century and since then reported from almost all states (Renukaradhya *et al.* 2002).The true prevalence of brucellosis in animal as well as human in India is not known. It has been estimated that the true prevalence may be 20 to 25 times higher than the reported, which may be due to misdiagnosis and underreporting of cases. The evidence for prevalence of brucellosis on basis of serosurvey has been reported for a number of domestic animals besides poultry and wild animals (Table 9.1). Prevalence of brucellosis in animals has been reported to vary from as low as 0.13 per cent (Chatterjee *et al.* 1986) to as high as 44 per cent (Zaki *et al.* 1975). In general, incidence of brucellosis has been found to be higher among cattle than buffaloes (Maansi 1999). A serological survey of brucellosis in cattle and buffalo was performed by Isloor *et al.* (1998) in 23 states of India which showed an overall prevalence rate of antibodies of 1.9 per cent in cattle and 1.8 per cent in buffalo in 19 of 23 states. They also showed a seropositivity of 4.1 per cent in cattle in 47 organised farms in contrast to 0.7 per cent seropositivity in cattle owned by individual farmers in Karnataka.

Table 9.1 : Prevalence of Brucellosis in Man and Animals in India

Animal Species	*Seropositivity*	*Isolation of Brucella*
Cattle	+	+
Buffalo	+	+
Sheep	+	+
Goat	+	+
Swine	+	+
Equine	+	+
Camel	+	+
Dog	+	+
Poultry	+	+
Wild animals	+	+
Man	+	+

Samples predominantly from large herds with a history of abortion and infertility showed a highly variable seroprevalence ranging from 6.6 per cent in Madhya Pradesh (Mehra *et al.*, 2000) to 60 per cent in Assam (Chakraborty *et al.*, 2000). Mehra *et al* (2000) reported 6.5 per cent prevalence in cattle from organized farms, compared to 5.1 per cent prevalence in cattle in the unorganized sector. National survey of bovine brucellosis (1994-2001) showed national average of brucellosis as 5 per cent in cattle and 3 per cent in buffaloes (Renukaradhya *et al.,* 2002). In a similar national survey of sheep and goat brucellosis, Isloor *et al.* (1998) showed a cumulative incidence of 7.9 per cent in sheep and 2.2 per cent in goats. Serological evidence of *B. ovis* infection in 6 out of 102 rams has been reported in Himachal Pradesh (Katoch *et al.* 1996). Seroprevalence of brucellosis in pigs is 3.2 per cent in Madhya Pradesh (Soni and Pathak 1969), 11.3 per cent in Tamil Nadu (Kumar and Rao 1980) and 6.3 per cent in Karnataka (Krishnappa *et al.* 1981) and 9.5 per cent in 756 pigs slaughtered in Karnataka (Thoppil 2000). Brucellosis has also been reported from dairy farm in Goa region (Barbuddhe *et al.* 2004). Recently, serological evidence has been reported for brucellosis in Andaman and Nicobar Islands (Jai-Sunder *et al.* 2005). Serological evidence has also been reported in Mithuns (Rajkhowa *et al.* 2005) and Yaks (Bandyopadhyay *et al.* 2008).

B. abortus biotypes I and III have been isolated from cattle (Chatterjee *et al.* 1995) besides biotype IV (Batra *et al.* 1989). Though biotype I have been found to predominate in cattle in organized farms, biotype III has been usually reported to infect the cattle in the village population (Anon 1986). Occasionally, *B. melitensis* biotype I have also been isolated from cattle (Hemashettar *et al.* 1987). *B. melitensis* biotypes I, II and III have been isolated from sheep and goats (Sharma *et al.* 1995) besides *B. abortus* biotype I (Panjarathinum and Gulrajani 1974). Of the three biotypes of *B. melitensis*, biotype I have been found to infect majority of the sheep and goat population (Sen and Sharma 1972). *B. canis* was isolated from dogs in Chennai (Pillai *et al.* 1991) while isolation of *B. suis* biotype II from a sow was reported from Tamil Nadu (Kumar and Rao 1980). Subsequently, isolation of *B. suis* biotype II from an aborted foetus of goat was reported (Reddy and Rao 1984). *B. suis* biotype I was isolated from dog in Madras (Pillai *et al.* 1990). The only isolation report of *B. abortus* and *B. melitensis* from horses is that of Polding in 1947 (Polding 1947). Isolation of *B. ovis* has not been reported from India. Biotypes of *Brucella* isolated from man and animals in India are shown in Table 9.2

Table 9.2 : Biotypes of *Brucella* spp. Isolated from Man and Animals in India

Species	*Biotypes*	*Animal*
B. abortus	1, 3, 4, 6	Cattle
	1, 3	Buffalo
	1	Sheep
	1	Goat
	1, 3	Man
	#	Equine
B. melitensis	1	Cattle
	1, 2, 3	Sheep
	1, 2, 3	Goat
	1, 2, 3	Man
	#	Equine
B. suis	2	Goat
	2	Pig
	1	Dog
B. canis	—	Dog

Human brucellosis cases are rarely reported. Mathur (1964) reported 8.5% seroprevalence of brucellosis among dairy personnel in contact with infected animals and isolated *Brucella* from seven cases and a seropositivity of 4.2% among aborted women were found (Randhawa *et al.* 1974). Rana *et al.* (1985) showed a seropositivity of 27.7 per cent among veterinarians in Delhi. In Gujrat, 8.5% prevalence of *Brucella* agglutinins was recorded in human cases (Panjarathinam and Jhala 1986). In a study by Hemashettar and Patil (1994), 24 (8.2%) veterinary workers showed *Brucella* specific antibodies in significant titres. High seroprevalence rate has also been noted in specific risk groups such as abattoir workers (Chadda *et al.* 2004, Barbuddhe *et al.* 2000). Handa *et al.* (1998) identified 4 (3.3%) cases with acute brucellosis in a group of 121 patients with fever of unknown origin (FUO). In Haryana, 34% prevalence of human brucellosis was recorded among veterinarians, attendants and compounders in contact with animals (Chauhan 1999). Thakur and Thapliyal (2002), in a study, observed a prevalence rate of

4.97% in samples obtained from persons exposed to animals with a markedly higher prevalence of 17.39% among field veterinarians. Sen *et al.* (2002) identified 28 (6.8%) seropositive cases in a group of 414 patients with FUO, while Kadri *et al.* (2000) identified 28 (0.8%) seropositive cases in a group of 3,532 patients with FUO.

A study by Mudaliar *et al.* (2003) showed the presence of *Brucella* antibodies in 5.33 per cent of animal handlers of which 4.51 per cent were dairy farm workers and 14.63 per cent were veterinary doctors. Mantur *et al.* (2004) showed a seroprevalence of 1.6% by SAT and confirmed by isolating *B. melitensis* in 43 of the 93 children referred to the microbiology laboratory of the Patil Medical College in Bijapur during a period of 13 yr. Most of them were shepherds and had the habit of consuming fresh goat milk. They also reported brucellosis in 495 adults with a prevalence rate of 1.8% by testing blood samples of 26,948 adults in Bijapur during a period of 16 years from 1988 to 2004 and isolated *B. melitensis* from 191 cases (Mantur *et al.* 2006). Recently, Agasthya *et al.* (2007) reported brucellosis in high risk group individuals with disease prevalence at 41.23 per cent in veterinary inspectors, 30.92 per cent in veterinary assistants, 12.37 per cent in veterinary officers, 6.18 per cent in veterinary supervisors, 6.18 per cent in Group-D workers, 2.06 per cent in shepherds and 1.03 per cent in butchers. Similarly, Bedi *et al.* (2007), too, reported brucellosis in animal handlers of Punjab.

ECONOMIC IMPACT

The earlier report of Mathur and Sharma (1974) on economic loss due to brucellosis among bovines was estimated about Rs. 311.47 millions. However, the impact of the disease on national economy due to brucellosis in cattle and buffalo as reported by Schwabe (1984) was to the tune of Rs. 240 million every year. This amounts to more than half percent of total value of all meat and milk products produced in the country. The annual loss due to human brucellosis was estimated to be 30 million man-days. Kunen (1994) estimated that the losses due to brucellosis cost India at least Rs. 350 million annually in terms of food animals and man-days of labour lost.

PREVENTION AND CONTROL

Prevention of human brucellosis is dependent primarily on control of this disease among animals. Control of animal brucellosis is feasible by:

Prevention of exposure of animals to infection which can be achieved by preventing free grazing and movement along with frequent mixing of flocks of sheep and goats, unrestricted trade, use of local cattle yards and fairs for trading, sending dry animals back to villages for maintenance, use of semen from unscreened bulls for artificial insemination and poor farm hygiene, and elimination of infected animals from the herd. The detection of truly infected animals assumes paramount importance in brucellosis control programme. The campaign is easy to operate with high success in small farms with control over movement of animals. A test and slaughter of infected animals or extensive vaccination with approved vaccine, depending on the situation, may be used. This requires a quick, cheap and reasonably sensitive screening test besides a good confirmatory test. In case of cattle, RBPT is used as screen test followed by testing positive sera with CFT for confirmation. The milk ring test (MRT) could be used for identifying infected dairy herd with good results followed by sero-testing individual animals. Its major drawbacks are that this cannot be used on dry animals and its efficacy is doubtful in sheep and goats.

At present, mass immunization with recommended doses of approved vaccines is the only way to bring down the incidence of brucellosis in areas with high prevalence. For cattle, *B. abortus* S-19, a live attenuated vaccine, given at the age of 3 to 6 months (in certain cases up to 8 months) has been recommended. In spite of certain drawbacks, it has been used with satisfactory results. When used routinely to attain coverage of 80% of population, there is a gradual decline in incidence leading to herd immunity. Where eradication is the aim, vaccination should be stopped once the incidence falls below 0.2% and the infected animals must be eliminated.

A live attenuated vaccine, the *Brucella* RB51 strain lacks S-LPS, has much lower pathogenicity in vaccinates, considered only mildly abortifacient and presumed to have much lower pathogenicity in humans in response to accidental exposure. In addition, the *B. abortus* RB51 vaccine has a substantial advantage in animal disease control programmes because it does not elicit an antibody response against S-LPS and does not, therefore, interfere with results of serological testing.

For sheep and goats, *B. melitensis* Rev-1, a live attenuated vaccine is highly effective and is used to vaccinate small ruminants' world over. Immunization of young recently weaned rams (weaner rams) with the *B. melitensis* Rev-1 vaccine has also been recommended for control of *B. ovis* in some countries (Waring 2005). Like the strain 19 vaccine, this vaccine, too, causes abortions in pregnant animals and short-term shedding of the Rev-1 strain in milk (Banai 2002) leading to human infections with *B. melitensis* Rev-1 (Refai 2002, Banai 2002, Bardenstein *et al.* 2002). The probability of success in flocks where contact with other flocks is frequent remains poor. Under such circumstances, all the animals coming in contact should be tested.

In case of swine, control of brucellosis poses difficulty because there is no satisfactory test to identify neither individual animal nor a satisfactory vaccine. It is, therefore, advisable to slaughter the herd. To date, no effective vaccines against *B. canis* have been identified for use in any animal species.

In India, effective control of the brucellosis requires a national plan. A major obstacle in the control of this disease has been the disposal of positive animals. In brucellosis free countries, test and elimination of positive animals slaughter is proved to be effective. However, in our country the existing socioeconomic conditions do not advocates this policy. The alternative method of "Test and Segregation" is perhaps the only method, which is practical and feasible in our country. The positive reactors should be transferred to a separate farm, which should be like closed herd, once animals brought inside, will not go out till death. Strict hygienic measures should be taken while handling these animals and their products. These animals are not used for reproductive purpose and if lactating, then their milk must be pasteurized/boiled before use.

FUTURE PROSPECTS

Inspite of availability of a battery of diagnostic tests, vaccines - both live and attenuated progress in diagnosis, and necessary technical know-how for the formulation and execution of control and eradication programmes under different socio-cultural and epidemiological situations, a lot more needs to be done. The available vaccines are far from ideal. Vaccine for all species is not available. Prompt reporting of brucellosis to health authorities is extremely important as no vaccine for use in humans exists. Human vaccine development remains a challenge. In areas where brucellosis is enzootic, good animal husbandry practice is a critical component to prevent transmission both among same and/or different species of animals and between animal and human. Cheeses and other foods made from unpasteurized dairy products from countries where brucellosis is enzootic should be avoided, and meat should not be consumed from animals that appear to be sick at the time of slaughter.

REFERENCES

Agasthya, A.S., Isloor, S. and Prabhudas, K. (2007). Brucellosis in high risk group individuals. *Indian J. Med. Microbiol.* **25** : 28-31.

Anon (2008). Material safety data sheet—infectious substances, *Brucella* spp. Available at: www.phac-aspc.gc.ca/msds-ftss/msds23e.html. Accessed Mar 5, 2008.

Anon (1986). Joint FAO/WHO expert committee on brucellosis. VIth Report. WHO TRS No. 740, WHO, Geneva.

Banai, M. (2002). Control of small ruminant brucellosis by use of *Brucella melitensis* Rev.1 vaccine: laboratory aspects and field observations. *Vet. Microbiol.* **90** : 497–519.

Bandyopadhyay, S., Sasmal, D., Dutta, T.K., Ghosh, M.K., Sarkar, M., Sasmal, N.K. and Bhattacharya, M. (2008). Seroprevalence of brucellosis in yaks (*Poephagus grunniens*) in India and evaluation of protective immunity to S19 vaccine. *Trop. Anim. Hlth. Prod.*

Barbuddhe, S.B., Chakurkar, E.B., Bale, M.A., Sundaram, R.N.S and Bansode, R.B. (2004). Prevalence of brucellosis in organized dairy farms in Goa region. *Indian J. Anim. Sci.* **74** : 1030-31.

Barbuddhe, S.B., Kumar, P., Malik, S.V.S., Singh, D.K. and Gupta, L.K. (2000). Seropositivity for intracellular bacterial infections among abattoir associated personnels. *J. Communicable Dis.* **32** : 295-9.

Bardenstein, S., Mandelboim, M., Ficht, T. A., Baum, M and Banai, M. (2002). Identification of the *Brucella melitensis* vaccine strain Rev.1 in animals and humans in Israel by PCR analysis of the *Pst*I site polymorphism of its omp2 gene. *J. Clin. Microbiol.* **40** : 1475–80.

Batra, H.V., Chand, P., Ganju, L., Mukherjee, R. and Sadana, J.R. (1989). Dot-enzyme linked immunosorbent assay for the detection of antibodies in bovine brucellosis. *Res. Vet. Sci.* **46** : 143-46.

Bedi, J.S., Sharma, J.K., Gill, J.P.S., Aulakh, R.S., Sharma, C.S. and Gupta, V.K. (2007). Seroepidemiological survey of *Brucella* agglutinins in animal handlers in Punjab, India. *Indian J. Anim. Sci.* **77** : 1283-85.

Brew S.D., Perret, L.L., Stack, J.A., MacMillan, A.P. and Staunton, N.J. (1999). *Vet. Rec.* **144** : 483.

CDC, Office of Inspector General, Department of Health and Human Services. (2005). Possession, use, and transfer of select agents and toxins. Final rule. *Federal Register*. **70** : 13293–325.

Chadda, V.S., Soni, P.K., Gupta, A., Gupta, B.K., Chadda, S. and Nayak, K.C. (2004). Incidence of brucellosis in arthritis and chronic low back pain in high risk group. *J. Assoc. Physicians of India*. **52** : 338.

Chakraborty, M., Patgiri, G.P. and Barman, N.N. (2000). Application of delayed-type hypersensitivity test (DTH) for the diagnosis of bovine brucellosis. *Indian Vet. J.* **77** : 849–51.

Chatterjee. A., De, B.N., Mondol, P., Bidyant, J., Chakraborty, N.K., Nandy, A.K. and Sen, G. P. (1986). Studies on sero-prevalence of bovine brucellosis in rural areas of West Bengal. *Indian Vet. J.* **63** : 95-100.

Chatterjee, A., Mondol, P., De, B.N. and Sen, G.P. (1995). Cultural isolation of *Brucella* in relation to serum agglutinin level. *Indian Vet. J.* **72** : 211-15.

Chauhan, R.S. (1999). Brucellosis in India and its impact on export of buffalo meat. *J. Anim. Prod.* **31** : 316-17.

Corbel, M.J. (1997). Brucellosis: an overview. *Emer. Infect. Dis.* **3** : 213–21.

Cutler, S.J., Whatmore, A.M. and Commander, N.J. (2005). Brucellosis-new aspects of an old disease *J. Applied Microbiol.* **98** : 1270-81.

Eckman, M.R. (1975). Brucellosis linked to Mexican cheese. *JAMA*. **232** : 636-37.

Ewalt, D.R., Payeur, J.B., Martin, B.M., Cummins, D.R. and Miller, W.G. (1994). Characteristics of a *Brucella* species from a bottlenose dolphin (*Tursiops truncates*). *J. Vet. Diag. Invest.* **6** : 448-52.

Handa, R., Singh, S., Singh, N. and Wali, J.P. (1998). Brucellosis in North India : results of a prospective study. *J. Comm. Dis.* **30** : 85-87.

Hemashettar, B.M., Patil, C.S., Jaikumar, K., Devraj, M. and Nagalotimath, S.J. (1987). Isolation of *Brucella melitensis* biotype I from a cow and two of its attendents. *Indian Vet. J.* **64** : 822-25.

Hollew, R.B. (2006). Canine brucellosis: outbreaks and compliance. *Theriogenology.* **66** : 575–87.

Isloor, S., Renukaradhya, G.J. and Rajashekhar, M. (1998). A serological survey of bovine brucellosis in India. *Rev. Sci. Tech., Off. Int. Epiz.* **17** : 781-5.

Jai-Sunder Rai, R.B., Kundu, A., Chatterjee, R.N., Senani, S. and Jeyakumar. (2005). Incidence and prevalence of livestock diseases of Andaman and Nicobar Islands. *Indian J. Anim. Sci.* **75** : 1041-43.

Kadri, S.M., Rukhsana, A., Laharwal, M.A. and Tanvir, M. (2000). Seroprevalence of brucellosis in Kashmir (India) among patients with pyrexia of unknown origin. *J. Indian Med. Assoc.* **98** : 170-1.

Katoch, R.C., Joshi, V.B., Sharma, M., Batta, M.K. and Nagal, K.B. (1996). Seroprevalence of *Brucella ovis, Brucella melitensis* and *Chlamydia psittaci* in rams. *Indian J. Anim. Sci.* **66** : 1130-31.

Krishnappa, G., Zaki, S. and Keshavamurthy, B.S.K. (1981). Serological evidence of swine brucellosis in and around Bangalore. *Mysore J. Agri. Sci.* **15** : 77–80.

Kumar, R. and Rao, C.V.N. (1980). Porcine brucellosis in Tamil Nadu. *Indian Vet. J.* **57** : 1–4.

Kunen, A.V. (1994). Brucellosis In: *Infectious diseases, diagnosis and management in clinical practice*. Ed. Atmakurivinaya Kunen. CBS Publishers, New Delhi. 448-49.

Maansi (1999). Sero-epidemiology of brucellosis in animals and man in Tarai region. M. V. Sc. Thesis submitted to G. B. Pant. Univ. Agril. Technol., Pantnagar.

Malik, G.M. (1997). A clinical study of brucellosis in adults in the Asir region of southern Saudi Arabia. *American Journal of Tropical Medicine and Hygiene.* **56** : 375-77.

Mantur, B.G., Akki, A.S., Mangalgi, S.S., Patil, S.V., Gobbur, R.H. and Peerapur, B.V. (2004). Childhood brucellosis–a microbiological, epidemiological and clinical study. *J. Trop. Pediatrician.* **50** : 153-57.

Mantur, B.G., Biradar, M.S., Bidri, R.C., Mulimani, M.S., Veerappa Kariholu, P., Patil, S.B. and Mangalgi, S.S. (2006). Protean clinical manifestations and diagnostic challenges of human brucellosis in adults: 16 years' experience in an endemic area. *J. Med. Microbiol.* **55** : 897-903.

Mantur, B.G., Mangalgi, S.S. and Mulimani, B. (1996). *Brucella melitensis:* A sexually transmissible agent? *Lancet.* **347** : 1763.

Mathur, A.C. and Sharma, G.L. (1974). Studies on the estimates of the economic losses caused by brucellosis among bovines and its control in India. *Indian J. Anim. Sci.* **44** : 654-61.

Mathur, T.N. (1964). *Brucella* strains isolated from cows, buffaloes, goats, sheep and human beings at Karnal : Their significance with regard to the epidemiolgy of brucellosis. *Indian J. Med. Res.* **52** : 1231-40.

McDonald, W.L., Jamaludin, R., Mackereth, G., Hansen, M., Humphrey, S., Short, P., Taylor, T., Swingler, J., Dawson, C.E., Whatmore, A.M., Stubberfield, E., Perrett, L.L. and Simmons, G. (2006). Characterisation of a *Brucella* sp. strainas a marine mammal type despite isolation from a patient with spinal osteomyelitis in New Zealand. *J. Clin. Microbiol.* **44** : 4363-70.

Mehra, K.N., Dhanesar, N.S. and Chaturvedi, V.K. (2000). Seroprevalence of brucellosis in bovines in Madhya Pradesh. *Indian Vet. J.* **77** : 571–73.

Memish, Z.A. and Balkhy, H.H. (2004). Brucellosis and International Travel. *Journal of Travel. Med.,* **11** : 49-55.

Mudaliar, S., Bhore, A. and Pandit, D. (2003). Detection of antibodies to *Brucella abortus* in animal handlers. *Indian J. Med. Sci.* **57** : 181-86.

Noviello, S., Gallo, R., Kelly, M., Limberger, R.J., Angelis, K., Cain, L., Wallace, B. and Dumas, N. (2004). Laboratory-acquired brucellosis. *Emerg. Infect. Dis.* **10** : 1848-50.

Panjarathinam, R. and Jhala, C.I. (1986). Brucellosis in Gujrat state. *J. Pathol. Microbiol.* **29** : 53-60.

Panjarathinam, R. and Gulrajani, T.S. (1974). Studies on brucellosis. II. Isolation of *Brucella* organism in milk of cows, sheep and goats. *Indian J. Anim. Hlth.* **13** : 29-35.

Paulsen, I.T., Seshadri, R., Nelson, K.E., Eisen, J.A., Heidelberg, J.F., Read, T.D., Dodson, R.J., Umayam, L., Brinkac, L.M., Beanan,M.J., Daugherty, S.C., Deboy, R.T., Durkin, A.S., Kolonay, J.F., Madupu, R., Nelson, W.C., Ayodeji, B., Kraul, M., Shetty, J., Malek, J., Van Aken, S.E., Riedmuller, S., Tettelin, H., Gill, S.R., White, O., Salzberg, S.L., Hoover, D.L., Lindler, L.E., Halling, S.M., Boyle, S.M. and Fraser, C.M. (2002). The *Brucella suis* genome reveals fundamental similarities between animal and plant pathogens and symbionts. *Proceedings of National Academy of Sciences USA.* **99** : 13148–53.

Pillai M T, Nendunchelliyan S and Raghvan N. 1991. Serological and bacteriological detection of *Brucella canis* infection of dogs in Madras. *Indian Vet. J.* **68** : 399-401.

Pillai M T, Nendunchelliyan S and Raghvan N. 1990. Brucellosis in a dog caused by *B. suis* biovar I in Madras. *Cherion.* **19** : 97-8.

Polding J B. 1947. Brucellosis in India. *Indian J. Vet. Sci.* 147-55.

Rajkhowa S, Rahman H, Rajkhowa and Bujarbaruah K.M. 2005. Seroprevalence of brucellosis in Mithuns (*Bos frontalis*) in India. *Preven. Vet. Medi.* **69** : 145-51.

Rana, U.V.S., Sehgal, S. and Bhardwaj, A.M. (1985). A sero-epidemiological study of brucellosis among workers of veterinary hospital and slaughter house of Delhi. *Intl. J. Zoon.* **12** : 74-79.

Randhawa, A.S., Kalra, D.S. and Kapur, M.P. (1974). Some sero-epidemiologic observations on brucellosis in humans and animals. *Indian J. Med. Sci.* **28** : 133-8.

Reddy, P.R.C. and Rao, P.V.R.C. (1984). A note on isolation of *Brucella suis* from foetus of a she-goat. *Kerala J. Vet. Sci.* **15** : 173-74.

Refai, M. (2002). Incidence and control of brucellosis in the Near East region. *Vet. Microbiol.* **90** : 81-110.

Renukaradhya, G.J., Isloor, S. and Rajasekhar, M. (2002). Epidemiology, zoonotic aspects, vaccination and control/eradication of brucellosis in India. *Vet. Microbiol.* **90** : 183-95.

Ross, H.M., Jahans, K.L., MacMillan, A.P., Rei, R.J, Thompson, P.M. and Foster, G. (1996). *Brucella* species infection in North Sea seal and cetacean populations. *Vet. Rec.* **138** : 647-48.

Rotz, L.D., Khan, A.S., Lillibridge, S.R., Ostroff, S.M. and Hughes, J.M. (2002). Public health assessment of potential biological terrorism agents. *Emer. Infect. Dis.* **8** : 225–30.

Scheftel, J. (2003). *Brucella canis*: potential for zoonotic transmission. *Compendium Continuing Education for Pract Veterinarians*. **25** : 846–853.

Sen G.P. and Sharma G.L. 1972. Speciation of seventy eight Indian strains of *Brucella*, an epidemiological study. *Indian J. Anim. Sci.* **45** : 537.

Sen, M.R., Shukla, B.N. and Goyal, R.K. (2002). Seroprevalence of brucellosis in and around Varanasi. *J. Communicable Dis.* **34** : 226-27.

Sharma, M., Batta, M.K., Asrani, R.K., Katoch, R.C., Joshi, V.B. and Nagal, K.B. (1995). *Brucella melitensis* abortions among organized sheep farms in north-west states in India. *Indian J. Anim. Sci.* **65** : 874-75.

Schwabe, C.W. (1984). *Vet. Med. and Human Hlth.* Waverly Press Inc. Mount Royal Guilford Avenues, Baltimore, M. D. 21202. US. 16-39.

Sohn, A.H., Probert, W.S., Glaser, C.A., Gupta, N., Bollen, A.W., Wong, J.D., Grace, E.M. and McDonald, W.C. (2003). Human neurobrucellosis with intracerebral granuloma caused by a marine mammal *Brucella* spp. *Emerg. Infect. Dis.* 9 : 485-88.

Soni, J.L. and Pathak, P.N. (1969). Serological investigations into porcine brucellosis. *Indian Vet. J.* **46** : 191-95.

Thakur, S.D. and Thapliyal, D.C. (2002). Seroprevalence of brucellosis in man. *J. Communicable Dis.* **34** : 106-9.

Thoppil, S.T. (2000). Serodiagnosis of brucellosis in pigs and man and differentiation of cross reactions due to *Yersinia enterocolitica* O:9. Master of Veterinary Science thesis submitted to the University of Agricultural Sciences, Bangalore, India.

Wanke, M.M. (2004). Canine brucellosis. *Anim. Reprod. Sci.* **82–83** : 195–207.

Waring, S.C. (2005). Brucellosis. In : Kahn CM, Line S, Eds. *Merck Veterinary Manual*. 9th ed. Whitehouse Station, NJ: Merck. 2546.

Zaki, S., Murty, B.S.K., Rao, S., and Nanjiah, R.D. (1975). Serological incidence of brucellosis in sheep and goats in Karnataka. *Current Research.* **4** : 196-97.

10

CURRENT TRENDS IN MOLECULAR DIAGNOSIS OF BRUCELLOSIS

Sanjay Kumar

Brucellosis is a worldwide zoonotic disease caused by facultative intracellular bacteria of the genus *Brucella*, which are widely distributed in both humans and animals, especially in the developing world. The routine identification and differentiation of *Brucella* species is a time-consuming and labor-intensive process that places personnel at risk for laboratory-acquired infection. In order to overcome these difficulties, PCR-based assays has been explored for the rapid detection and confirmation of *Brucella* species.

Several PCR-based assays have been developed for the identification of *Brucella* to improve diagnostic capabilities. For some purposes, such as diagnosis of human brucellosis or contamination of food products, the simple identification of *Brucella* is adequate. In these cases, a genus-specific PCR assay is sufficient. The main genetic targets utilized for these applications are the *Brucella BCSP31* gene and the 16S-23S rRNA operon. Other instances, for example, state-sponsored brucellosis eradication program and for epidemiological purposes, *Brucella* species and strain specific identification respectively is helpful. Typically, differential PCR-based assays tend to be more complex and consequently more difficult to perform. Several strategies have been explored to differentiate among *Brucella* species and strains, including locus specific multiplexing (*e.g.* AMOS-PCR based on IS*711*), PCR-RFLP (*e.g.* the *omp*2 locus), arbitrary-primed PCR, ERIC-PCR and more recently Bruce-ladder PCR to name a few. This article reviews some of the major advancements in molecular diagnosis for brucellosis. While the progress to date is impressive, more research is still needed in the areas of molecular subtyping and direct analysis of a variety of clinical samples.

Brucellosis is caused by a facultative intracellular bacterium of the genus *Brucella*, and it is one of the most frequent bacterial zoonoses in low-income countries, where the control programs have not succeeded in eradicating this neglected zoonosis. This disease is spread worldwide with areas of high endemicity seen in the Mediterranean, India, Middle East, Asia and South and Central America, which result in severe economic losses (Corbel, 1997, Lopez, 1989). The genus *Brucella* consists of six recognized species, designated on the basis of differences in pathogenicity and host preference: *B. melitensis* (goats and sheep), *B. abortus* (cattle and bison), *B. suis* (infecting primarily swine but also hares, rodents, and reindeer), *B. ovis* (sheep), *B. canis* (dogs), and *B. neotomae* (wood rats) (Corbel, 1988). The discovery of *Brucella* in a wide variety of marine mammals has led to the proposal of two new species: *B. ceti* (cetaceans) and *B. pinnipedialis* (pinnipeds) (Foster *et al.*, 2007). *Brucella* spp. is regarded as class III pathogens. In 1954, *B. suis* became the first agent weaponized by the U.S. in the days of its offensive biological warfare program. The most common mode of brucellosis transmission is the consumption of unpasteurized dairy products. Brucellosis is also transmitted through direct skin contact and is an occupational hazard for farmers, veterinarians, butchers and laboratory workers. Person-to-person transmission is not epidemiologically significant. Aerosols containing *Brucella* are considered to be highly infectious. It is estimated that inhalation of 10 to 100 bacteria is sufficient to trigger disease in humans.

Laboratory diagnosis includes isolation and identification of *Brucellae* from clinical samples, detection of antigen, demonstration of genome and demonstration of *Brucella* specific antibodies. Blood culture provides definite proof of brucellosis but may not provide a positive result. *Brucellae* are relatively slow growing and the culture result may not become available for several days or weeks. Identification of *Brucella* strains is done using standard classification test, including Gram stain, a modified Ziehl-Neelsen stain, growth characteristic, oxidase activity, urease activity, H_2S production, dye tolerance (basic fuchsin and thionin) and seroagglutination (Alton *et al.*, 1988). There are currently a wide variety of serological tests that can be used for the diagnosis of human and bovine brucellosis. The serological tests like Rose Bengal Plate Agglutination Test (RBPT), standard tube agglutination test (SAT), Coombs test, immunocapture agglutination test (Orduna *et al.*, 2000), latex agglutination, complement fixation test, ELISA, lateral flow assay, dipstick assay, fluorescence polarization assay (FPA) (Lucero *et al.*, 2003), have been applied in the diagnosis of brucellosis. Indirect enzyme-linked immunosorbent assay typically uses smooth LPS lipopolysaccharide and cytoplasmic proteins as antigens. The serological responses following infection with smooth *Brucella* species are predominantly directed against the S-LPS [smooth LPS (lipopolysaccharide)]. Thus, in humans as well as in animals, the diagnosis of brucellosis is usually based on the detection of specific antibodies against S-LPS (Alton *et al.*, 1988, Wright and Nielsen, 1990). Proteins of *Brucella abortus* have been considered important for diagnostic purposes. Several workers described different immunodominant protein antigens useful as a marker of active infection in humans and bovine brucellosis have been used for the diagnosis of brucellosis (Goldbaum *et al.*, 1993, Hemmen *et al.*, 1995, Kumar *et al.*, 2007a, Kumar *et al.*, 2007b, Kumar *et al.*, 2008, Stevens *et al.*, 1994). A dipstick assay (Casao *et al.*, 2003) offers a rapid reliable diagnostic alternative in acute brucellosis. The rapid and simple assays like *Brucella* IgM and IgG lateral flow and latex agglutination (Abdoel *et al.*, 2007) have been developed.

Laboratory detection of *Brucella* and species identification is time-consuming, requires skilled technicians, and is not straightforward, and some reagents are not commercially available. In addition, handling of this microorganism represents a high risk for laboratory personnel, since most *Brucella* strains are highly pathogenic for humans (Bricker, 2002, Navarro *et al.*, 2004). To surmount these problems, nucleic acid amplification has been explored for the rapid detection and confirmation of *Brucella*. Since 1987, numerous PCR-based assays for *Brucella* have been developed and published. The earliest PCR-based assays developed for *Brucella* concentrated on genus-specific loci for identification. The advantage of these types of assays is that they tend to have a simple design and are very robust. Such tests are useful for screening or for identification when species or biovar designations are not critical. The first published PCR based diagnostic assay was reported by Fekete *et al.* 1990. This assay was based on the amplification of a 635-bp sequence from a gene encoding a 43-kDa outer membrane protein of *B. abortus* strain S19. The next *Brucella* gene target to be explored was the 16S rRNA gene (Hermen and De, 1992). Successful amplification of a predicted 800 bp amplicon from *B. abortus* and other species of *Brucella* demonstrated that the sequences were highly conserved and that the test could be extended to the entire genus. In 1992, a new PCR assay was published based on the gene encoding *BCSP31* (Baily *et al.*, 1992). This gene encodes an antigenic periplasmic protein of unknown function. It is conserved in all species and biovar of *Brucella* examined, except in *Brucella ovis*. The PCR yielded a 223 bp amplicon and the assays were found to be robust, sensitive and specific for *B. abortus* and *B. melitensis*.

For some purposes, identification of *Brucella* at the species level is not immediately necessary to initiate action. However, there are many instances where the *Brucella* species involved is relevant to the initiation of an appropriate action. For example, brucellosis eradication programs are typically species-specific and the associated regulatory actions are species dependent. Furthermore, differential assays are particularly useful for epidemiological trace back to its source of infection. In the species specific identification the work of Bricker and Halling, (1994), is remarkable where they exploited the multi-copy element IS*711*, the number and placement of the IS elements in *Brucella* species are typically conserved. The assay was named the AMOS-PCR assay for the *Brucella* species it can identify and differentiate. The multiplex design consists of one common primer anchored in the IS element and a species-specific primer that binds to the unique sequence flanking that insertion site. The assay primers were chosen so that species discrimination was determined by the size of the amplicon. In 1995, Cloeckaert *et al.*, developed a PCR assay based on the *omp*2A and *omp*2B gene sequences. He greatly enhanced the discriminatory power of the PCR assay by incorporating restriction endonucleases cleavage of the amplicon after amplification. As a result, most *Brucella* species and some biovars could be identified and differentiated. Da Costa *et al.* (1996) examined six *Brucella* genes by PCR-RFLP: *BCSP31*, 16S rRNA, *gro*EL, *dna*k, *dna*J and *htr*A. Other laboratories reported success with the published protocol Sreevatsan *et al.* (2000), Adone *et al.* (2001) or a modified version (Redkar *et al.*, 2001). Probert *et al.* (2004) described a real-time multiplex PCR assay using the same targets used by Redkar *et al.*, (2001), which allow the confirmation of bacterial isolates as *Brucella* spp., *B. abortus*, or *B. melitensis* within 2 to 3 h. Garcia-Yoldi *et al.*, (2006) developed a multiplex PCR (Bruce-ladder) for the identification and differentiation of all *Brucella* spp. and the vaccine strains *B. abortus* S19, RB51 and *B. melitensis* Rev 1. This multiplex PCR was evaluated in seven different European laboratories. The Bruce-ladder PCR worked equally well irrespective of the cultural conditions, DNA extraction methods, or thermocyclers used. The same results were obtained in seven different laboratories with brucellae obtained from the five continents and from humans and both domestic and wild animals, demonstrating without a doubt the reproducibility and robustness of the PCR assay. More recently, Hinic and co-workers (2008) describe the establishment of a PCR assay using seven individual reactions for the rapid detection of the *Brucella* genus, and the differentiation between six recognized *Brucella* species. The same primer pairs can be used in both real-time and conventional PCR. For the rapid, sensitive and accurate detection of *Brucella* spp., the multiple insertion elements, IS711, which is stable in both number and position in the *Brucella* chromosomes, was chosen as a target (Moreno *et al.*, 2002, Ouahrani *et al.*, 1993, Vemulapalli *et al.*, 1999). The PCRs for species differentiation were based on unique genetic loci of

B. melitensis, B. abortus, B. suis, B. ovis, B. canis, and *B. neotomae.* The unique genetic markers for the differentiation of *B. melitensis, B. abortus, B. suis,* and *B. ovis* were identified by in silico comparisons of published genome sequences with the Artemis Comparison Tool (ACT) (Carver *et al.,* 2005). For the differentiation of *B. neotomae* and *B. canis,* unique deletions described by Rajashekara *et al.* (2004) were used. This is very simple and easily performed assay represents a highly specific approach for the identification of the *Brucella* genus as well as the differentiation between six *Brucella* species.

With respect to biowarfare or other emergency conditions, it may be critical to perform analyses directly in the field. Therefore, efforts have been made to develop methods for analyzing infected or contaminated materials directly. Sample preparation is key to success since most of these sources are rich in the PCR inhibitors. PCR has been applied to tissues mainly aborted fetuses and associated maternal tissues (Centikya *et al.,* 1999, Cortez *et al.,* 2001, Fekete *et al.,* 1992, Gallien *et al.,* 1998), blood (Guarino *et al.,* 2000), milk (Leal *et al.,* 2000, Romero and Lopez, 1999, Tantillo *et al.,* 2001), nasal secretions (Sreevastan *et al.,* 2000) and semen (Amin *et al.,* 2001). In endemic areas, human brucellosis, particularly when caused by *B. melitensis,* is a serious health concern. The requirements for a diagnostic medical test are different from the requirements for testing livestock. To date, nearly all PCR-based diagnostics for human brucellosis target peripheral blood as the sample source. Begining with Matar and associates (Matar *et al.,* 1996), the preferred assay for human use is the BCSP31-based, genus-specific assay developed by several workers (Baily *et al.,* 1992, Casanas *et al.,* 2001, Morata *et al.,* 1999, Morata *et al.,* 1998, Queipo *et al.,* 1999, Queipo *et al.,* 1997, Zerva *et al.,* 2001). A simple PCR-ELISA was employed for the rapid diagnosis of human brucellosis directly from peripheral blood (Vrioni *et al.,* 2004). Queipo-Ortuno and associates (2005b) reported for the first time the use of real-time PCR to detect *Brucella* DNA in human clinical samples which targeted a 223 bp gene sequence encoding an immunogenetic membrane protein (BCSP31) specific for the *Brucella* genus. The same year Queipo-Ortuno *et al.* (2005a) compare the diagnostic yield of an LC-PCR (Light cycler real-time-PCR) with serum samples and a PCR-ELISA assay with whole blood samples for the diagnosis of human brucellosis. More recently 16S rRNA based fluorescence in situ hybridization (FISH) assay was developed that facilitates rapid and specific detection of all human pathogenic species of *Brucella* and that can be applied directly to positive blood cultures (Wellinghausen *et al.*, 2006).

Over the past decade, there has been major advancement in all aspects of molecular diagnostics with regard to human and animal brucellosis. PCR-based tests are proving to be faster and more sensitive than traditional methods and assays will only improve further in the future. So far acceptance of molecular diagnostics had been slow. However, threats of biological warfare and agroterrorism may accelerate the process. More research is needed in the areas of molecular subtyping and direct analysis of clinical samples.

REFERENCES

Abdoel, T.H., Pastoor, R., Smits, H.L. and Hatta, M. (2007). Laboratory evaluation of a simple and rapid latex agglutination assay for the serodiagnosis of typhoid fever. *Trans. R. Soc. Trop. Med. Hyg.* **10** : 1032-1038.

Adone, R., Ciuchini, F., La Rosa, G., Marianelli, C. and Muscillo, M. (2001). Use of polymerase chain reaction to identify *Brucella abortus* strain RB51 among *Brucella* field isolates from cattle in Italy. *J. Vet. Med. B. Infect. Dis. Vet. Public Hlth.* **48** : 107-113.

Alton, G.G., Jones, L.M., Angus, R.D. and Verger, J.M. (1988). Techniques for brucellosis laboratory. Institut National de la Recherche Agronomique, Paris.

Amin, A.S., Hamdy, M.E. and Ibrahim, A.K. (2001). Detection of *Brucella melitensis* in semen using Polymerase chain assay. *Vet. Microbiol.* **83** : 3 7-44.

Baily, G.G., Krahn, J.B., Drasal, B.S. and Stoker, N.G. (1992). Detection of *Brucella melitensis* and *Brucella abortus* by DNA amplification. *J. Trop. Med. Hyg.* **95** : 271-275.

Bricker, B.J. and Halling, S.M. (1994). Differentiation of *Brucella abortus* bv. 1, 2 & 4, *Brucella melitensis, Brucella ovis* and *Brucella suis* bv. 1 by PCR. *J. Clin. Microbiol.* **32** : 2660-2666.

Bricker, B.J. (2002). PCR as a diagnostic tool for brucellosis. *Vet. Microbiol.* **90** : 435–446.

Carver, T.J., Rutherford, K.M., Berriman, M., Rajandream, M.A., Barrell, B.G. and Parkhill, J. (2005). ACT: the Artemis Comparison Tool. *Bioinformatics.* **21** : 3422–3423.

Casanas, M.C., Queipo-Ortuno, M.I., Rodriguez-Torres, A., Orduna, A., Colmenero, J.D. and Morata, P. (2001). Specificity of a Polymerase chain reaction assay of a target sequence on the 31-kilodalton *Brucella* antigen DNA use to diagnose human brucellosis. *Eur. J. Clin. Microbiol. Infect. Dis.* **20** : 127-131.

Casao, M.A., Smits, H.L., Navarro, E. and Solera, J. (2003). Clinical utility of a dipstick assay in patients with brucellosis: correlation with the period of evolution of the disease. *Clin. Microbiol. Infect.* **9(4)** : 301-315.

Cetinkya, B., Ongor, H., Muz, A., Ertas, H.B., Kalender, H. and Erdogan, H.M. (1999). Detection of *Brucella* species DNA in the stomach content of aborted sheep fetuses by PCR. *Vet. Rec.* **144** : 239-240.

Cloeckaert, A., Verger, J.M., Grayon, M. and Grepinet, O. (1995). Restriction site polymorphism of the genes encoding the major 25kDa and 36 kDa outer membrane proteins of *Brucella. Microbiol.* **141** : 2111-2121.

Corbel, M.J. (1997). Brucellosis: an overview. *Emerg. Infect. Dis.* **3** : 213*B. canis*-221.

Corbel, M.J. (1988). International committee on the systematic bacteriology subcommittee on the taxonomy of *Brucella. Int. J. Syst. Bacteriol.* **38** : 450–452.

Cortez, A., Scarcelli, E., Soares, R.M., Heinemann, M.B., Sakamoto, S.M., Genovez, M.E., Ferreira, F. and Richtzenhain, L.J. (2001). Detection of *Brucella* DNA from aborted bovine fetuses by polymerase chain reaction. *Aust. Vet. J.* **79** : 500-501.

Da Costa, M., Guillou, J.P., Garin-Bastuji, B., Thieubaud, M. and Dubray, G. (1996). Specificity of six gene sequences for the detection of the genus *Brucella* by DNA amplification. *J. Appl. Bacteriol.* **81** : 267-275.

Fekete, A., Bantle, J.A. and Halling, S.M. (1992). Detection of *Brucella* by polymerase chain reaction in bovine fetal and maternal tissues. *J. Vet. Diagn. Invest.* **4** : 79-83.

Fekete, A., Bantle, J.A., Halling, S.M. and Sanborn, M.R. (1990). Preliminary development of a diagnostic test for *Brucella* using polymerase chain reaction. *J. Appl. Bacteriol.* **69** : 216-227.

Foster, G., Osterman, B.S., Godfroid, J., Jacques, I. and Cloeckaert, A. (2007). *Brucella ceti* sp. nov. and *Brucella pinnipedialis* sp. nov. for

Brucella strains with cetaceans and seals as their preferred hosts. *Int. J. Syst. Evol. Microbiol.* **57** : 2688–2693.

Gallien, P., Dorn, C., Alban, G., Staak, C. and Protz, D. (1998). Detection of *Brucella* species in organs of naturally infected cattle by polymerase chain reaction. *Vet. Rec.* **142** : 512-514.

Garcia-Yoldi, D., Marín, C.M., De Miguel, M.J., Munoz, P.M., Vizmanos, J.L. and Lopez-Goni. I. (2006). Multiplex PCR assay for the identification and differentiation of all *Brucella* species and the vaccine strains *Brucella abortus* S19 and RB51 and *Brucella melitensis* Rev1. *Clin. Chem.* **52** : 779–781.

Goldbaum, F.A., Leoni, J., Wallach, J.C. and Fossati, C.A. (1993). *J. Clin. Microbiol.* **31** : 2141–2145.

Guarino, A., Serpe, L., Fuso, G., Scaramuzzo, A. and Gallo, P. (2000). Detection of *Brucella* species in buffalo whole blood by gene-specific PCR. *Vet. Rec.* **147** : 634-636.

Hemmen, F., Weynants, T., Scarcez, T., Letesson, J. and Saman, E. (1995). *Clin. Diagn. Lab. Immunol.* **2** : 263–267.

Hermen, L. and De Ridder, H. (1992). Identification of *Brucella* spp. by using the polymerase chain reaction. *Appl. Environ. Microbiol.* **55** : 2099-2101.

Hini, V., Brodard, I., Thomann, A., Cvetni, Z., Makaya, P.V., Frey, J. and Abril, C. (2008). Novel identification and differentiation of Brucella melitensis, *B. abortus, B. suis, B. ovis, B. canis, and B. neotomae* suitable for both conventional and real-time PCR systems. *J. Microbiol. Methods.* **75** : 375-378.

Kumar, S., Tuteja, U. and Batra, H.V. (2007a). Generation and characterization of murine monoclonal antibodies to recombinant 26-kDa periplasmic protein of *Brucella abortus*. 2007. *Hybridoma* **26** : 322-327.

Kumar, S., Tuteja, U. and Batra, H.V. (2007b). Generation and characterization of murine monoclonal antibodies to genus-specific 31-kilodalton recombinant cell surface protein of *Brucella abortus*. *Hybridoma* **26** : 211-216.

Kumar, S., Tuteja, U., Kumar, A. and Batra, H.V. (2008). Expression and purification of the 26 kDa periplasmic protein of *Brucella abortus*: a reagent for the diagnosis of bovine brucellosis. *Biotechnol. Appl. Biochem.* **49** : 213-218.

Leal-Klevezas, D.S., Martinez-Vazquez, I.O., Garcia-Cantu, J., Lopez-Merino, A. and Martinez-Soriano, J.P. (2000). Use of polymerase chain reaction to detect *Brucella abortus* biovar I in infected goats. *Vet. Microbiol.* **75** : 91-97.

Lopez, M. (1989). Brucellosis in Latin America. P.151-161. In Young EJ, and Corbel MJ (ed.), Brucellosis: Clinical and Laboratory aspects. CRC Press, Inc., Boca Raton, Fla.

Lucero, N.E., Escobar, G.I., Ayala, S.M., Silva Paulo, P. and Nielsen, K. (2003). Fluorescence polarization assay for diagnosis of human brucellosis. *J. Med. Microbiol.* **52** : 883-887.

Matar, G.M., Khneisser, I.A. and Abdelnoor, A.M. (1996). Rapid laboratory confirmation of human brucellosis by PCR analysis of a target sequence on the 31 kilodalton *Brucella* antigen DNA. *J. Clin. Microbiol.* **34** : 477-478.

Morata, P., Ortuno Mi., Reguera, J.M., Ordonez, M.A., Cardenas, A. and Colmenero, J.D. (2003). Development and evaluation of a PCR-ELISA assay for diagnosis of human brucellosis. *J. Clin. Microbiol.* **41** : 144-148.

Morata, P., Queipo-ortuno, M.I., Reguera, J.M., Reguera, J.M., Garcia-Ordonez, M.A., Pichardo, C. and Colmenero, J.D. (1999). Post treatment follow-up of brucellosis by PCR assay. *J. Clin. Microbiol.* **37** : 4163-4166.

Morata, P., Queipo-ortuno, M.I. and Colmenerom, J.D. (1998). Strategy for optimizing DNA amplification in a peripheral blood PCR assay used for diagnosis of human brucellosis. *J. Clin. Microbiol.* **36** : 2243-2246.

Moreno, E., Cloeckaert, A. and Moriyón, I. (2002). *Brucella* evolution and taxonomy. *Vet. Microbiol.* **90** : 209–227.

Navarro, E., Casao, M.A., Solera, J., 2004. Diagnosis of human brucellosis using PCR. *Expert Rev. Mol. Diagn.* **4** : 115–123.

Orduna, A., Almaraz, A., Prado, A., Gutierrez, M.P., Garcia-Pascual, A., Duenas, A., Cuervo, M., Abad, R., Hernández, B., Lorenzo, B., Bratos, M.A. and Torres, A.R. (2000). Evaluation of an immunocapture-agglutination test (Brucellacapt) for serodiagnosis of human brucellosis. *J. Clin. Microbiol.* **38** : 4000-4005.

Ouahrani, S., Michaux, S., Widada, J.S., Bourg, G., Tournebize, R., Ramuz, M., Liautard, J.P. (1993). Identification and sequence analysis of IS6501, an insertion sequence in *Brucella* spp.: relationship between genomic structure and the number of IS6501 copies. *J. Gen. Microbiol.* **139** : 3265–3273.

Probert, W.S., Schrader, K.N., Khuong, N.Y., Bystrom, S.L. and Graves, M.H. (2004). Real-Time Multiplex PCR assay for detection of *Brucella* spp., *B. abortus* and *B. melitensis*. *J. Clin. Microbiol.* **42** : 1290-1293.

Queipo-Ortuno, M.I., Colmenero, J.D., Baeza, G. and Morata, P. (2005a). Comparison between Light Cycler Real-Time Polymerase Chain

Reaction (PCR) assay with serum and PCR-enzyme-linked immunosorbent assay with whole blood samples for the diagnosis of human brucellosis. *Clin. Infect. Dis.* **40** : 260-264.

Queipo-Ortuno, M.I., Colmenero, J.D., Reguera, J.M., García-Ordonez, M.A., Pachón, M.E., Gonzalez, M. and Morata, P. (2005b). Rapid diagnosis of human brucellosis by SYBR Green I-based real-time PCR assay and melting curve analysis in serum samples. *Clin. Microbiol. Infect.* **11** : 713-718.

Queipo-Ortuno, M.I., Garcia-Ordonez, M.A., Colmenero, J.D. and Morata, P. (1999). Hydrogen peroxide improves the efficacy of a peripheral blood PCR assay for diagnosis of human brucellosis. *Biotechniques*. **27** : 248-252.

Queipo-Ortuno, M.I., Morata, P., Ocon, P., Manchado, P. and Colmenero, J.D. (1997). Rapid diagnosis of human brucellosis by peripheral blood PCR assay. *J. Clin. Microbiol.* **35** : 2927-2930.

Rajashekara, G., Glasner, J.D., Glover, D.A. and Splitter, G.A. (2004). Comparative whole genome hybridization reveals genomic islands in *Brucella* species. *J. Bacteriol.* **186** : 5041-5051.

Redkar, R., Rose, S., Bricker, B. and DelVecchio, V. (2001). Real-time detection of *Brucella abortus, Brucella melitensis* and *Brucella suis*. *Mol. Cell. Probes*. **15** : 43-52.

Romero, C. and Lopez-Goni, I. (1999). Improved method for purification of bacterial DNA from bovine milk for detection of *Brucella* spp. by PCR. *Appl. Environ. Microbiol.* **65** : 3735-3737.

Sreevastan, S., Bookout, J.B., Ringpis, F., Perumuaalla, V.S., Isloor, S. and Barathur, R.R. (2000). A multiplex approach to molecular detection of *Brucella abortus* and/or Mycobacterium bovis infection in cattle. *J. Clin. Microbiol.* **38** : 2602-2610.

Stevens, M. G., Olsen, S. C. and Cheville, N. F. (1994). *Infect. Immun.* **62** : 4646–4649.

Tantillo, G., Di Pinto, A., Vergara, A. and Buonavoglia, C. (2001). Polymerase chain reaction for the direct detection of *Brucella* sp. In milk and cheese. *J. Food Prot.* **64** : 164-167.

Vemulapalli, R., McQuiston, J.R., Schurig, G.G., Sriranganathan, N., Halling, S.M. and Boyle, S.M. (1999). Identification of an IS711 element interrupting the wboA gene of Brucella abortus vaccine strain RB51 and a PCR assay to distinguish strain RB51 from other Brucella species and strains. 1999. *Clin. Diagn. Lab. Immunol.* **6** : 760-764.

Vrioni, G., Gartzonika, C., Kostoula, A., Boboyianni, C., Papadopoulou, C. and Levidiotou, S. (2004). Application of a polymerase chain reaction enzyme immunoassay in peripheral whole blood and serum specimens for diagnosis of acute human brucellosis. *Eur. J. Clin Microbiol. Infect. Dis.* **23** : 194-199.

Wellinghausen, N., Nöckler, K., Sigge, A., Bartel, M., Essig, A. and Poppert, S. (2006). Rapid detection of *Brucella* spp. in blood cultures by fluorescence *in situ* hybridization. *J. Clin. Microbiol.* **44** : 1828-1830.

Wright, P.F. and Nielsen, K.H. (1990) In : Advances in Brucellosis Research (Adams, L.G., ed.), pp. 305–320, Texas A&M University Press, College Station, TX.

Zerva, L., Bourantas, K., Mitka, S., Kansouzidou, A. and Legakis, N.J. (2001). Serum is the preferred clinical specimen for diagnosis of human brucellosis by PCR. *J. Clin. Microbiol.* **39** : 1661-1664.

11

BOVINE TUBERCULOSIS: A ZOONOTIC THREAT AND ITS NATURAL RESERVOIRS

JPS Gill

Tuberculosis (TB), one of the most widespread infectious diseases, is the leading cause of death due to a single infectious agent among adults in the world. Bovine tuberculosis is a chronic bacterial disease of cattle and is a significant zoonosis that can spread to humans through inhalation of aerosols or the ingestion of unpasteurized milk. In developed countries, eradication programs have reduced or eliminated tuberculosis in cattle, and human disease is now rare but it is difficult to eradicate reservoirs in wildlife. Bovine tuberculosis still exists in less developed countries, and severe economic losses due to livestock deaths, chronic disease and trade restrictions. Bovine tuberculosis is caused by *Mycobacterium bovis*, a Gram positive, acid-fast bacterium in the *Mycobacterium tuberculosis* complex of the family Mycobacteriaceae.

Amongst the members of the Mycobacterium tuberculosis complex (MTBC), *M. tuberculosis* is mainly a human pathogen, whereas *M. bovis* the causative agent of bovine tuberculosis has an exceptionally wide host range and is the principal agent responsible for tuberculosis in domestic and wild mammals. Susceptible species include cattle, humans, non-human primates, goats, cats, dogs, pigs, buffalo, badgers, possums, deer and bison. Bovine tuberculosis is a well-known zoonotic disease which affects cattle world-wide. *M. bovis* also infects humans, causing zoonotic TB through ingestion, inhalation and, less frequently, by contact with mucous membranes and broken skin. The Office International des Epizooties has classified bovine tuberculosis as a List B disease, a disease which is considered to be of socio-economic and public health importance within countries and is of significance to the international trade of animals and animal products. The introduction of pasteurization has alleviated the public health risk of bovine tuberculosis in many countries, but it continues to cause production losses when poorly controlled. So, most developed nations have embarked on campaigns to eradicate *M. bovis* from the cattle population or at least to control the spread of infection.

The complex interactions between humans, domestic and wild animals make favourable environment for the emergence of new diseases. The reservoirs of *M. bovis,* the causative agent of tuberculosis in animals which is also communicable to human beings, also exist in wildlife. The presence of these wildlife reservoirs is the direct result of spillover from domestic livestock, human factors such as translocation of wildlife, supplemental feeding of wildlife and wildlife populations reaching densities beyond normal habitat carrying capacities due to human intervention.

M. bovis infection has been confirmed in a wide range of mammals' hosts throughout the world. Among the wild animals, monkeys, deer and elephants suffer from tuberculosis and probably maintain the sylvatic cycle of tuberculosis whereas domestic animals, mainly cattle maintain the infection in the agricultural and farm lands. Usually domestic animals and wild animals do not come in contact with each other, but transmission of *M. bovis* from domestic animals to wild life and vice versa continued over the millennia. It is a cycle that kept the disease going among animals and also in those human populations that came in close contact with *M. bovis* infected animals due to reasons such as agriculture, animal husbandry or hunting related activities.

Epidemiologic investigations reveal that the organism may be ingested or inhaled. Extra pulmonary lesions may occur associated with consumption of infected milk, but due to introduction of milk pasteurization and the practice of boiling milk, the digestive route of infection became less important. The airborne infection usually occurs among meat industry and slaughterhouse workers, where the infection is still prevalent in cattle. Main causes of concern related to *M. bovis* in industrialized countries are: epizootics in domesticated and wild mammals and latent infection in immigrants.

Mandatory pasteurization of milk has decreased the prevalence of human tuberculosis due to *M. bovis* in developed countries. In some countries eradication has been prevented by several factors one of which is the presence of a wildlife reservoir of *M. bovis*. Though *M. bovis* has an exceptionally wide host range, but until recent years there was little concern about infection in species other than cattle and man. Diversification of farming enterprises has led to cognizance of the need for control in other domestic animals, notably deer. *M. bovis* has been isolated from a wide range of wildlife species, in addition to domestic animals. There has also been recognition that self-maintaining infection is present in wildlife hosts in some countries-notably the European badger in the United Kingdom and Ireland, the Australian brush-tailed possum in New Zealand, and various species of ungulates in limited areas of a number of countries. Various wild animal species play an important role in the maintenance of *M. bovis* in wildlife communities and the spread to domestic animals. Badgers (*Meles meles*), brushtail possums (*Trichosurus vulpecula*), deer (*Odocoileus virginianus*), bison (*Bison bison*) and African buffalo (*Syncerus caffer*) are examples of wildlife that are maintenance hosts of *M. bovis*. The importance of these hosts has been highlighted by the growing realization that these animals can represent the principal source of infection for both domestic animals and protected wildlife species.

The potential of each wild animal population as a reservoir of infection for domestic animals is determined by the nature of the disease in each wild animal species, the routes of transmission for domestic animals and the risk of domestic animals encountering an infectious dose. Mere presence of infection in a wild animal population does not itself give evidence of a significant wildlife reservoir. The key concepts used in deciding whether an infected wild animal population is involved in the epidemiology of tuberculosis in domestic livestock is illustrated by reference to six well-researched cases: the feral pig (*Suis scrofa*) and feral Asian water buffalo (*Bubalus bubalis*) in Australia, white tailed deer (*Odocoileus virginianus*) in Michigan, and the brushtail possum (*Trichosurus vulpecula*) and other species, such as the ferret (*Mustela furo*), in New Zealand. A detailed analysis of *M. bovis* infection in the Eurasian badger (*Meles meles*) in Ireland and their role as a reservoir of infection for cattle has been reported. In recent years, tuberculosis in farmed cervidae has become a disease of economic as well as public health importance in several countries.

In Great Britain evidence suggests that *M. bovis* is endemic among European badgers (*Meles meles*), and that tuberculous badgers are implicated as significant sources of infection for domestic cattle. The risk of transmission of infection between a wildlife population and domestic animals will be determined by both the epidemiology of the disease and the ecology of the host. In the UK, surveys by the UK Ministry of Agriculture, Fisheries and Food (MAFF) have identified *M. bovis* infection in deer (*Cervus* sp., *Capreolus* sp., *Dama* sp.), red fox (Vulpes vulpes), mink (*Mustela vison*), feral ferret (*Mustela furo*), mole (*Talpa europaea*), brown rat (*Rattus norvegicus*) and feral cat (*Felis catus*). However, the potential contribution to cattle herd breakdowns, of reservoirs of *M. bovis* infection in mammals other than the badger is poorly understood and is the subject of current research. The pattern of infection in the population and potential risks to cattle, are profoundly influenced by badger social organization and behaviour. The pattern of land use and cattle farming practices in the UK brings badgers into close contact with domestic animals and provides conditions that may enhance the likelihood of disease.

In New Zealand, brushtail possums (*Trichosurus vulpecula*), first taken to New Zealand in the mid-19th century now occupy over 90% of New Zealand land mass and serve as a source of *M. bovis* for domestic livestock. In Michigan, USA free-ranging white-tailed deer (*Odocoileus virginianus*) represent the first reservoir of *M. bovis* in free-living wildlife in the United States. White-tailed deer, the primary reservoir and maintenance host of tuberculosis, are highly valued by the public, and particularly hunters, for cultural and economic reasons. Since 1995, significant progress has been made in defining and reducing the reservoir of tuberculosis in deer. As yet, no other wildlife species has been shown to play an epidemiologically important role in the disease cycle. Deer to cattle transmission of *M. bovis* has been documented. Tuberculosis caused by *M. bovis* has also been a problem in captive wildlife and in recently domesticated animals such as farmed deer. Wildlife reservoirs of *M. bovis* represent a serious challenge to the eradication of *M. bovis*. The presence of wildlife reservoirs is the direct result of spill-over of *M. bovis* from domestic livestock and efforts to eradicate *M. bovis* from domestic livestock are impeded by spill-back from wildlife reservoirs.

In South Africa, African buffaloes (*Syncerus caffer*) are considered as the most important maintenance host for *M. bovis*. African buffaloes not only transmit the disease to predators and scavengers that feed on them, but also serve as a source of infection to other wildlife species through environmental contamination. The infection is primarily spread between buffaloes via the respiratory route, but it is not known whether shedding of *M. bovis* in nasal and oral excretions may lead to contamination of ground and surface water and facilitate the transmission to other animal species. Once the infection spills over into a wild animal species with maintenance host potential, conventional measures are no longer sufficient to provide effective control. In several countries, it was shown that an infected wildlife reservoir that interacts with livestock causes frequent herd breakdowns and substantial economic losses to the agricultural sector. Experimentally infected deer can transmit *M. bovis* to cattle through sharing of feed. Livestock producers in areas where tuberculosis is endemic in free-ranging white-tailed deer should implement management practices to prevent access of wildlife to feed intended for livestock.

The outbreak of tuberculosis in free-ranging wildlife populations thus poses a huge challenge on long-term management and control strategies to prevent spillover into other wildlife, especially endangered, wildlife species and domestic livestock. Many susceptible species, including man, are spillover hosts in which infection is not self-maintaining. In countries where there is transmission of infection from endemically infected wildlife populations to cattle or other farmed animals, eradication is not feasible and control measures must be applied indefinitely.

Expansion of ecotourism-based industries, changes in land-use practices and escalating competition for resources have increased contact between free-ranging wildlife and humans. Although human presence in wildlife areas may provide an important economic benefit through ecotourism, exposure to human pathogens may represent a health risk for wildlife. There are reports on introduction of a primary human pathogen into free-ranging wildlife and described outbreaks of Mycobacterium tuberculosis, a human pathogen, in free-ranging banded mongooses (*Mungos mungo*) in Botswana and suricates (*Suricata suricatta*) in South Africa.

The test and slaughter policies of tuberculosis control, effectively used with livestock, are insufficient where wildlife reservoirs exist. It will not be possible to eradicate *M. bovis* from livestock until transmission between wildlife and domestic animals is halted. Control of *M. bovis* in this group of animals is dependent on the judicious use of diagnostic tests and the application of sound disease control principles. The advances in the development of bovine tuberculosis vaccines for cattle and farmed deer may offer valuable insights into the use of vaccination for the control of tuberculosis in a range of captive wildlife species. Such an endeavor will require a collaborative effort between agricultural, wildlife, environmental and political interests.

12

CURRENT STATUS OF *ESCHERICHIA COLI* 0157 : H7 AN EMERGING FOOD BORNE PATHOGEN

Y. Singh

In last two decades, Enterohaemorrhagic *Escherichia coli* (EHEC) have emerged as an important foodborne enteropathogen of humans which often leads to bloody diarrhea, and occasionally to kidney failure. The most notorious serotype of EHEC responsible for 85-90% cases of Haemorrhagic Colitis (HC), Haemolytic Uremic Syndrome (HUS) and Thrombotic Thrombocytopenic Purpura (TTP) is *E. coli* 0157:H7 which belongs to a subgroup of VTEC. This strain was isolated for the first time in 1975 from a woman in California with grossly bloody diarrhea. But this organism as a group of Enterohaemorrhagic *E. coli* came into existanse only after 1982 when it was recognized for the first time as a cause of Haemorrhagic Colitis in two major foodborne outbreaks in Oregon and Michigan states of America.

The other non-0157 serotypes that cause remaining 5-15% human diseases are 010, 026, 055, 069, 0111, 0128, 0145 and 0172. Bovines are perceived to be their natural reservoirs. The majority of human EHEC including both 0157:H7 and non-0157:H7 strains, outbreaks for which a same source has been identified includes the consumption of cattle products especially improperly cooked ground hamburger. Besides, raw milk and yogurt have also been implicated in various outbreaks.

In the years since the discovery of these pathogens, *E. coli* 0157:H7 has become increasingly prominent in the developed countries like UK, Canada, Japan, Germany and other parts of the world. In United States alone, it causes an estimated 20,000 illness and 250 deaths each year. Many of the questions that faced by the investigators of original outbreak in 1982 remain unanswered today. Prominent question among these is the question of why this pathogen suddenly emerged as a public health problem. Is *E. coli* 0157:H7 a completely new pathogen which suddenly appeared in the food supply or is this pathogen which was present but remain unrecognized prior to 1982? If *E. coli* 0157:H7 infection is truly increasing in incidence, what factors are favouring its emergence and more importantly, what can be done to check the spread of this microbe?

EPIDEMIOLOGY

Escherichia coli O157:H7 was first recognized as a cause of human illness in two separate outbreaks of hemorrhagic colitis in Michigan and Oregon in 1982 (Riley *et al.*, 1983). The organisms were transmitted in both cases by undercooked beef. Increasing numbers of diseases related to *E. coli* O157:H7 have been reported since 1982, most have been sporadic (Ostroff *et al.* 1989), but many institutional and community-wide outbreaks (Swerdlow *et al.*, 1992) have occurred in nursing homes, schools and day care centers or have been related to eating at fast food restaurants (Bell *et al.*, 1994), drinking untreated municipal water or fresh-pressed apple cider (Swerdlow *et al.*, 1992), or swimming in lake water (Keene *et al.*, 1994).

It is estimated that 0.6% to 2.4% of all cases of diarrhea and 15% to 36% of all cases of bloody diarrhea or hemorrhagic colitis are associated with *E. coli* O157:H7. The minimum estimated attack rates of *E. coli* O157:H7 among persons who consumed the suspected food product were 3.5% in a community outbreak and 8% in a junior high school outbreak. These estimated attack rates include only cases in which patients had bloody diarrhea or a positive stool culture; thus, "possible" cases or those with milder symptoms were excluded. In a nursing home outbreak, the estimated attack rates from both food-borne and person-to-person transmission were 33% among the nursing home residents and 13% among the staff. The attack rate was reported to be as high as 67% (42 of 63 persons) in a kindergarten outbreak involving unpasteurized milk. Most reported cases of *E. coli* O157:H7 infection have occurred in the United States, Canada, and Great Britain, but cases have also been documented in Japan, Australia, South Africa, Europe, Argentina, and Chile. *Escherichia coli* O157:H7 has been detected in most areas of the United States; the largest numbers of isolations have been found in Washington State, Oregon, Minnesota, and Massachusetts.

Escherichia coli O157 : H7 infections occur in all age groups, and the young are most often affected. The annual incidence rate in children less than 5 years of age (6.1 cases per 100,000 persons) compared with an overall incidence rate (2.1 cases per 100,000 persons) is higher. *Escherichia coli* O157:H7 generally affects both sexes equally. The rate of *E. coli* O157:H7 infection follows a seasonal pattern, with a peak incidence from June through September. Sixty percent of *E. coli* O157:H7 infections and 73% cases of the hemolytic-uremic syndrome and thrombotic thrombocytopenic purpura presented with bloody diarrhea between June and September, and patients affected during the summer months were younger than those seen during the rest of the year (Ostroff *et al.*, 1989). Food-borne transmission of *E. coli* O157:H7 is the most important means of infection. Transmission has primarily been linked to undercooked meat, and, during the 1982 outbreaks, the organism was cultured from a suspected lot of hamburger patties (Riley *et al.* 1983). Sources other than undercooked hamburger meat include heat-processed meat patties; roast beef; ham, turkey, cheese, sandwiches and potatoes. Unpasteurized milk has been implicated as the vehicle for two cases of the hemolytic-uremic syndrome and for a kindergarten outbreak of *E. coli* O157:H7 infection. *E. coli* O157:H7 was isolated from the feces of healthy cows who had supplied raw milk consumed by the patients affected in the outbreak. Even fresh-pressed, unpreserved apple cider, a seemingly unlikely vehicle, was implicated in one outbreak. The isolation of *E. coli* O157:H7 from milk and from the feces of healthy cattle and the fact that hamburger is a major vehicle associated with food-borne outbreaks of *E. coli* O157:H7 infection (Riley *et al.* 1983) suggest that cattle are an important reservoir for the pathogen.

Water-borne transmission has been implicated in two outbreaks, and transmission by person-to-person contact or by fomites has been suggested in sporadic cases and outbreaks. Secondary person-to-person contact can be an important method of spread in institutional settings, especially day care centers and nursing homes, but it is less common in community-wide outbreaks. Nosocomial *E. coli* O157:H7 infections have also been reported (Yannelli *et al.*, 1990). Incidence rates of 1-3:100,000 are reported. Rates are highest during July-October. The main reservoir for *E. coli* O157 is the intestine of healthy cattle. The bacteria can survive in faeces and soil. Carcasses can become contaminated through contact with intestinal contents at slaughter. The infectious dose of *E. coli* O157 appears to be very low, probably fewer than 100 organisms.

SURVEILLANCE

E. coli O157:H7 infection is nationally reportable in the USA and Great Britain, and is reportable in most US states. HUS (hemolytic-uremic syndrome) is also reportable in most US states.

SPREAD OF INFECTION

A major source of infection is undercooked ground beef; other sources include consumption of unpasteurized milk and juice, raw sprouts, lettuce, and salami, and contact with infected live animals. Disease caused by *E. coli* O157:H7 is known as the "hamburger disease" because of its association with eating home-made hamburgers. Waterborne transmission occurs through swimming in contaminated lakes, pools, or drinking inadequately treated water. The organism is easily transmitted from person-to-person.

Where does *E. coli* come from? As of today this is a mystery that no one has been able to solve. *E. coli* O157:H7 is found on cattle farms and can live in the intestines of healthy cattle. The toxin requires highly specific receptors on the cells surface in order to attach and enter the cell. Species such as cattle, swine, and deer which do not carry these receptors may harbor toxigenic bacteria without any ill effect, shedding them in their feces, from which they may be spread to humans. It is thought that cattle subjected to stress are more likely to have *E. coli.* Because of these abnormally small enclosures, these cattle may defecate and urinate onto each other and their hides are covered with this filth when they are led to slaughter. In the slaughter houses, the cattle are stunned and hung from hooks on a conveyor line, where the first thing done is the removal of their hides. Occasionally these conveyor belts move in jerky motions causing swaying which may cause the contaminated hides to flap against the exposed meat of the animal carcass or that of a neighboring carcass. It takes only a very minute amount of contamination to infect the meat. Sometimes an entire animal carcass falls unto the filthy floor of the slaughter house and it is hung back on the line with insufficient or even no cleaning whatsoever. Sometimes during the cutting of the carcass, the intestines of the animal are accidentally sliced and their contents explode over the exposed meat. Thus the meat can become contaminated during slaughter and butchering, and organisms can be thoroughly mixed into beef when it is ground into hamburger. Another potential vector of *E. coli* O157:H7 is filth flies (which includes house flies, *Musca domestica*). Filth flies have been shown to be vectors of *E. coli* O157:H7 using PCR.

PATHOGENICITY

E. coli O157:H7, which was first identified in 1982, is a particularly nasty version. The pathogenesis of *E. coli* 0157, other EHEC and VTEC is complex and is encoded by a number of plasmid, bacteriophage and chromosomal genes. Like enteropathogenic *E. coli* (EPEC), EHEC contain virulence plasmid that promote non-intimate attachment and a pathogenicity island encoding both intimate attachment and signaling apparatus to induce attaching effacement of the mammalian enterocyte. Most strains of EHEC have a 60 mDa virulence plasmid. This plasmid may have a role in initial attachment to mucosal surfaces of colonic epithelium. The majority of the untoward consequences of VTEC infection result from production of one or both types of verotoxin *viz.* VT1 and VT2. These verotoxins are immunologically indistinguishable from shiga toxin and therefore are also known as shiga like toxins (SLT). However, VT1 is more identical to shiga toxin while VT2 group is more heterogenous collection of toxins showing 50-60% genetic homology with VT1. Besides, a third vero cell cytotoxin of 64 kDa has also been identified which is not neutralized by antiserum against shiga toxin. The genes controlling the production of VT1 and VT2 are bacteriophage encoded. This toxin has capacity to bind the receptors on human kidney, brain and gut cells and kills them. Not all people have the receptors, which explain why some people and animals, including cattle that get O157:H7 become very ill and some don't.

CLINICAL MANIFESTATIONS

Infection with *E. coli* O157:H7 presents with a wide spectrum of clinical manifestations, including severe abdominal cramps with little or no fever and watery diarrhea that often progresses to grossly bloody diarrhea. Infection can be asymptomatic or can present with only nonbloody diarrhea. Extraintestinal involvement, including cardiac and neurologic manifestations, has been reported, and infection can be associated with the hemolytic-uremic syndrome and thrombotic thrombocytopenic purpura. The disease can be fatal and seen in three forms.

Asymptomatic Infection and Nonbloody Diarrhea

Cases of asymptomatic *E. coli* O157:H7 infection has occasionally been detected in outbreaks, but the incidence rates are difficult to estimate because stool samples from asymptomatic persons are rarely obtained for culturing.

Hemorrhagic Colitis

Hemorrhagic colitis caused by *E. coli* O157 : H7 is a clinical syndrome that consists of abdominal cramps; diarrhea that progresses to become bloody; radiologic or endoscopic evidence of colonicmucosal edema, erosion, or hemorrhage; and the absence of conventional enteric organisms in the stool. After the outbreaks of hemorrhagic colitis in Michigan and Oregon and subsequent similar outbreaks, *E. coli* O157 : H7 have been recognized as an important etiologic agent for hemorrhagic colitis. Hemorrhagic colitis may be the only manifestation of *E. coli* O157:H7 infection or it may result into development of the hemolytic-uremic syndrome. Thirty-eight percent to 61% of such infections result in hemorrhagic colitis, and surveillance studies have found *E. coli* O157:H7 in 27% to 36% of sporadic cases of hemorrhagic colitis. Infection with *E. coli* O157:H7 usually begins with the sudden onset of severe abdominal cramps, which are followed within hours by watery diarrhea that progresses to grossly bloody stools. Upper gastrointestinal symptoms, such as nausea and vomiting, occur early and may be prominent. The incubation period ranges from 1 to 9 days (mean, 3.1 to 3.9 days) during community outbreaks and from 1 to 14 days (mean, 4 to 8 days) in institutional settings.

Hemolytic-Uremic Syndrome

The hemolytic-uremic syndrome is a distinct entity characterized by microangiopathic hemolytic anemia, thrombocytopenia, and renal failure. Many factors have been implicated in the development of this syndrome, including genetics, pregnancy, drugs (such as oral contraceptives and estrogen therapy), toxins, chemicals, viruses, and bacteria. On the basis of epidemiologic, clinical, and laboratory data, two major subgroups of the syndrome have been identified: typical (or epidemic) and atypical (or sporadic). The syndrome occurs predominantly in infants and young children and is the most common cause of acute renal failure in children; the mortality rate is 5% to 10%, and persistent disability occurs in one third of survivors. Most patients with the hemolytic-uremic syndrome have nonbloody or bloody diarrhea which is the most common presenting symptom. Other presenting symptoms include abdominal cramps, vomiting, fever, lethargy, seizure, pallor and respiratory distress. The cecum and ascending colon are most commonly involved and often show hemorrhage and necrosis. Common neurologic manifestations include irritability and lethargy, but serious complications, such as seizure and coma, could occur.

Thrombotic Thrombocytopenic Purpura

Thrombotic thrombocytopenic purpura (TTP) is characterized by thrombocytopenia, microangiopathic hemolytic anemia, fever, renal failure, and neurologic symptoms. TTP is thought to represent a more extensive form of the clinical spectrum of vascular diseases that produces the hemolytic-uremic syndrome, and the criteria for diagnosis of thrombotic thrombocytopenic purpura are the same as those for the hemolytic-uremic syndrome, with the addition of fever and new-onset neurologic deficit. Infection with *E. coli* O157:H7 has been implicated in some cases of thrombotic thrombocytopenic purpura, and this condition has served as a clue in the recognition of outbreaks of *E. coli* O157:H7 infection. Although such progression is rare, as many as 8% of patients (3 of 37) with hemorrhagic colitis associated with *E. coli* O157:H7 infection progressed to TTP in one outbreak. The progression of HUS to TTP in children with *E. coli* O157:H7 infection has not been reported.

DIAGNOSIS

The sample is cultured on sorbitol MacConkey (SMAC) agar, or the variant cefeximine potassium tellurite sorbitol-MacConkey agar (CT-SMAC). On SMAC agar O157 colonies appear colourless due to their inability (unlike other *E. coli* serotypes) to ferment sorbitol. Non-sorbitol fermenting colonies are tested for the somatic O157 antigen before being confirmed as *E. coli* O157. Screening specimens on sorbitol-containing MacConkey culture medium and then testing the non-sorbitol-fermenting colonies for *E. coli* O157:H7 by using biochemical parameters and by serotyping with O157 and H7 antisera can be laborious and time-consuming. Antisera to both H7 and O157 are now commercially available, so that after screening with sorbitol-MacConkey medium, the sorbitol-negative colonies can be rapidly confirmed with O serum and H serum in the slide agglutination test. Investigators have shown that the commercially available latex slide agglutination tests for O157 serum are an efficient and reliable alternative to conventional serotyping with the standard-tube agglutination test (Chapman, 1989). However, colonies that agglutinate should be confirmed serologically, using agglutination or direct immunofluorescent antibody tests (Tison, 1990).

Another sensitive method of diagnosing *E. coli* O157:H7 infection is to look for Shiga-like toxins. These toxins have been detected in *E. coli* culture broth filtrate and in stool extracts. Other methods for detecting toxins include genetic probes and immunospecific assays, which are simpler and more sensitive than culture techniques. Deoxyribonucleic acid hybridization assays using synthetic nucleotides or fragments of structural genes specific for the toxins can also be used to detect Shiga-like toxin-producing *E. coli*. Gene probes are sensitive and specific. These specific DNA probes are able to detect colonies of Shiga-like toxin-producing *E. coli* present in numbers as small as 1 in 1200 colonies. Gene probes are diagnostically useful, but the cost and concern associated with radioactive safety have limited their widespread applicability.

Various enzyme-linked immunosorbent assays using polyclonal and monoclonal antibodies against Shiga-like toxins I and II to detect the presence of toxins in culture or fecal extract have also been developed. On the basis of its specific binding to the globotriaosyl ceramide natural receptor, a modified enzyme-linked immunosorbent assay for the rapid detection of Shiga-like toxin I has been reported, in which toxin bound to the globotriaosyl ceramide receptor has been detected by enzyme-linked immunosorbent assay with monoclonal antibodies against Shiga-like toxin I.

Another genetic technique involves polymerase chain reaction (PCR) amplification to test for the presence of

Shiga-like toxin genes (Gunzer *et al.*, 1992; Pollard *et al.*, 1990). Because PCR can detect organisms in low numbers, it can detect Shiga-like toxin production when culture fails (Brain *et al.*, 1992). In addition, like other methods for detecting the presence of Shiga-like toxin, PCR can identify Shiga-like toxin-producing *E. coli* other than O157:H7. Techniques for the direct detection of Shiga-like toxin sequences in stool and food specimens have also been reported (Brain *et al.*, 1992), overcoming the difficulty of high-frequency loss of toxin genes with repeated cultures.

Additional phenotypic and genotypic assays have been developed to assist in epidemiologic studies. These schemes include Shiga-like toxin genotyping, plasmid DNA profiling, bacteriophage typing, restriction digests of plasmid, restriction fragment length polymorphism with a bacteriophage probe, electrophoresis of plasmids and multilocus enzyme electrophoretic typing, pulsed-field gel electrophoresis of restriction fragment length polymorphism, and patterns of antibiotic susceptibilities.

In summary, the most common method for diagnosing *E. coli* O157:H7 infection in current clinical practice is to culture stool specimens for the organisms using sorbitol-MacConkey agar. The sorbitol-negative colonies can be serotyped using commercially available anti-sera to O157. In addition, DNA probes and PCR for toxin genes are used to detect Shiga-like toxin in stools at some reference laboratories.

PREVENTIVE MEASURES

E. coli O157:H7 will continue to be an important public health concern as long as it contaminates meat. Application of HACCP should be mandatory at meat processing plants. Other preventive measures mainly involve adequate hygiene to prevent contamination of food and person-to-person spread. It particularly applies to farms, abattoirs and those working in healthcare, nurseries and food provision. Correct food preparation including washing of raw vegetables, adequate cooking of meat especially beefburgers and pasteurisation of dairy products is also important. Keep cooked and uncooked meats separately and store uncooked meat on the bottom shelf of the fridge to avoid dripping raw meat juices on to other food. Never put cooked food back on a plate which has had fresh uncooked meat on it. Thoroughly wash all salads and vegetables that are to be eaten raw. Avoid eating and drinking unpasteurised milk and dairy products. Do not swim in water that may be contaminated. Regarding personal hygienic measures, thoroughly wash hands after using the toilet, handling raw meat, before meals and after contact with animals. Ensure children wash their hands with warm water and soap after contact with animals, particularly while on farm visits. If someone has *E. coli* infection, wash all dirty clothes, bedding and towels in the washing machine on the hottest cycle possible. Clean toilet seats, toilet bowls, flush handles, taps and wash hands, basins after use, with detergent and hot water, followed by a household disinfectant. Person having *E. coli* infection should not prepare food for others.

In January 2007 Canadian bio-pharmaceutical company Bioniche had developed a bovine vaccine capable of reducing O157:H7 in cattle by over 99%. On March 4, 2009, the United States Department of Agriculture (USDA) granted a conditional license for the first *E. coli* O157 vaccine for cattle in the U.S.

CONCLUSIONS

Infection with *E. coli* O157:H7 presents with many clinical manifestations and should be included in the differential diagnosis for any patient with new-onset bloody diarrhea. Development of the hemolytic-uremic syndrome or thrombotic thrombocytopenic purpura should raise strong suspicion of *E. coli* O157:H7 infection and should lead to prompt evaluation. If infection is confirmed, it should be reported to public health officials.

The increasing frequency of recognized cases may be due in part to heightened awareness of the organism, especially in regions with previous outbreaks; it may also reflect an epizootic infection among cattle, the principal animal reservoir for *E. coli* O157 : H7. The potentially high morbidity and mortality associated with this infection warrant better preventive measures. As the properties and actions of Shiga-like toxins and the pathogenesis of *E. coli* O157:H7 infections are being elucidated, many questions remain unanswered and provide areas for future research. Epidemiologic studies may evaluate the geographic variation in prevalence of *E. coli* O157:H7 infection and the significance of animal reservoirs with respect to the apparent increase in frequency of infection. Several Shiga-like toxin-producing *E. coli* other than those with the O157:H7 serotypse have been associated with human diseases and may become increasingly important. It is also of clinical importance to determine host factors for infection with this organism, such as age and gastric activity, and to identify susceptibility for disease progression to the hemolytic-uremic syndrome using factors such as age, blood-group antigens, and antibiotic therapy. Other factors, such as strain characteristics and inoculum size, may affect the outcome of the infection and require further examination. Toxin production is believed to be the primary etiologic event of *E. coli* O157 : H7 infection, but detailed pathogenic sequences still need to be characterized. These include the intracellular mechanism for the inhibition of protein synthesis; receptor binding; and determinants mediating cellular adhesion and bowel colonization (such as an attachment-effacement mediated by a chromosomal-encoded *eae* gene product, an outer membrane protein called intimin).

Rapid, convenient, and cost-effective diagnostic methods that are specific and sensitive for *E. coli* O157:H7 are necessary for prompt detection of infections. Such methods may involve serologic tests, immunologic assays, genetic tools, or PCR amplification.

REFERENCES

Bell, B.P., Goldoft, M., Griffin, P.M., Davis, M.A., Gordon, D.C., Tarr, P.I. (1994). A multistate outbreak of *Escherichia coli* O157:H7-associated bloody diarrhea and hemolytic-uremic syndrome from hamburgers. *J A M A*. **272** : 1349-53.

Brian, M.J, Frosolono, M., Murray, B.E., Miranda, A., Lopez, E.L., Gomez, H.F (1992). Polymerase chain reaction for diagnosis of enterohemorrhagic *Escherichia coli* infection and hemolytic-uremic syndrome. *J. Clin. Microbiol.* **30** : 1801-6.

Chapman, P.A. (1989). Evaluation of commercial latex slide test for identifying *Escherichia coli* O157. *J Clin Pathol.* **42** : 1109-10.

Gunzer, F., Bohm, H., Russman, H., Bitzan, M., Aleksic, S. and Karch, H. (1992). Molecular detection of sorbitol-fermenting *Escherichia coli* O157 in patients with hemolytic-uremic syndrome. *J. Clin. Microbiol.* **30** : 1807-10.

Keene, W.E., McAnulty, J.M., Hoesly, F.C., Williams, L.P. Jr, Hedberg, K., Oxman, G.L (1994). A swimming-associated outbreak of hemorrhagic colitis caused by *Escherichia coli* O157 : H7 and *Shigella sonnei. N Engl J. Med.* **331** : 579-84.

Ostroff, S.M., Kobayashi, J.M. and Lewis, J.H. (1989). Infections with *Escherichia coli* O157:H7 in Washington State. The first year of statewide disease surveillance. *J A M A.* **262** : 355-9.

Ostroff, S.M., Hopkins, D.P., Tauxe, R.V., Sowers, E.G. and Strockbine, N.K. (1988.). Surveillance of *Escherichia coli* O157 isolation and confirmation, United States, *M M W R CDC Surveill Summ.* **40** : 1-6.

Pollard, D.R., Johnson, W.M., Lior, H., Tyler, S.D., Rozee, K.R. (1990). Rapid and specific detection of verotoxin genes in *Escherichia coli* by the polymerase chain reaction. *J. Clin. Microbiol.* **28** : 540-5.

Riley, L.W., Remis, R.S., Helgerson, S.D., McGee, H.B., Wells, J.G., Davis, B.R (1983). Hemorrhagic colitis associated with a rare *Escherichia coli* serotype. *N Engl. J. Med.* **308** : 681-5.

Swerdlow, D.L., Woodruff, B.A., Brady, R.C., Griffin, P.M., Tippen, S., Donnell, H.D. Jr (1992). A Waterborne outbreak in Missouri of *Escherichia coli* O157:H7 associated with bloody diarrhea and death. *Ann Intern Med.* **116** : 812-19.

Tison, D.L. (1990). Culture confirmation of *Escherichia coli* serotype O157:H7 by direct immunofluorescence. *J Clin. Microbiol.* **28** : 612-3.

Yannelli, B., Domenico, P. and Cunha, B.A. (1990). Quadri SM. Nosocomial *Escherichia coli* O157:H7 diarrhea [Letter]. *Am J. Infect. Contrl.* **18** : 341-2.

13

ARCOBACTER SPP. AN EMERGING FOOD BORNE PATHOGEN : ITS DIAGNOSIS, PREVENTION AND CONTROL

H.V. Mohan and R.S. Rathore

Developments such as increasing globalization of the food industry, new technologies, products and changes in the susceptibility of population to disease have all highlighted the problem of food-borne emerging pathogens. Foodborne zoonotic pathogens are of great concern with regard to consumer protection. During the past decade, improvements in the isolation techniques in veterinary medicine led to discovery of *Arcobacter* spp. as animal and human pathogen. *Arcobacter* species are Gram-negative spiral-shaped organisms belonging to the family *Campylobacteraceae* that can grow microaerobically or aerobically. The association of *Arcobacter butzleri, Arcobacter cryaerophilus* and *Arcobacter skirrowii* with humans and animals has been clearly established. These bacteria have been detected world wide in products of animal origin and in healthy animals as well as in surface water. Although evidence was found for the connection of *Arcobacter* spp. with human and animal illness, *Arcobacter* spp. can be pathogens, opportunistic pathogens and commensals. Their potential as zoonotic foodborne and waterborne agents, the routes of transmission and the pathogenic mechanisms of these bacteria are largely unknown. Antibiotic resistance is present in *Arcobacter* strains to significant levels. The abundant presence of four *Arcobacter* species in foods of animal origin and the recovery of these bacteria from surface and drinking water suggest an important role of these bacteria as foodborne or waterborne agent and as zoonotic agent. In view of control measures to be used to prevent or to eliminate the hazard of *Arcobacter* spp. in food, several treatments have been evaluated for their effectiveness. Measures aimed at reduction or eradication of *Arcobacter* from the human food chain should be encouraged.

ETIOLOGY

In 1991, the genus *Arcobacter,* which together with *Campylobacter* was included in the family *Campylobacteraceae,* was proposed (Vandamme and De 1991). *Arcobacters* are Gram-negative, non-sporeforming rods, generally 0.2–0.9 mm wide and 0.5–3 mm long. The bacteria are curved to S-shaped rods. They are motile and have one unsheathed single polar flagellum at one or both ends of the cells. *Arcobacters* are able to grow under aerobic and anaerobic conditions over a wide temperature range (15–42°C). Optimal growth occurs under microaerobic conditions (3–10% O_2) and the bacteria do not require hydrogen. Presently the genus *Arcobacter* includes six species: *Arcobacter nitrofigilis,* a nitrogen-fixing bacterium associated with the roots of *Spartina alterniflora* a marsh plant, *Arcobacter butzleri, Arcobacter cryaerophilus* and *Arcobacter skirrowii* frequently associated with animals and occasionally with humans; and two recently described species, *Arcobacter cibarius,* isolated from chicken carcasses and *Arcobacter halophilus,* a second environmental species isolated from a hyper saline lagoon.

Like *Campylobacter,* routine identification of *Arcobacters* is difficult because these organisms have fastidious growth requirements and are relatively inert biochemically. Moreover, since *Arcobacter* and *Campylobacter* species show several morphological and biochemical similarities, incorrect detection and identification of *Arcobacters* might occur by relying on conventional plating methods and phenotypic tests. These drawbacks emphasize the need for rapid, reliable and sensitive molecular techniques for the specific detection of *Arcobacter* spp. in food products.

Most important phenotypical traits for differentiation between *Arcobacter* spp., and *Campylobacter* spp. (according to On, 1996)

Characteristic	*Arcobacter*	*Campylobacter*
Aerobic growth at 25 °C	+	-
Catalase	+	+
Oxidase	+	+
Urease	-	-
Hippurate hydrolysis	-	+

PATHOGENSIS AND VIRULENCE FACTORS

Production of toxins or other virulence factors has not been demonstrated but adhesive and/or invasive properties were apparent. Fernandez *et al.* (1995) using HEp-2 cell culture and rat ileal loop assay proposed that invasion was a pathogenicity mechanism. Wesley *et al.* (1995, 1996) reported that *A. butzleri* colonized the neonate piglet intestines and hence suggests an invasive potential. Villarruel-Lopez *et al.* (2003) investigated the cytotoxic effects of *Arcobacter* strains isolated from retail meats. A total of 38 isolates induced cell elongation, indicating entrotoxin production and 18 isolates induced vacuole formation. Meanwhile, 39 isolates led to both vacuolization and elongation in Vero cells.

ANIMAL INFECTIONS

Arcobacter organisms were first isolated from aborted bovine and porcine fetuses as well as from control placentas by Ellis and others in the 1970's. *Arcobacter* spp. have been isolated from uterine and oviduct tissues and from placental samples of sows with reproductive problems (Van Driessche *et al.*, 2004). Aerotolerant *Campylobacter*-like organisms have been isolated from aborted and normal porcine fetuses, sows with reproductive problems and from clinically healthy specific pathogen-free pigs (Suarez *et al.*, 1997). In boars, *Arcobacters* have been recovered from preputial swabs, but not from semen (De Oliveira *et al.*, 1999). Apart from *A. nitrofigilis*, the other species of *Arcobacter* spp. have been isolated from various animal diseases including abortion, septicemia, mastitis, gastritis and enteritis.

LIVESTOCK AS A RESERVOIR FOR *ARCOBACTER*

Different recent studies reported *Arcobacter* spp. occurrence in feces of livestock animals detected by different isolation methods and molecular techniques. Poultry in particular might be a significant reservoir of *Arcobacter* spp. *Arcobacter* spp. was isolated from 44% of porcine, 40% of bovine, 16% of ovine and 15% of equine faecal samples (Van Driessche *et al.*, 2003). Kabeya *et al.* (2003) examining the distribution of *Arcobacter* spp. among livestock in Japan. *Arcobacter* spp. was isolated from 3.6 and 10% of the cattle and swine fecal samples, respectively, along with 14.5% of chicken cloacal swabs. *A. butzleri* was the most prevalent species.

OCCURRENCE IN FOODS OF ANIMAL ORIGIN

Arcobacter spp. is frequently isolated from products of animal origin (chickens, pork, beef and lamb). The highest prevalence is found in chickens, followed by pork and beef. In Japan 23% of chickens, 7% of pork and 2.2% of beef samples from retail shops were positive for *A. butzleri*, *A. cryaerophilus* and *A. skirrowii* (Kabeya *et al.*, 2004). Among *Arcobacter* spp. isolated from meat samples, *A. butzleri* was found most, followed by *A. cryaerophilus* (Kabeya *et al.*, 2004). The bacteria were detected on almost all slaughterhouse carcasses tested during a large-scale study in Belgium and up to several thousand bacteria were present per gram of neck skin prior to evisceration (Houf *et al.*, 2002). Although a high prevalence of *Arcobacter* species on chicken meat is reported worldwide, the bacteria are rarely detected in the intestinal contents of these animals. It was therefore assumed that contamination of meat probably arises from other sources and occurs during processing.

OCCURRENCE IN WATER

Apart from poultry and other meat, *Arcobacter* spp. (mostly *A. butzleri*) was isolated from a drinking water reservoir (Jacob *et al.*, 1993), river or surface water, ground water and sewage.

Thus consumption of contaminated water is a likely source of exposure to *Arcobacters. A. butzleri* can easily attach to water distribution pipe surfaces (stainless steel, copper and plastic), which makes regrowth in the water distribution system a possibility. This can become a significant problem in drinking water and food processing plants with respect to public health.

AS POTENTIAL PATHOGEN IN HUMANS

In recent years *A. butzleri* and *A. cryaerophilus* have been isolated from the faeces of patients with diarrhoea or recurrent abdominal pain in USA, Canada, Australia, South Africa, Thailand, Italy, France and Germany.

A. butzleri was recovered from 2.4% of diarrhoeal stool samples collected from Thai children during a survey of paediatric gastro-enteritis (Taylor *et al.*, 1991). Morethan 50% of 22 patients with *A. butzleri* associated diarrhoea suffered from abdominal pain and nausea; fever, chills and vomiting and malaise were other frequently reported features (Kiehlbauch *et al.*, 1991). On *et al.* (1995) isolated *A. butzleri* from bacterimia in a new born in the United Kingdom. *A. butzleri* has been isolated from 22 patients with severe diarrhoea (Wesley *et al.*, 1996). *A. butzleri* has been cultured from human cases of enteritis, healthy patients and patients with chronic underlying disease (Dediste *et al.*, 1998).

Vandenberg *et al.* (2004) reported that *A. butzleri* was the fourth most common *Campylobacter*-like organism isolated from 67,599 stool specimens and also they suggested that *A. butzleri* displays microbiologic and clinical features similar to those of *Campylobacter jejuni;* however, *A. butzleri* is more frequently associated with persistent, watery diarrhoea. *A. butzleri* and *C. jejuni* were isolated in 0.14% and 5.81% respectively. And among the non diarrhoeic stool specimens, *A. butzleri* and *C. jejuni* were isolated in 0.06% and 1.65% respectively. This indicates that *A. butzleri* was more frequently isolated from diarrhoeic stool specimens than from non diarrhoeic stool specimens.

STATUS IN INDIA

Kownhar *et al.* (2007) reported 3 *Arcobacter* spp., 16 *Campylobacter jejuni*, from 200 HIV infected patients with diarrhoeal symptoms at AIDS Hospital in southern India. This may be an indication of the association of *Arcobacter* infections with immunodeficient patients.

In a study made by Seleshe Nigatu, (2007) isolation rate of *Arcobacter butzleri* and *A. skirrowii* from poultry, pigs and cattle faecal sample were 6.67%, 21.67%, 11.67% and 0%, 5.0%, 1.67% respectively. In the same study reported isolation rate of *A. butzleri* in human diarrhoeic patients and healthy persons (non diarrhoeic) were 8.0% and 4.0% respectively and isolation rate of *A. butzleri* in food samples like neck region chicken flesh including skin and milk from clinically healthy cattle were 12% and 6.0% respectively.

Arcobacter spp. were isolated from 2% of human diarrhoeal stool samples, 10% of cattle, 8% of poultry, 12% of porcine faecal samples and 1.66% of raw milk, 10% of chicken meat, 5% of beef and 5% of pork samples (Mohan, 2008).

DIAGNOSIS

(*a*) By Conventional Cultural Method

Standardized methods do not exist for the isolation of *Arcobacter* species, nevertheless common procedures have developed by many workers. *Arcobacters* were first recovered from bovine and porcine fetal tissues cultured in semisolid Elling-hausen-McCullough-Johnson–Harris (EMJH) isolation medium containing 5-fluorouracil, which was originally designed for the isolation of *Leptospira* (Ellis *et al.*, 1977). De Boer *et al.* (1996) developed an *Arcobacter* selective enrichment broth (ASB) and an *Arcobacter* selective semisolid medium (ASM) for the recovery of *Arcobacter* from food. Atabay and Corry (1998) described the *Arcobacter* enrichment broth which incorporated with CAT selective supplement for the recovery of *A. butzleri, A. cryaerophilus* and *A. skirrowii*. Houf *et al.* (2001)

described a further selective broth and agar medium with selective antibiotic supplement.

Gonzalez *et al.* (2000) developed combined PCR-culture technique for the rapid detection of *Arcobacter* spp. in chicken meat following a short selective enrichment of chicken samples. Using a variable 16S rRNA and 23S rRNA region, Houf *et al.* (2000) developed a species-specific multiplex PCR assay for the simultaneous detection and identification of *A. butzleri, A. cryaerophilus* and *A. skirrowii*. Atabay *et al.* (2002) used RAPD-PCR technique to reveal epidemiologic association among strains. While PCR-based methods seem to be advantageous in time saving, pulsed-field gel electrophoresis (PFGE) is generally considered to be the 'gold standard' for most of the relevant pathogens in food hygiene. Hume *et al.* (2001) used PFGE for genotyping *Arcobacter* spp. from nursing sows and growing pigs on three farms.

PREVENTION AND CONTROL MEASURES

A definitive link between *Arcobacter* spp. and human disease has not been established yet, but public health concerns have been raised. This is due to the fact that there are several opportunities that exist for human exposure to *Arcobacter*. A major focus is currently on raw meat products. Furthermore, unpasteurized dairy products may also pose a risk of *Arcobacter* transmission to the human population. Therefore, while the role of *Arcobacter* in human disease awaits further evaluation, a precautionary approach is advisable. Measures aimed at reduction or eradication of *Arcobacter* from the human food chain should be encouraged. The faecal carriage of foodborne pathogens among livestock animals at slaughter is strongly correlated with the hazard of carcasses contamination at the slaughter line. In order to reduce the risk represented by zoonotic agents to the consumer health, it is essential to reduce contamination of carcasses during the slaughtering processes. Therefore, the maintenance of slaughter hygiene is consequently of central importance in meat production. It can be measured in daily practice by "in-process-controls" and regular microbiological monitoring of carcasses as a verification system according to the HACCP principles. Moreover, preventive measures, such as implementation of codes of good manufacturing practices (GMP), increased care during hiding and evisceration should be encouraged. Since *Arcobacter* spp. are non-spore formers, standard cooking regimes (heat treatment to 70 °C) will kill the organism. Moreover, beside a standard isolation procedure for *Arcobacter* spp. detection, further studies would be needed to estimate the prevalence of *Arcobacter* spp. in patients with diarrhoea and to illuminate the pathogenic role and potential virulence factors of *Arcobacter* spp. Furthermore, additional information on the epidemiology of these microorganisms is necessary.

REFERENCES

Atabay, H.I. and Corry, J.E.L. (1998). Evaluation of a new *Arcobacter* enrichment medium and comparison with new media developed for enrichment for *Campylobacter spp. Int. J. Food Microbiol.* **41** : 53-58.

Atabay, H.I., Bang, D.D., Aydin, F., Erdogan, H.M. and Madsen, M. (2002). Discrimination of *Arcobacter butzleri* isolates by Polymerase chain reaction-mediated DNA fingerprinting. *Lett. Appl. Microbiol.* **35** : 141-145.

De Boer, E., Tilburg, J.J.H.C., Woodward, D.L., Loir, H. and Johnson, W.M. (1996). A selective medium for the isolation of *Arcobacter* from meats. *Lett. Appl. Microbiol.* **23** : 64-66.

Dediste, A., Aeby, A., Ebraert, A. and Vlaes, L. (1998). *Arcobacter* in stools: Clinical features, diagnosis and antibiotic susceptibility. In Lastovica A.J. Newwell, D.G., Lastovia, E.E. (Eds) Campylobacter, Helicobacter and related organisms. Cape Town: Institute of Child Health Pages 436-439.

De Oliveira, S.J., Wesley, I.V., Baetz, A.L., Harmon, K.M., Kader, I.T.A. and de Uzeda, M. (1999). *Arcobacter cryaerophilus* and *Arcobacter butzleri* isolated from preputial fluid of boars and fattening pigs in Brazil. *J. Vet. Diagnostic Investigation.* **11** : 462-464.

Ellis, W.A., Neill, S.D., O' Brien, J.J., Ferguson. H.W. and Hanna, J. (1977). Isolation of Spirillum/Vibrio-like organisms from bovine fetuses. *Vet. Record.* **100** : 451-452.

Fernandez, H., Eller, G., Paillacar, J., Gajardo, T. and Riquelme, A.C. (1995). Toxigenic and invasive capacities: possible pathogenic mechanisms in *Arcobacter cryaerophilus. Mem. Inst. Oswaldo Cruz, Rio de Janeiro.* **90** : 633-634.

Gonzalez, I., Garcia, T., Antonlin, A., Hernandez, P.E. and Martin, R. (2000). Development of a combined PCR-Culture technique for the rapid detection of *Arcobacter* spp. in chicken meat. *Lett. Appl. Microbiol.* **30** : 207-212.

Houf, K., Tutenel, A., De Zutter, L., Van Hoof, J. and Vandamme, P. (2000). Development of a multiplex PCR assay for the simultaneous detection and identification of *Arcobacter butzleri, Arcobacter cryaerophilus* and *Arcobacter skirrowii. FEMS Immunol Med Microbiol.*, **49** : 337-45.

Houf, Kurt., Luc, A., Devriese, Lieven, De zutter., Hoof, Van Jan., and Vandamme, Peter. (2001). Susceptibility of *Arcobacter butzleri, Arcobacter cryaerophilus,* and *Arcobacter skirrowii* to antimicrobial agents used in selective media. *J. Clin. Microbiol.* **39** : 1654–1656.

Houf, K., De Zutter, L., Van Hoof, J. and Vandamme, P. (2002). Occurrence and distribution of *Arcobacter* species in poultry processing. *J. Food Protect.* **65** : 1233-1239.

Hume, M.E., Harvey, R.B., Stanker, L.H., Droleskey, R.E., Poole, T.L. and Zhang, H.B. (2001). Genotypic variation among *Arcobacter* isolates from a farrow-to-finish swine facility. *J. Food Protect.* **64** : 645–651.

Jacob, J., Loir, H. and Feuerpfeil, I. (1993). Isolation of *Arcobacter butzleri* from drinking water reservoir in Eastern Germany. *Zbl. Hyg.* **193** : 557-562.

Kabeya, H., Maruyama, S., Morita, Y., Kubo, M., Yamamoto, K., Arai, S., Izumi, T., Kobayashi, Y., Katsube, Y. and Mikami, T. (2003). Distribution of *Arcobacter* species among livestock in Japan. *Vet. Microbiol.* **93** : 153-158.

Kabeya, H., Maruyama, S., Morita, Y., Ohsuga, T., Ozawa, S., Kobayashi, Y., Abe, M., Katsube, Y. and Mikami, T. (2004). Prevalence of *Arcobacter* species in retail meats and antimicrobial susceptibility of the isolates in Japan. *Int J. Food Microbiol.* **90** : 303-308.

Kiehlbauch, J.A., Plikaytis, B.D., Swaminathan, B., Cameron, D.N. and Wachsmuth, I.K. (1991). Restriction fragment length polymorphisms in the ribosomal genes for species identification and subtyping of aerotolerant *Campylobacter* species. *J. Clin. Microbiol.* **29** : 2362.

Kownhar, H., Shankar, E.M., Rajan, R., Vengatesan, A. and Rao, U.A. (2007). Prevalence of *Campylobacter jejuni* and enteric bacterial pathogens among hospitalized HIV infected versus non-HIV infected patients with diarrhoea in southern India. *Scand. J. Infect. Dis.* **39** : 862-866.

Mohan, H.V. (2008). Detection of *Arcobacter* spp. in man, animals and foods of animal origin by using culture and PCR techniques. M.V.Sc Thesis submitted to Deemed University, IVRI, Izatnagar.

On, S.L.W., Stacey, A. and Smyth, J. (1995). Isolation of *Arcobacter butzleri* from neonate with Bacteraemia. *J. Infect.* **31** : 225-227.

On, S.L.W (1996). Identification methods for *Campylobacters, Helicobacters,* and related organisms. *Clin. Microbiol. Reviews* **9** : 405– 422.

Seleshe Nigatu (2007). Detection of *Campylobacter jejuni* and *Arcobacter* species from various sources by conventional and molecular techniques. M.V.Sc Thesis, Deemed University, IVRI, Izatnagar.

Suarez, D.L., Wesley, I.V. and Larson, D.J., (1997). Detection of *Arcobacter* species in gastric samples from swine. *Vet. Microbiol.* **57** : 325-336.

Taylor, D.N., Kiehlbauch, J.A., Tee, W, Pitarangsi, C. and Echeverria, P. (1991) Isolation of group 2 aerotolerant *Campylobacter* species from Thai children with diarrhoea. *J. Infect. Dis.* **163** : 1062-7.

Vandamme, P. and De ley, J. (1991). Proposal for a new family *Campylobacteraceae. Int. J. of systematic Bacteriology.* **41** : 451-455.

Vandenberg, O., Dediste, A., Houf, K., Ibekwem, S., Souayah, H., Cadranel, S., Douat, N., Zissis, G., Butzler, J.P. and Vandamme, P. (2004). *Arcobacter* species in humans. *Emerg. Infect. DIs.* **10** : 1863-1867.

Van Driessche, E., Houf, K., Van Hoof, J., De Zutter, L. and Vandamme, P. (2003). Isolation of *Arcobacter* species from animal feces. *FEMS Microbiol. Letters.* **229** : 243-248.

Van driessche, E., Houf, K., Van groenweghe, F., De zutter, L., Vandamme, P. and Van Hoof, J. (2004). Occurrence and strain diversity of *Arcobacter* species in Belgian pigs. *Res. Microbial.* **155** : 662-666.

Wesley, I.V., Schroder-Tucker, L., Baetz, A.L., Dewhurst, F.E. and Paster, B.J. (1995). *Arcobacter butzleri*-specific 16S rRNA based probes. *J. Clin. Microbiol.* **33** : 1691-1698.

Wesley, I.V., Baetz, A.L., and Larson, D.J. (1996). Infection of cesarean-derived colostrum-deprived 1-day-old piglets with *Arcobacter butzleri, Arcobacter cryaerophilus and Arcobacter skirrowii. Infect. Immun.* **64** : 2295–2299.

14

TRENDS IN DETECTION OF *CAMPYLOBACTER* FROM FOODS

Ashok Kumar, K.N. Bhilegaonkar and R.K. Agarwal

Campylobacteriosis has now become one of the most commonly reported bacterial gastroenteritis in humans in many countries (Moore *et al.*, 2005). Several species of campylobacters are encountered in animals, birds and man, but mainly *C. jejuni* and *C. coli*; occasionally *C. lari* and more recently *C. upsaliensis* have been found to be involved in human cases. These species grow at 42°C and thus have been grouped as thermophilic organisms. Another important member of genus *Campylobacter* is *C. fetus*, which grows at 37°C and causes bovine venereal campylobacteriosis.

The spectrum of disease in case of *Campylobacter* infection may range from mild, self- limiting non-inflammatory diarrhoea to severe, inflammatory, bloody diarrhoea with pyrexia, abdominal cramps, bacteraemia and faecal leukocytes (Sack *et al.*, 2001). Besides enteritis, other clinical manifestations associated with *Campylobacter* infection are Guillain Barre Syndrome (GBS), reactive arthritis, haemolytic uraemic syndrome and rarely meningitis in human (Shoenfeld *et al.*, 1996). *Campylobacter* can also cause enteritis in several species of domestic animals like dogs, cattle, sheep, pigs, etc. The cases of bovine mastitis and abortion or stillbirth in ewes and cattle have also been observed (Skirrow, 1994).

METHODS OF DETECTION

1. Isolation and Identification

The development of a culture medium for isolation of *Campylobacter* from human faeces by Skirrow (1977) helped to firmly establish its role in human disease. Earlier *Campylobacter* detection was reliant on membrane filtration of faecal samples on to non-selective media, a laborious and cumbersome method, which was less suitable for environmental specimens, owing to the presence of contaminating organisms. This led to the development of enrichment and selective media suitable for the isolation of *Campylobacter* from foods and environmental samples.

The samples collected for isolation of *Campylobacter* should be kept at 4°C or on ice. Cary-Blair transport medium may be used for transportation of samples to laboratory. The samples can be directly inoculated on to selective media for isolation of *Campylobacter* spp. However, where the number of organisms is less, enrichment of the samples is required. Thioglycollate broth, Brucella broth, Preston broth and *Campylobacter* enrichment broth, etc. are some media used for enrichment of the samples. The selective media used for isolation of *Campylobacter* usually consist of a basal medium, blood, growth and selective supplements. Ferrous sulphate, sodium metabisulphite and sodium pyruvate (FBP) are commonly used growth supplements. Different combinations of various antimicrobial agents like vancomycin, bacitracin, novobiocin, rifampicin, polymyxin B, colistin, trimethoprim, cephalothin, cyclohexamide and amphotericin B have been successfully tried. Various media *viz.* Skirrow's selective medium, Butzler selective medium, Blaserwang's medium and Preston medium, etc are commercially available. Sometimes blood free media are also used.

Incubation is done at 42-43°C for thermophilic group and 37°C for *C. fetus* for a period of about 48 hours under microaerophilic conditions, which may be obtained in an anaerobic jar by evacuation/replacement method or using

Campylobacter gas generating, envelop with catalyst. Use of selective media containing oxygen-quenching agents such as hemin and charcoal further facilitates the isolation (Martin *et al.*, 2002). Colonies of *Campylobacter* are flat, light, opaque and nearly always tend to spread along the growth line. Campylobacters are gram-negative organisms, which are spirally curved with tapering ends. They are oxidase positive, Gram negative and S-shaped or spiral in morphology. Characteristic cork screw like motility can be seen under dark field microscopy. The inability of thermophilic *Campylobacter* to grow at 25°C distinguishes them from *C. fetus*. *C. jejuni* can be differentiated from *C. coli* by its ability to hydrolyse the hippurate. Both *C. jejuni* and *C. coli* are susceptible to nalidixic acid where as *C. lari* is resistant.

2. Phenotyping

Biotyping, serotyping and phage typing, etc. have been used for phenotyping of *campylobacter* isolates. Serotyping of organisms has been the most widely used phenotypic procedure. It includes the Penner scheme which is based on heat-stable (HS) antigens (Penner and Hennessy 1980) and Lior scheme using heat-labile (HL) antigens (Lior *et al.*, 1982).

3. Cellular Fatty Acid Profiles

The fatty acid (FA) composition of bacterial cells may significantly differ between taxa, and its determination and analysis have been found to be useful for classifying and identifying many bacteria (Priest and Austin 1993). The technique has been used to differentiate various species of *Campylobacter* (Blaser *et al.*, 1980; Cutis 1983; Moss *et al.*, 1984).

4. Protein Profiles

The protein content of a living cell is determined by its genomic content; analysis of the protein composition thus reflects the genetic organization of an organism, and this can be determined by using electrophoresis. Five types of protein profiling have been applied for identification of campylobacters, each differing principally in the types of proteins that are extracted and/or detected. Profiles of acid-phenol-extracted proteins have been used to differentiate various species of *Campylobacter* (Fernie and Park 1977); and aerotolerant campylobacters (now classified as *Arcobacter* spp.) from other *Campylobacter* species (Hanna *et al.*, 1983).

Differences between the outer membrane protein (OMP) composition of *C. jejuni* subsp. *jejuni, C. coli,* and *C. fetus* subsp. *fetus* had been demonstrated by Dunn *et al.* (1987) by means of immunoblotted two-dimensional gel electrophoregrams of sarcosyl-insoluble proteins.

Multilocus enzyme electrophoresis patterns may also discriminate between certain *Campylobacter* species. Isolates are characterized by the relative electrophoretic mobility of a large number of water-soluble cellular enzymes. Because of the net electrostatic charge, the rate of migration of a protein during electrophoresis are determined by its amino acid sequence, and the mobility variants of an enzyme can be directly equated with alleles at the corresponding structural gene locus (Selander *et al.*, 1986).

5. Serological Tests

The development of both poly and monoclonal antibodies specific for campylobacters has facilitated the development of a number of antibody-based tests. Falsen (1983) described an immunodiffusion assay that correctly identified *C. fetus, C. jejuni/ coli, C. mucosalis* and *C. sputorum*. Extensive modifications of this system have been described by Falsen *et al.* (1988) who delineated 14 immunotyping groups, and by Vandamme *et al.* (1991) who described 16 immunotyping groups.

A number of specific antibodies that can be used to identify particular species have been described. Taylor and Chang (1987) produced an antibody specific for outer membrane proteins (OMPs) of *C. jejuni* subsp. *jejuni, C. coli,* and *C. lari,* detectable by either ELISA or immunoblot. Griffiths *et al.* (1992) developed a series of antibodies capable of discriminating between *C. jejuni, C. coli, C. lari* and *C. upsaliensis* by employing dot ELISA. A flourescein-labelled antibody raised against a defined, recombinant membrane protein was useful for identifying *C. jejuni* strains in Western blot (immunoblot) assay, although weak reactions with *C. coli* were observed (Stucki *et al.*, 1995). Several studies have described the use of lectins, the proteins that bind specific carbohydrate groups, in typing *C. coli* and *C. jejuni, C. hyintestinalis, C. lari* and *C. sputorum* bv. *fecalis* (Gill and Corbel, 1986; Corbel and Gill, 1987).

Antibody-mediated agglutination of campylobacterial cellular antigens as a means of identification has been exploited by three commercially available systems (Campyslide, BBL Microbiology Systems and Merica Diagnostics). Each uses latex particles coated with immunoglobulins raised against different *Campylobacter* species. These systems are designed principally for presumptive but rapid identification of the thermophilic enteropathogenic campylobacters (On, 1996). A commercial enzyme-linked immunosorbent assay (ELISA) (ProSpecT Microplate assay; Alexon-Trend, USA) was developed for the detection of *C. jejuni* and *C. coli* directly in faecal samples from humans with gastroenteritis (Tolcin *et al.*, 2000).

6. Nucleic Acid Probes

A number of probes have been developed and used for identification of campylobacters. Zhou and Wang (1989) used non-radioactively labeled probes to detect thermophilic *Campylobacter*. The probes used were 12.8 Kb cloned DNA fragment for *C. jejuni* and a mixture of total genomic DNA from *C. coli* and *C. jejuni*. Taylor and Hiratsuka (1990) used 1.5 Kb DNA-probe for *C. jejuni* and 1.8 Kb DNA probe for *C. jejuni* and *C. coli*. Wang and Taylor (1993) used 1.2 Kb DNA fragment from *C. jejuni gyr*A gene. Total genomic DNA from *C. jejuni, C. coli, C. lari* and *C. upsaliensis* labeled with dioxigens was used by Burnens and Nicolet (1992) for detection of *Campylobacter* from diarrhoeic cats and dogs. As oligonucleotide probes are highly specific and easy to synthesize in large quantities, they are well suited for use in clinical laboratories. The targets for oligonucleotide probe have mostly been 16SrRNA (Olsen *et al.*, 1995). The method using strain- and genus-specific oligonucleotide probes has been developed to detect and enumerate specific *Campylobacter* strains in mixed populations. Strain-specific oligonucleotide probes were designed for the short variable regions (SVR) of the *fla*A gene in individual *C. jejuni* strains. A 16S rRNA *Campylobacter* genus-specific probe was also used. Both types of probes were used to investigate populations of campylobacters by colony lift hybridization (Elvers *et al.*, 2008).

One of the important diagnostic methods developed for identification of *Campylobacter* in clinical, environmental samples and chicken products is fluorescence in situ hybridization (FISH) (Poppert *et al.*, 2008). FISH is a microscopic method that uses fluorescently labeled oligonucleotide DNA probes that bind specifically to unique target sites on ribosomal RNA.

7. Polymerase Chain Reaction (PCR)

PCR is now one of the common techniques applied for detection of and discrimination between species of *Campylobacter*. Because of the strong conservation in the regions of 16S rRNA, this gene has widely been exploited for the detection of campylobacters (Persson and Olsen, 2005). Detection of *C. jejuni* and *C. coli* targeting the flagellin A gene of *C. jejuni* and *C. coli* specific for these two species was successfully used by Oyofo *et al.*, (1992). Giesendorf *et al.* (1992) reported PCR assay for the detection of campylobacters in foods particularly in chicken products after enrichment of the samples for 18 h in Preston enrichment broth. The *hip* (hippurase) gene has been used to differentiate *C. jejuni* from *C. coli* (Linton *et al.*, 1997). Lawson *et al.* (1999) developed a panel of PCR-ELISA assays, which they used in a large-scale survey for detection of *Campylobacter* species in human gastroenteritis. Use of PCR-ELISA has increased the specificity and sensitivity of detection. The paramagnetic beads have also been utilized for isolating *Campylobacter* from chicken caecal contents and faecal samples prior to PCR (Rudi *et al.*, 2004). Several genes appeared to be responsible for virulence and considered useful to know the pathogenic potential of *Campylobacter*. The PCR-based methods have been used to detect such virulence genes in *C. jejuni* (Rizal *et al.*, 2008).

There has recently been interest in the use of RNA as the molecular target for viability assessment. The most commonly used amplification techniques for detecting RNA are reverse transcriptase PCR (RT-PCR) and nucleic acid sequence based amplification (NASBA). NASBA with the use of molecular probes (Real-Time NASBA) has been found to be convenient and rapid for the detection of *C. jejuni* and *C. coli* in food samples (Churruca *et al.*, 2007). The introduction of real-time PCR methods has facilitated the development of quantitative PCR assays for the detection of *Campylobacter* in foods (Sails *et al.*, 2003), milk and water (Yang *et al.*, 2003).

8. Flagellin Typing (*Fla* Typing)

The flagellin gene locus of *C. jejuni* contains two flagellin genes (*fla*A and *fla*B), which are arranged in tandem and are separated by approximately 170 nucleotides. This locus is suitable for restriction fragment length polymorphism (RFLP) analysis of a PCR product because both highly conserved and variable regions are present at this locus (Meinsermann *et al.*, 1997). According to Ayling *et al.* (1996) at least seven *fla* typing procedure have been developed. Because *fla* typing profiles can be readily stored in electronic databases (Nachamkin *et al.*, 1996), many isolates can be easily compared and global studies are feasible. However, before such comparisons are possible, international standardization of at least the primers and restriction enzymes used are essential.

9. Pulsed-Field Gel Electrophoresis (PFGE)

Digestion of bacterial chromosomes by restriction enzymes that cleave the DNA infrequently has proved to be a useful typing technique for many bacteria (Tenover *et al.*, 1995; Finney, 1993). The fragmented DNA can be separated by using special electrophoretic conditions under which the orientation of the electrical field is changed in a pulsed manner and the variations in the presence of relevant restriction sites result in genotypic profiles (also called macrorestriction profiles) (Owen *et al.*, 1995;

Stanley *et al.*, 1995). PFGE for different species of *Campylobacter* has been used by many workers (Fujita *et al.*, 1995, Bourke *et al.*, 1996). The restriction enzymes, which have been seen to give satisfactory result, are *Sma*I, *Kpn*I, *Apa*I and *Bss*HII. *Xho*I appears to be useful for *C. upsaliensis* (Bourke *et al.*, 1996).

10. Ribotyping

The multiple copies of the rRNA gene loci (coding for 5S, 16S and 23S rRNA) are present at different positions on the *Campylobacter* chromosome and have been found to be suitable target for subtyping purpose. This technique is useful for determining the species of *Campylobacter* isolates that are difficult to analyze phenotypically (Kiehlbauch *et al.*, 1991). The technique includes the digestion with restriction enzymes followed by gel electrophoresis and southern blot hybridization with a probe specific for rRNA genes. The enzymes used in ribotyping studies for chromosomal digestion varies. The *Pst*I, *Hae*III, *Hind*III and *pvu*II have been used alone, in pairs, or even in combinations consisting of three enzymes (Owen *et al.*, 1995). The differences in the restriction enzymes and probes used generally hamper direct comparisons of the ribotype profiles obtained in different laboratories (Wassenaar *et al.*, 2000).

11. Random Amplification of Polymorphic DNA (RAPD) Analysis

Random amplified polymorphic DNA (RAPD) methods have been developed for *Campylobacter* spp. by using various primers and reaction conditions (Mazurier *et al.*, 1992, Acik and Cetinkaya, 2006). The primers are often selected arbitrarily (Owen and Hernandez, 1993). RAPD analysis of *C. jejuni* and *C. coli* has frequently used 10-mer primers (Madden *et al.*, 1996; Ertas *et al.*, 2004).

12. Amplified Fragment Length Polymorphism (AFLP) Analysis

AFLP analysis has been used to subtype *C. jejuni* (Kokotovic and On, 1999). AFLP fingerprints produced by complete digestion of chromosomal DNA with two restriction enzymes, one with 4-bp recognition site and other with a 6-bp recognition site has been shown to have potential for strain identification, as well as high-resolution differentiation of genetically related bacterial strains (Duim *et al.*, 1999). The primers used are labeled and resultant labeled PCR products are analyzed on denaturing polyacrylamide gels. With this technique, Godschalk *et al.* (2006) have shown that bacterial GBS markers are limited in number and located in the LOS (lipo-oligosaccharide) biosynthesis, which corroborated the current consensus that LOS mimicry may be the prime etiologic determinant of GBS.

13. Microarray Technology

DNA microarray has been used to compare interstrain, intraspecific variations in bacteria at the genomic level, referred to as genomotyping (Dorrell *et al.*, 2006). An electronic oligonucleotide microarray technique has been developed for detection and differentiation of the viable *Campylobacter* species (Zhang *et al.*, 2006). This development consisted of four major components: identification of single nucleotide polymorphisms (SNPs) within the *hsp* 60 gene as species markers, design of fluorescently labeled SNP-based reporters, development of an electronic microarray detection, and application of the integrated technique for analysis of *Campylobacter* species in food samples. A unique capability of this technique is the specific detection of viable cells and not dead ones. This is achieved by using mRNA of the 60 kDa heat-shock protein as the viability marker. The identification of two unique SNPs closely located at positions 291 and 294 of the *hsp* 60 gene enabled the differentiation of the three *Campylobacter* species. Very little sequence diversity has been reported between housekeeping genes from different *C. jejuni* strains, particularly between human isolates (Dingle *et al.*, 2001; Suerbaum *et al.*, 2001). Therefore, *C. jejuni* appears to be an ideal organism for genomotyping as per the report of Dorrell *et al.*, (2006) who have used a microarray approach to reveal extensive genetic diversity within *C. jejuni*.

SUMMARY

Although considerable progress has been made in the development of rapid and accurate methods for identifying campylobacters, it is nonetheless apparent that significant improvements are still required. The development of selective media and several selective supplements have no doubt increased the sensitivity of detection by conventional methods but the limitations cannot be overlooked. The use of molecular techniques has narrowed the limitations of the conventional detection methods and serves as easy and important tool for detection of campylobacters. But, even the molecular techniques have certain disadvantages so widely acceptable standard protocols for rapid and specific detection, typing and subtyping methods are mandatory.

REFERENCES

Acik, M.N. and Cetinkaya, B. (2006). Random amplified polymorphic DNA analysis of *Campylobacter jejuni* and *Campylobacter coli* isolated from healthy cattle and sheep. *J. Med. Microbial.* **55** : 331-334.

Ayling, R.D., Woodward, M.J., Evans, S. and Newell, D.G. (1996). Restriction fragment length polymorphism of polymerase chain reaction products applied to the differentiation of poultry campylobacters for epidemiological investigations. *Res. Vet. Sci.* **60** : 168-172.

Blaser, M.J., Moss, C.W. and Weaver, R.E. (1980). Cellular fatty acid composition of *Campylobacter fetus*. *J. Clin. Microbiol.* **11** : 448-451.

Bourke, B., Shreman, P.M., Woodward, D., Lior, H. and Chan, V.L. (1996). Pulsed-field gel electrophoresis indicates genotypic hererogenity among *Campylobacter upsaliensis* strains. *FEMS Microbiol. Lett.* **143** : 57-61.

Burnens, A.P. and Nicolet, J. (1992). Detection of *Campylobacter upsaliensis* in diarrhoeic dogs and cats, using a selective medium with cefoperazone. *Am. J. Vet. Res.* **53** : 48-51.

Churruca, E., Girbau, C., Martinez, I., Mateo, E., Alonso, R. and Fernandez-Astorga, A. (2007). Detection of *Campylobacter jejuni* and *Campylobacter coli* in chicken meat samples by real-time nucleic acid sequence-bases amplification with molecular beacons. *Int. J. Food Microbiol.* **117** : 85-90.

Corbel, M.J. and Gill, K.P.W. (1987). Lectin agglutination of thermophilic *Campylobacter* species. *Vet. Microbiol.* **15** : 163-173.

Cutis, M.A. (1983). Cellular fatty acid profiles of campylobacters. *Med. Lab. Sci.* **40** : 333-348.

Dingle, K.E., Colles, F.M., Wareing, D.R., Ure, R., Fox, A.J., Bolton, F.E., Bootsman, H.J., Willems, R.J., Urwin, R. and Maiden, M.C. (2001). Multilocus sequence typing system of *Campylobacter jejuni. J. Clin. Microbiol.* **39** : 14-23.

Dorrell, N., Mangan, J.A., Laing, K.G., Hinds, J., Linton, D., Al-Ghusein, H., Barrell, B.G., Parkhill, J., Stoker, N.G., Karlyshev, A.V., Butcher, P.D. and Wern, B.W. (2006). Whole Genome Comparison of *Campylobacter jejuni* Human isolates using a Low-Cost Microarray Reveals Extensive Genetic Diversity. *Genome Res.* 10.1101/gr.185801.

Duim, B., Wassenaar, T.M., Rigter, A. and Wagenaar, J. (1999). High-resolution genotyping of *Campylobacter* strains isolated from poultry and humans with amplified fragment length polymorphism fingerprinting. *Appl. Environ. Microbiol.* **65** : 2369-2375.

Dunn, B.E., Blaser, M.J. and Snyder, E.L. (1987). Two dimensional gel electrophoresis and immunoblotting of *Campylobacter* outer membrane proteins. *Infect. Immun.* **55** : 1564-1572.

Elvers, K.T., Helps, C.R., Wassenaar, T.M., Allen, V.M. and Newell, D.G. (2008). Development of a strain-specific molecular method for quantitating individual Campylobacter strains in mixed populations. *Appl. Environ. Microbiol.* **74** : 2321-31.

Ertas, H.B., Çetinkaya, B., Muz, A. and Ongor, H. (2004). Genotyping of broiler-originated *Campylobacter jejuni* and *Campylobacter coli* isolates using *fla* typing and random amplified polymorphic DNA methods. *Int. J. Food Microbiol.* **94** : 203–209.

Falsen, E. (1983). Immunodiffusion as an aid in routine identification of uncommon aerobic Gram-negative bacteria, p.477-483. In H. Leclere (ed.), Gram negative bacteria of medical and public health importance: taxonomy, identification, and applications. Les editions de l'Institute National de la Sante et de la Recherche Medicale, Paris, France.

Falsen, E., Nehls, I. and Borjesson, A. (1988). Immunotyping campylobacters. Taxonomic implications, p. 56-59. In Kaijser B and Falsen E (ed.), *Campylobacter* Infections. University of Goteborg, Goteborg, Sweden.

Fernie, D. and Park, R.W.A. (1977). The isolation and nature of campylobacters (microaerophilic vibrios) from laboratory and wild rodents. *J. Med. Microbiol.* **10** : 325-329.

Finney, M. (1993). Plused-field electrophoresis, p. 2.5.9-2.5.17. *In* Ausubel, F.M, Brent, R., Kingston, R.E., Moore, D.D., Seidman, J.G., Smith, J.A. and Struhl, K. (ed.), Current protocols in molecular biology, vol. 1. Currents Protocols Greene-Wiley, New York.

Fujita, M., Fujimoto, S., Morooka, T. and Amako, K. (1995). Analysis of strains of *Campylobacter fetus* by pulsed-filed gel electrophoresis. *J. Clin. Microbiol.* **33** : 1676-1678.

Giesendorf, B.A.J., Quint, W.G., Henkens, M.H., Stegeman, H., Huf, F.A. and Niesters, H.G. (1992). Rapid and sensitive detection of *Campylobacter* spp. in chicken products by using the polymerase chain reaction. *Appl. Environ. Microbiol.* **58** : 3804-3808.

Gill, K.P.W. and Corbel, M.J. (1986). Lectin agglutination for the differentiation of *Campylobacter fetus* serotypes. *Vet. Rec.* **118** : 158.

Godschalk, P.C.R., Bergman, M.P., Gorkink, R.F.J., Simons Guss, van den Braak, N., Lastovica, A.J., Endtz, H.P., Verbrugh, H.A. and van Belkum, A. (2006). Identification of DNA sequence variation in *Campylobacter jejuni* strains associated with the Guillain-Barre syndrome by high-throughput AFLP analysis. *BMC Microbiol.* **6** : 32.

Griffiths, P., Moreno, G.S. and Park, R.W.A. (1992). Differentiation between thermophilic *Campylobacter* species by species-specific antibodies. *J. Appl. Bacteriol.* **72** : 467-474.

Hanna, J., Neill, S.D., O'Brien, J.J. and Ellis WA (1983). Comparison of aerotolerant and reference strains of *Campylobacter* species by polyacrylamide gel electrophoresis. *Int. J. Syst. Bacterial.* **33** : 143-146.

Kiehlbauch, J.A., Plikaytis, B.D., Swaminathan, B., Cameron, D.N. and Wachsmuth, I.K. (1991). Restriction fragment length polymorphisms in the ribosomal genes for species identification and subtyping of aerotolerant *Campylobacter* species. *J. Clin. Microbiol.* **29** : 1670-1676.

Kokotovic, B. and On, S.L.W. (1999). High-resolution genomic fingerprinting of *Campylobacter jejuni* and *Campylobacter coli* by analysis of amplified fragment length polymorphisms. *FEMS Microbiol. Lett.* **173** : 77-84.

Lawson, A.J., Logan, J.M., O'Neill, G.L., Desai, M. and Stanley, J. (1999). Large-scale survey of *Campylobacter* species in human gastroenteritis by PCR and PCR-enzyme linked immunosorbent assay. *J. Clin. Microbiol.* **37** : 3860-3864.

Linton, D., Lawson, A.J., Owen, R.J. and Stanley, J. (1997). PCR detection, identification to species level, and fingerprinting of *Campylobacter jejuni* and *Campylobacter coli* direct from diarrheic samples. *J. Clin. Microbiol.* **35** : 2568-2572.

Lior, H., Woodward, D.L., Edgar, J.A., Laroche, L.J. and Gill, P. (1982). Serotyping of *Campylobacter jejuni* by slide agglutination based on heat-labile antigenic factors. *J. Clin. Microbiol.* **15** : 761-768.

Madden R.H., Moran, L. and Scates, P. (1996). Sub-typing of animal and human *Campylobacter* spp. using RAPD. *Lett. Appl. Microbiol.* **23** : 167-170.

Martin, K.W., Mattick, K.L., Harrison, M. and Humphrey, T.J. (2002). Evaluation of selective media for *Campylobacter* isolation when cycloheximide is replaced with amphotericin B. *Lett. App. Microbiol.* **34** : 124–129.

Mazurier, S., van der Giessen, A., Heuvelman, K. and Wernars, K. (1992). RAPD analysis of *Campylobacter* isolates: DNA fingerprinting without the need to purify DNA. *Lett. Appl. Microbiol.* **14**: 260-262.

Meinsermann, R.R., Helsel, L.O., Fields, P.I. and Hiett, K.L. (1997). Discrimination of *Campylobacter jejuni* isolates by *fla* gene sequencing. *J Clin Microbiol.* **35** : 2810-2814.

Moore, J.E., Corcoran, D., Dooley, J.S.G., Fanning, S., Lucey, B,, Matsuda, M., McDowell, R., O'Riordan. L., O'Rourke, M., Rao, J.R., Rooney, P.J., Sails, A. and Whyte, P. (2005). *Campylobacter. Vet Res.* **36** : 351-382.

Moss, C., Kai, A., Lambert, M.A. and Patton, C. (1984). Isoprenoid quinone content and cellular fatty acid composition of *Campylobacter* species. *J. Clin. Microbiol.* **19** : 772-776.

Nachamkin, I., Ung, H. and Patton, C.M. (1996). Analysis of the HL and O serotypes of *Campylobacter* strains by the flagellin gene typing system. *J. clin. Microbiol.* **34** : 277-281.

Olsen, J.E., Aabo, S., Hill, W., Notermans, S., Wernars, K., Granum, P.E., Popovic, T., Rasmussen, H.N. and Olsvik, O. (1995). Probes and polymerase chain reaction for detection of food-borne bacterial pathogens. *Int. J. Food Microbiol.* **28** : 1-78.

On, S.L.W. (1996). Identification methods of Campylobacters, Helicobacters, and related organisms. *Clin. Microbiol. Rev.* **9** : 405-422.

Owen, R.J. and Hernandez, J. (1993). Ribotyping and arbitrary primer PCR-fingerprinting of Campylobacters. *Soc. Appl. Bacteriol. Tech. Ser.* **31** : 265-285.

Owen, R.J., Sutherland, K., Fitzgerald, C., Gibson, J., Borman, P. and Stanley, J. (1995). Molecular subtyping scheme for serotyping HS1 and HS4 of *Campylobacter jejuni. J. Clin. Microbiol.* **33** : 872-877.

Oyofo, B.A., Thronton, S.A., Burr, D.H., Trust, T.J., Pavlovskis, O.R. and Guerry, P. (1992). Specific detection of *Campylobacter jejuni* and

Campylobacter coli by using the polymerase chain reaction. *J. Clin. Microbiol.* **30** : 2613-2619.

Penner, J.L. and Hennessy, N. (1980). Passive haemagglutination technique for serotyping *Campylobacter fetus* subsp. *jejuni* on the basis of soluble heat-stable antigens. *J. Clin. Microbiol.* **12** : 732-737.

Persson, S. and Olsen, K.E. (2005). Multiplex PCR for identification of *Campylobacter coli* and *Campylobacter jejuni* from pure cultures and directly on stool samples. *J. Med. Microbiol.* **54** : 1043-1047.

Poppert, S., Haas, M., Yildiz, T., Alter, T., Bartel, E., Fricke, U. and Essig, A. (2008). Identification of Thermotolerant *Campylobacter* Species by Fluorescence *In situ* Hybridization. *J. Clin. Microbiol.* **46** : 2133–2136.

Priest, F. and Austin, B. (1993). Modern bacterial taxonomy, 2nd ed. Chaman and Hall, London.

Rizal Anjana, Kumar, Ashok and Vidyarthi, A.S. (2008). Prevalence of pathogenic genes in *Campylobacter jejuni* isolated from poultry and human. Proc. International Symposium on food safety, quality assurance and global trade: Concern and strategies and VII Annual Conference of Indian Association of Veterinary Public Health Specialists. Pantnagar, November 7-9, 2008, Abst. No. YSA 153, Pp. 85.

Rudi, K., Hoidal, H.K., Katla, T., Johansen, B.K., Nordal, J. and Jakobsen, K.S. (2004). Direct real-time PCR quantification of *Campylobacter jejuni* in chicken fecal and cecal samples by integrated cell concentration and DNA purification. *Appl. Environ. Microbiol.* **70** : 790-797.

Sack, D.A., Lyke, C., McLauglin, C. and Suwanvanichkij, V. (2001). Antibacterial Resistance in Shigellosis, Cholera and Campylobacteriosis. WHO/CDS/CSR/ DSR/ 2001.8. Geneva: World Health Organization.

Sails, A.D., Fox, A.J., Bolton, F.J., Wareing, D.R. and Greenway, D.L. (2003). A real-time PCR assay for the detection of *Campylobacter jejuni* in foods after enrichment culture. *Appl. Environ. Microbiol.* **69** : 1383-1390.

Selander, R.K., Caugant, D.A., Ochman, H., Musser, J.M., Gilmour, M.N. and Whittam, T.S. (1986). Methods of multilocus enzyme electrophoresis for bacterial population genetics and systematics. *Appl. Environ. Microbiol.* **51** : 873-884.

Shoenfeld, Y., George, J. and Peter, J.B. (1996). Guillain-Barre as an autoimmune disease. *Int. Arch.Allergy and Immunol.***109** : 318-326.

Skirrow, M.B. (1994). Diseases due to *Campylobacter, Helicobacter* and related organisms. *J. Comp. Path.* **111** : 113-149.

Skirrow, M.B. (1977). *Campylobacter* enteritis: a "new" disease. *BMJ.* **2** : 9-11.

Stanley, J., Linton, D., Sutherland, K., Jones, C. and Owen, R.J. (1995). High-resolution genotyping of *Campylobacter coli* identifies clones of epidemiologic and evolutionary significance. *J. Infect. Dis.* **172** : 1130-1134.

Stucki, U., Frey, J., Nicolet, J. and Burnens, A.P. (1995). Identification of *Campylobacter jejuni* on the basis of a species-specific gene that encodes a membrane protein. *J. Clin. Microbiol.* **33** : 855-859.

Suerbaum, S., Lohrengel, M., Sonnevend, A., Ruberg, F. and Kist, M. (2001). Allelic diversity and recombination in *Campylobacter jejuni. J. Bacteriol.* **183** : 2553-2559.

Taylor, D.E. and Chang, N. (1987). Immunoblot and enzyme-linked immunosorbent assays of *Campylobacter* species. *Mol. Cell. Probes.* **1** : 261-274.

Taylor, D.E. and Hiratsuka, K. (1990). Use of non-radioactive probes for detection of *Campylobacter jejuni* and *Campylobacter coli* in stool specimens. *Mol. Cell Probes* **4** : 261-71.

Tenover, F.C., Arbeit, R.D., Goering, R.V., Mickelsen, P.A., Muruay, B.E., Persing, D.H. and Swaminathan, B. (1995). Interpreting chromosomal DNA restriction patterns produced by pulsed-field gel electrophoresis: criteria for bacterial strain typing. *J. Clin. Microbiol.* **33** : 2233-2239.

Tolcin, R., LaSalvia, M.M., Kirkley, B.A., Vetter, E.A., Cockerill, F.R. and Procop, G.W. (2000). Evaluation of the Alexon-trend ProSpecT *Campylobacter* microplate assay. *J. Clin. Microbiol.* **38** : 3853-3855.

Vandamme, P., Falsen, E., Rossau, R., Hoste, B., Segers, P., Tytgat, R. and De Ley, J. (1991). Revision of *Campylobacter, Helicobacter,* and *Wolinella* taxonomy: emendation of generic descriptions and proposal of *Arcobacter* gen. Nov. Int. *J. Syst. Bacteriol.* **41** : 88-103.

Wang, Y. and Taylor, D.E. (1993). Modified colony hybridization using whatman 54 filter paper. *Biotechniq.* **14** : 746-748.

Wassenaar, T.M. and Newel, D.G. (2000). Genotyping of *Campylobacter* sp. *Appl. Environ. Microbiol.* **66** : 1-9.

Yang, C., Jiang, Y., Huang, K., Zhu, C. and Yin, Y. (2003). Application of real-time PCR for quantitative detection of *Campylobacter jejuni* in poultry, milk and environmental water. *FEMS Immunol. Med. Microbiol.* **38** : 265-271.

Zhang, H., Gong, Z., Pui, O., Liu, Y. and Xing-Fang, Li (2006). An electronic DNA microarray technique for detection and differentiation of viable *Campylobacter* species. *Analyst* **13** : 907-915.

Zhou, Y.T. and Wang, S.Q. (1989). Application of a biotin – labeled DNA probe to detect *Campylobacter. Zbl. Bakt.* **272** : 186-190.

15

FOODBORNE LISTERIOSIS IN INDIA : AN UPDATE

S.B. Barbuddhe and S.V.S. Malik

Listeria monocytogenes is a foodborne pathogen that can cause serious invasive illness, mainly in certain well-defined high-risk groups, including elderly and immunocompromised patients, pregnant women, newborns and infants. Potential sources of the organism in these operations include the environment, food handlers, and incoming raw ingredients or processed products that have become contaminated after the lethality treatment at the manufacturing facility. In India, the pathogen has been isolated from humans, animals, a variety of foods including milk and milk products, meat and meat products and vegetables. In India, studies on molecular epidemiological aspects of *Listeria monocytogenes* are largely lacking. Therefore, we do not know the genetic variability of strains isolated and their epidemic potential. The molecular characterization of *Listeria* isolates from India should help to establish the characteristics of the strains responsible for epidemics, and allow the developing of new diagnostic tools and molecular typing. This would not only help in better understanding of the sources of infection and their risk assessment, routes of transmission of the infective agent, influencing factors, clinical forms and virulence characteristic of the pathogenic isolates of *Listeria* in order to diagnose the infection rapidly and reliably but also in instituting the effective control measures.

The Gram-positive bacterium *Listeria monocytogenes* is a ubiquitous pathogen that thrives in diverse environments such as soil, water, various food products, humans and animals. The disease caused by this bacterium, listeriosis, is acquired by ingesting contaminated food products and mainly affects immunocompromised individuals, pregnant women and newborns. Listeriosis manifests as gastroenteritis, meningitis, encephalitis, mother-to-fetus infections and septicaemia, resulting in death in 25–30% of cases. The diverse clinical manifestations of infection with *L. monocytogenes* reflect its ability to cross three tight barriers in the human host. Following ingestion, *L. monocytogenes* crosses the intestinal barrier by invading the intestinal epithelium, thereby gaining access to internal organs. During severe infections, crossing the blood–brain barrier results in infection of the meninges and the brain, and in pregnant women, crossing the fetoplacental barrier leads to infection of the fetus.

The genus *Listeria* consists of a group of Gram-positive bacteria of low G+C content. Six species, *L. monocytogenes, L. ivanovii, L. seeligeri, L. innocua, L. welshimeri,* and *L. grayi,* have been identified. Recently, a new species, *L. marthii* has been isolated from soil, standing water, and flowing water samples obtained from the natural environment. However, only *L. monocytogenes* and *L. ivanovii* are considered virulent. Human cases of *L. ivanovii* infection are rare, whereas *L. monocytogenes* is an important foodborne pathogen. *L. monocytogenes* has been isolated from a variety of food products. Meat, poultry, dairy, and vegetable products have all been implicated as vehicles of listeriosis. Since foodborne listeriosis was first reported in 1981, numerous foodborne outbreaks of *L. monocytogenes* have been documented worldwide (Farber and Peterkin, 1991; Jacquet *et al.,* 2002).

Serotyping has been widely used to characterize *L. monocytogenes* (Wiedmann, 2002). Although 13 serotypes have been identified, only 1/2a, 1/2b, and 4b are frequently isolated from clinical samples, with serotype 4b causing by far the most cases of human listeriosis (Raybourne, 2002; Borucki and Call, 2003). However, serotype 1/2a is the most prevalent serotype in food. Therefore, serotyping may have value as a virulence screening test.

CLINICAL SYNDROME

Although *L. monocytogenes* occasionally causes localized infections, the most frequent clinical manifestations of listeriosis are neuromeningeal infections and bacteremia, particularly in immunocompromised individuals. As pregnancy induces a selective decrease in some immunological reactions, listeriosis is also particularly dangerous for pregnant women, and more precisely for their fetuses. Fetal infection is usually severe and can result in miscarriage, stillbirth or neonatal listeriosis. Early- and late onset neonatal listeriosis has a poor prognosis with a high mortality rate and serious sequelae.

The incidence of listeriosis varies between 0.1 and 11.3/ 1,000,000 in different countries. Most reported cases present as life-threatening illness in one of three clinical syndromes: maternofetal listeriosis or neonatal listeriosis, blood stream infection, and meningoencephalitis. Besides the invasive forms, listeriosis may present as a febrile gastroenteritis and as cutaneous listeriosis. These presentations are self-limiting clinical conditions with non-specific symptoms and are therefore probably vastly underdiagnosed. Febrile gastroenteritis may affect persons with no known immunocompromising condition following ingestion of likely high numbers of organisms, after which the victim develops fever and diarrhoea within 24 h; the illness usually resolves spontaneously. Cutaneous listeriosis is an eczematous skin infection caused by direct exposure of intact skin to *L. monocytogenes,* typically in a veterinarian exposed to a diseased animal often after a listerial abortion. The incidence of listeriosis in certain populations at risk is listed in table 15.1

Table 15.1 : Incidence of Listeriosis in Certain Populations at Risk (Per 100,000 Individuals Per Year)

Normal population	0.7
Aged persons (s70 years)	2
Alcoholics	5
Diabetic people	5
Iron overload	5
Pregnant women	12
Cancer patients	15
Steroid therapy	20
Lupus erythematodes	50
Kidney transplant recipients	100
Chronic lymphatic leukemia	200
AIDS	600
Leukemia (acute monocytic + acute lymphoblastic)	1000

LISTERIA AS A FOOD-BORNE PATHOGEN

Listeria spp. is robust bacteria with wide distribution. Despite their poor survival in nutrient-deficient, unpolluted seawater and spring water, *Listeria* spp. readily replicate in nutrient-rich, contaminated waters, sewage, sludge, soil, foods, and animal hosts. Healthy cows can serve as reservoirs for *L. monocytogenes* and secrete the organism in milk. Contamination of milk may also occur through accidental contact with faeces and silage. Indeed, with mortality rates on average approaching 30%, *L. monocytogenes* far exceeds other common foodborne pathogens, such as *Salmonella enteritidis* (with a mortality of 0.38%), *Campylobacter* species (0.02–0.1%) and *Vibrio* species (0.005–0.01%) in terms of disease severity (Mead *et al.*, 1999). The list of food items which favours growth of *Listeria* and which are generally free are listed in Table 15.2.

The genes encoding the virulence-associated proteins PIPLC, LLO, Mpl, ActA and PC-PLC are located in a 9.6 kb virulence gene cluster (Gouin *et al.*, 1994), which is principally regulated by a pleiotropic virulence regulator, *prfA* (a 27 kDa protein encoded by *prfA*). In addition to these virulence associated genes and proteins, several other genes, such as *iap, bsh, vip, inlJ, auto, ami, bilA* are also involved in *L. monocytogenes* virulence and pathogenicity. The resistance of *L. monocytogenes* to acidic conditions and to bile salts makes it particularly adept at infecting the gastrointestinal tract (Hamon *et al.*, 2006).

Table 15.2 : List of Items Favouring and Generally Free of Listeriae

Food items which may contain L. monocytogenes	*Food items which in general free of listeriae*
Sausages (salami, pate.)	All kinds of food immediately after heating
Raw meat, in particular turkey and chicken	Pasteurized milk, yoghurt (industrial products)
Sandwiches	Hard cheese
Lettuce, raw mushrooms	Chocolate, marmalade, cookies
Raw milk and products made from this material	Raw carrots
Soft cheese	Raw apples
Fresh cheese (ricotta, feta)	Raw tomatoes
Seafood (mussels, salmon)	

THE INTRACELLULAR HABITAT

Listeriae can grow in the environment as well as in the extracellular space within a host. However, they belong to a group of bacteria that are able to penetrate into, and to survive and multiply within host cells (Fig. 15.1), not only in professional phagocytes but also in virtually every nucleated cell of the body. By means of factors such as internalin A and/or B the host cells are triggered to internalize the attached bacteria. Inside a host cell the pathogenic bacterium produces hemolysin and phospholipases and it can leave the phagocytic vacuole and enter the cytoplasm. Once in the cytosol, pathogenic strains will polymerize actin from the host cell cytoskeleton. This happens mainly at the apical tip of a bacterium so that the new actin filaments act like a driving force; the bacterium moves around in the host cell until it by chance gets under the surface of the host cell. This contact induces the host cell membrane to produce extrusions which penetrate a neighboring host cell. The second host cell can engulf these ramifications containing the living *L. monocytogenes*. Hence, the bacterium will lyse the double cell membrane and invade the cytoplasm of the second host cell. By this mechanism of cell-to-cell spreading the intracellular parasite avoids the host cell's defense mechanisms.

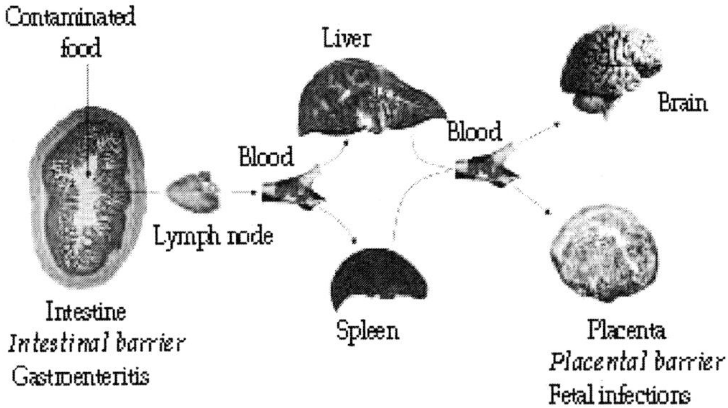

Fig. 15.1 : The intracellular habitat.

FOODBORNE LISTERIOSIS IN INDIA

Reports of listeriosis in India are scanty, either because of failure to identify the isolate, its rarity, improper isolation techniques, low incidence rate or lack of awareness. The epidemiological data available in the country to date is neither adequate nor reliable for assessing the extent of infection in human beings and animals, because it is based on conventional diagnostic tests which show considerable cross-reactivity. The disease largely remains undiagnosed and under reported, mainly because of the non-availability of a reliable, rapid and simple diagnostic test (Barbuddhe *et al.*, 2004).

The occurrence of listeric infections in the Indian subcontinent has been extensively reviewed by Malik *et al.* (2002). Listeriolysin O based ELISA (Barbuddhe *et al.*, 1999) and interferon-g assay (Barbuddhe *et al.*, 1998) has been developed for diagnosis of listeriosis in animals. *L. monocytogenes* has been isolated from cases of mastitis, reproductive disorders and septicaemia in animals (Shakuntala *et al.*, 2006; Rawool *et al.* 2007).

Listeria monocytogenes has been found to be one of the etiological factors in the causation of abortions and premature births (Bhujwala, *et al.*, 1973). At Chandigarh (Northern India), Krishna and co-workers (1966) working in Mumbai (Maharashtra) isolated *L. monocytogenes* from the cervix of 14% of 150 patients of bad obstetric history i.e., past history of abortions, miscarriages, still births or neonatal deaths. Isolation of *L. monocytogenes* has also been reported from 3 of 100 (Bhujwala, *et al.*, 1973) and 9 of 670 women with a bad obstetric history (Bhujwala and Hingorani, 1975) and 4 of 40 women with a history of abortions (Stephen *et al.*, 1978). *L. monocytogenes* was also isolated from a aborted foetus and blood of the mother (Bhujwala *et al.*, 1973). However, no isolations were made from 150 healthy controls that were either primigravidas or gave no past history of obstetric mishaps (Bhujwala, *et al.*, 1973; Bhujwala and Hingorani, 1975). Isolation of *L. monocytogenes* from cultured blood taken from 3 cases, one each of a 4 hr old baby, a one and half month old child, with congenital heart disease and digestive failure, and a one and half year old severely malnourished child have also been described (Gupta *et al.*, 1997). A perinephric abscess presenting as abdominal pain and caused by *L. monocytogenes* in a 5 yr old malnourished child has also been reported (Gomber *et al.*, 1998). Dhanashree *et al.* (2003) isolated *L. monocytogenes* from women with poor obstetrics history.

A virulence marker of *L. monocytogenes*, namely listeriolysin-O(LLO) has been employed as an antigen in an indirect ELISA and the separate IgG and IgM seropositivity for 238 humans (abattoir associated personnel, persons with various clinical conditions (mainly suspect venereal diseases), and dairy farm workers) has been reported (Barbuddhe *et al.*, 1999). Seropositivity for ALLO was observed in 16.8, 15.5, and 8.7% of abattoir associated personnels, 13.6, 31.8 and 36.4% of persons with clinical conditions, and 16.4, 32.7 and 10.9% of farm workers for the IgM, IgG and IgM plus IgG isotypes, respectively. Cerebrospinal fluid (CSF) obtained from patients with partially treated and culture-negative meningitis was subjected to PCR using 16S rDNA universal primers followed by restriction endonuclease digestion. In all, 43 patients and 7 controls were enrolled in this study. *L. monocytogenes* was detected from one sample (Pandit *et al.*, 2005).

A significant number of patients in our country have advanced renal insufficiency at initial presentation. This has led to an increasing use of temporary dialysis catheters. Catheter related bacteremia (CRB) is a significant complication associated with its use. *Listeria monocytogenes* was isolated from one of 16 catheters cultured for bacteria (Modi *et al.*, 2001).

ISOLATION FROM FOODS

L. monocytogenes was isolated from raw milk samples collected at Ranchi, Jharkhand (Yadava *et al.*, 1985). *Listeria* sp. was detected in raw milk and ice cream samples from retail outlets in Mumbai, Maharashtra (Pednekar *et al.*, 1997). Most of the isolates were of non-pathogenic species, with *L. grayi* predominating. However, pathogenic *L. monocytogenes* was isolated from 1 ice cream sample. *L. monocytogenes* was also isolated from 8.1% of raw milk samples in Bareilly, Uttar Pradesh (Bhilegaonkar *et al.*, 1997). Most of the isolates were pathogenic. No *L. monocytogenes* was isolated from pasteurized bulk milk tanks. Pathogenic *L. monocytogenes* isolates have been recovered from the meat and milk of goats, sheep and buffaloes (Barbuddhe *et al.*, 2000; Barbuddhe *et al.*, 2002).

The organism has been isolated from fish and fishery products from different parts of the world and interestingly the incidence rate reported from tropical fish is rather low (Karunasagar and Karunasagar, 2000). In India, only a few surveys have been conducted to assess the presence of *Listeria* sp. in seafoods. The presence of *L. monocytogenes* has been documented in the tropical environment (Jayasekaran *et al.*, 1996), but, since the incidence of *L. monocytogenes* in fish and fishery products is very low, the risk associated with consumption of these products is also low (Karunasagar and Karunasagar, 2000), however, failure to isolate *L. monocytogenes* from tropical seafood in India need to be confirmed for other tropical areas and reasons elucidated.

In India, studies on molecular epidemiological aspects of *Listeria monocytogenes* are lacking. Therefore, we do not know the genetic variability of strains isolated and their epidemic potential. What are the different serotypes prevalent in India? What is the genetic variability among different strains? In what respect do the Indian *Listeria* isolates differ from/resemble isolates from other nations? The molecular characterization of *Listeria* isolates from India should help to establish the characteristics of the strains responsible for epidemics, and allow the developing of new diagnostic tools and molecular typing. This would not only help in better understanding of the sources of infection and their risk assessment, routes of transmission of the infective agent, influencing factors, clinical forms and virulence characteristic of the pathogenic isolates of *Listeria* in order to diagnose the infection rapidly and reliably but also in instituting the effective control measures.

SOURCES OF TRANSMISSION

The main route of transmission of pathogen is by ingestion of food and water contaminated with faeces, urine, soil, and/or aborted material from infected animals. *Listeriae* have also been frequently isolated from animal faeces, and from various animal sources including meat and milk from cattle, buffaloes, sheep, goats and poultry. The faeces of healthy animals often contain *L.monocytogenes*, so cross-contamination with pathogenic species is likely to occur. *Listeria* spp. was also isolated from the respiratory tract of ducks suggesting that they may be commensals.

In humans, food-borne transmission is the prominent means of infection. A wide variety of food stuffs including milk, cheese, ice cream, raw meats, ready-to-eat poultry, unprocessed vegetables, raw fish, and fish products, have been shown to be frequently contaminated with *L. monocytogenes*. Handling of newborn calves and infected material may also result in the infection. Poor hygiene and environmental conditions, or continuous exposure to domestic animals at abattoirs may act as source of infection. The possible routes of transmission are depicted in the Figure 15.2.

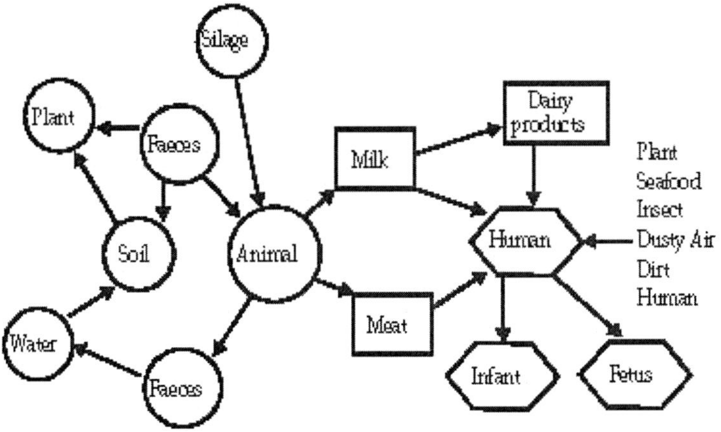

Fig. 15.2 : Possible routes for transmission of *L. monocytogenes* to humans (adapted from Ryser and Marth, 1991).

METHODS FOR DETECTION

Listeria monocytogenes is an important food-borne pathogen and is widely tested for in food, environmental and clinical samples. Identification traditionally involved culture methods based on selective enrichment and plating followed by the characterization of *Listeria* spp. based on colony morphology, sugar fermentation and haemolytic properties. These methods are the gold standard; but they are lengthy and may not be suitable for testing of foods with short shelf lives. Application of culture and serological methods in epidemiological studies is of limited value because of their low discriminatory power. As a result more rapid tests were developed based on antibodies (ELISA) or molecular techniques (PCR or DNA hybridization). While these tests possess equal sensitivity, they are rapid and allow testing to be completed within 48 h. More recently, molecular methods were developed that target RNA rather than DNA, such as RT-PCR, real time PCR or nucleic acid based sequence amplification (NASBA). These tests not only provide a measure of cell viability but they can also be used for quantitative analysis. In addition, a variety of tests are available for sub-species characterization, which are particularly useful in epidemiological investigations. Early typing methods differentiated isolates based on phenotypic markers, such as multilocus enzyme electrophoresis, phage typing and serotyping. These phenotypic typing methods are being replaced by molecular tests, which reflect genetic relationships between isolates and are more accurate. These new methods are currently mainly used in research but their considerable potential for routine testing in the future cannot be overlooked.

A rapid method involving matrix-assisted laser desorption ionization time-of-flight mass spectrometry (MALDI-TOF MS) have been developed that showed promise for identification of *Listeria* species and typing and even allowed for differentiation at the level of clonal lineages among pathogenic strains of *L. monocytogenes* (Barbuddhe *et al.*, 2008). MALDI-TOF MS technique examines the chemistry of major proteins, yielding profile spectra consisting of a series of peaks, a characteristic "fingerprint" mainly derived from ribosomal proteins. Specimens could be prepared in a few minutes from plate or liquid cultures and a spectrum could be obtained within one minute. Mass spectra derived from *Listeria* isolate showed characteristic peaks, conserved at both species- and lineage-level. MALDI-TOF MS fingerprinting may have potential for *Listeria* identification and subtyping, and may improve infection control measures (Barbuddhe *et al.*, 2008).

Given the high accuracy and speed with which molecular testing can be carried out, there is no doubt that most of these methods if not already applied, will be adopted by regulatory authorities and in food testing laboratories in the future. There are exciting new developments in molecular technologies such as the microarray technology which have great potential as the basis for future routine testing.

EPIDEMIOLOGICAL DATABASE

Electronic database libraries of the different PFGE profiles of human *Salmonella enterica*, *L. monocytogenes*, and STEC strains have been created in different countries. In these libraries, the PFGE profiles can be compared with each other much more quickly than by just the naked eye. This helps in more easily detecting possible infection clusters at an early stage of the outbreak. Under the aegis of Indo-German Collaborative project, a web based database, Indian Listeria Culture Collection (ILCD) of characterized strains has been created. The database contains geographical source of the strain, source of isolation (animal/ human), phenotypic and genotypic characteristics, and DNA fingerprint. This is an interactive web based database so that the data can be exchanged between laboratories electronically. The database can be viewed at http://www.icargoa.res.in/ilcd.

Control of *L. Monocytogenes* in the Food Processing Environment

It is not realistic to expect that food processing establishments can be continuously maintained free of *Listeria* species. Despite best efforts, *Listeria* are likely to be reintroduced into food processing environments that, if neglected, will eventually lead to contamination of RTE foods. Tompkin, (2002) outlined a six-step *Listeria* control program for food processing environments. These are: (1) prevention of the establishment and growth of *Listeria* species in niches or other sites that can lead to contamination of RTE foods; (2) implementation of a sampling program to assess how well the control program is working; (3) rapid and effective response when the sampling program yields positive results for *Listeria* species; (4) verification by follow-up sampling to ensure that the source of contamination has been identified and corrected; (5) short term assessment of the last 4-8 samplings to facilitate early detection of problems and trends; and (6) long-term assessment at appropriate intervals (quarterly, annually, etc.) to identify widely scattered contamination events and to measure overall progress towards continuous improvement. They emphasized that the design of the environmental sampling program and the response to positive findings by the sampling program determine the overall effectiveness of the *Listeria* control program in food processing environments.

In order to lower the incidence of *Listeria* spp. in raw food materials and farm-raised animals, it is important to adapt appropriate farming and husbandry practices that lessen *Listeria* contamination. Good manufacturing practices, appropriate cleaning, sanitation and hygiene programs, and temperature control required for prevention or inhibition of growth of the pathogen to high levels are critical for control of *L. monocytogenes* in the retail and food service sector.

CONCLUSIONS AND FUTURE PERSPECTIVES

The study of *L. monocytogenes* infection highlights the sophisticated relationship between this bacterium and its host, and reveals their long co-evolution and reciprocal adaptation. For decades, *L. monocytogenes* has been a tool for immunologists. It has now also become a paradigm in bacterial pathogenesis and cellular microbiology. The availability of the genome sequence of five *L. monocytogenes* serovars and *L. innocua, L. welshimeri* and soon of *L. ivanovii* will provide further insight into the molecular basis of the pathogenesis determinants of *Listeria* species. Comparative genomics could also reveal genetic loci that confer specific pathogenic traits to epidemic strains: for example, loci that facilitate adaptation to different environments and that influence the onset of infection. It should be noted that it is often difficult to unravel the function of virulence factors that are identified by post-genomic methods and reverse genetics. To this end, more sophisticated *in vivo* studies, such as measurement of cytokine production, non-invasive *in vivo* imaging techniques or infection of *ex vivo* tissue explants — need to be used to understand the role of these bacterial factors in the interplay between the bacterium and the host.

Research conducted on European and North American strains of *L. monocytogenes* prevalent in human and animal illnesses revealed surprisingly high genomic stability, and a relatively small number of unique regions for antigenic diversity and epidemiologically relevant attributes. Such findings serve to direct the focus of research efforts to a relatively small number of specific genomic regions, to elucidate their possible involvement in virulence and adaptive physiology attributes of epidemic-associated bacteria. The research on genome of *L. monocytogenes* will help to open new areas of research for Indian researchers.

REFERENCES

Barbuddhe, S.B., Malik, S.V.S., Chaudhari, S.P. and Gupta L.K. (1998). Kinetics of interferon gamma production and its comparison with anti-listeriolysin O detection in experimental bovine listeriosis. *Vet. Res. Commun.* **22** : 505 – 516.

Barbuddhe, S.B., Malik, S.V.S. and Kumar, P. (1999). High seropositivity against anti-listeriolysin O in humans. *Ann. Trop. Med. Parasitol.* **93** : 537-539.

Barbuddhe, S.B., Malik, S.V.S., Bhilegaonkar, K.N., Kumar, Prahlad and Gupta, L.K. (2000). Isolation of *Listeria monocytogenes* and anti-listeriolysin O detection in sheep and goats. Small Rum. *Res.* **38** : 151-155.

Barbuddhe S.B., Chaudhari S. P. and Malik S.V.S. (2002). The occurrence of pathogenic *Listeria monocytogenes* and antibodies against listeriolysin O in buffaloes. *J. Vet. Med. B* **49** : 181-184.

Barbuddhe, S.B., Malik, S.V.S. and Rawool, D.B. (2004). *Listeria monocytogenes* and listeriosis in India: current status. Abstract no. 158, presented at XV International Symposium on Problems of Listeriosis (ISOPOL XV), 12-16, Uppsala, Sweden.

Barbuddhe, S. B., Maier, T., Schwarz, G., Kostrzewa, M., Domann, E., Chakraborty, T. and Hain, T. (2008). Rapid identification and typing of *Listeria* species using matrix assisted laser desorption ionization-time of flight mass spectrometry. *Appl. Environ. Microbiol.* B5402-5407, 2008.

Bhilegaonkar, K.N., Kulshreshtha, S.B., Kapoor, K.N., Kumar, Ashok, Agarwal, R.K. and Singh, B.R. (1997). Isolation of *Listeria monocytogenes* from milk. *J. Food Sci. Technol.* **34** : 248-250.

Bhujwala, R.A., Hingorani, V. and Chandra, R.K. (1973). Genital listeriosis in Delhi: A Pilot study. *Indian J. Med. Res.* **61** : 1284-1287.

Bhujwala, R.A. and Hingorani, V. (1975). Perinatal listeriosis: A bacteriological and serological study. *Indian J. Med. Res.* **63** : 1503-1508.

Borucki, M.K. and Call, D.R. (2003) *Listeria monocytogenes serotype* identification by PCR, *J. Clin. Microbiol.* **41** : 5537.

Dhanashree B., Otta S.K., Karunasagar I., Goebel W. and Karunasagar I. (2003). Incidence of *Listeria* spp. in clinical & food samples in Mangalore, India. *Food Microbiol.* **20** : 447-453.

Farber, J.M. and Peterkin, P.I. (1991). *Listeria monocytogenes*, a food-borne pathogen, *Microbiol. Rev.* **55** : 476.

Gouin, E., Mengaud, J., and Cossart, P. (1994). The virulence gene cluster of *Listeria monocytogenes* is also present in *Listeria ivanovii,* an animal pathogen, and *Listeria seeligeri,* a nonpathogenic species. *Infect. Immun.,* **62** : 3550.

Gupta, R., Chandra, R.K. and Hingorani, V. (1997). Listeriosis: an opportunistic infection. *Indian Paediatrics.* **34** : 732-734.

Hamon, M., Bierne, H. and Cossart, P. (2006). *Listeria monocytogenes*: a multifaceted model. *Nat. Rev. Microbiol.* **4** : 423.

Jacquet, C. *et al.* (2002). Expression of *ActA, Ami, InlB,* and listeriolysin O in *Listeria monocytogenes* of human and food origin. *Appl. Environ. Microbiol.* **68** : 616.

Jayasekaran, G., Karunasagar, I. and Karunasagar, I. (1996). Incidence of *Listeria* sp. in tropical fish. Inter. J. Food Microbiol. **31** : 333-340.

Karunasagar, I. and Karunasagar, I. (2000). Listeria in tropical fish and fishery products. Inter. J. Food Microbiol. **62** : 177-181.

Karunasagar, I., Segar, K., Karunasagar, I. and Goebel, W. (1992). Incidence of Listeria species in tropical seafoods. In: Listeria 1992. Abstract 155, 11th International symposium on problems of listeriosis, 11-14 may 1992, Copenhagen.

Krishna, U., Desai, M.W. and Daftary, V.G. (1966). Listeriosis: A clinico-bacteriological study. *Journal of Obstetrics and Gynaecology of India.* **16** : 304-310.

Malik S.V.S., Barbuddhe S.B. and Chaudhari S. P. (2000). Listeric infections in man and animals in Indian subcontinent: a review. *Trop. Anim. Hlth. Prod.* **34** : 359-381.

Modi, G.K., Ray, D.S., Agarwal, S., Singh, S., Tiwari, S.C., Dash, S.C. and Agarwal, S.K. (2001). Temporary Dialysis Catheter Related Bacteremia-A Prospective Study. ABSTRACTS 32nd Annual Conference of Indian Society of Nephrology, September, 2001, Lucknow *Indian J. Nephrol.* **10** : 33/34.

Pandit, L., Kumar, S. Karunasagar, I. and Karunasagar, I. (2005). Diagnosis of partially treated culture-negative bacterial meningitis using 16S rRNA universal primers and restriction endonuclease digestion. *J. Med. Microbiol.* **54** : 539-42.

Pednekar, M.D., Kamat, A.S. and Adhikari, H.R. (1997). Incidence of Listeria species in milk and milk products. *Indian J.Dairy Sci.* **50** : 142-151.

Rawool, D.B., Malik, S.V.S., Shakuntala, I., Sahare, A.M. and Barbuddhe, S.B. (2007). Detection of multiple virulence associated genes in pathogenic *Listeria monocytogenes* from bovines with mastitis. *Inter. J. Food Microbiol.* **113** : 201-207.

Raybourne RB. (2002). Virulence testing of *Listeria monocytogenes*. *J. AOAC Int.* **85** : 516-523.

Shakuntala, I., Malik, S.V.S., Barbuddhe, S.B. and Rawool, D.B., (2006). Isolation of *Listeria monocytogenes* from buffaloes with reproductive disorders and its confirmation by polymerase chain reaction. *Vet. Microbiol.* **117** : 229-234.

Tompkin, R.B. (2002). Control of *Listeria monocytogenes* in the food-processing environment *J. Food Protect.* **65** : 709-725.

Wiedmann, M. (2002) Molecular subtyping methods for *Listeria monocytogenes*, *J. AOAC Int.* **85** : 524.

Yadava, R., Choudhary, S.P. and Narayan, K.G. (1985). Bacterial flora of market milk and its public health significance. *Indian Jour. Dairy Sci.* **38** : 23.

16

ZOONOTIC HELMINTH INFECTION : A PROFILE OF EMERGING AND RE-EMERGING ZOONOSES

D. Bhattacharya, Subhasish Bandyopadhyay, A.K. Bera, Samiran Bandyopadhyay, J. Deb & B. Biswas

The diseases and infections, which are naturally transmitted between vertebrate animals and human beings, are called zoonotic diseases and this phenomenon is called zoonosis. Rudolph Virchow coined the term zoonoses in 1855. Major impacts of zoonoses include illness, monetary loss, and adverse effect on morale of personnel, unfavourable publicity and medico-legal implications. Zoonotic infectious agents are responsible for more than 60 per cent of all human infections and 75 per cent of emerging infectious diseases. With the continuous growth of human population there is an ever increasing need to develop and maintain food products with a high protein content (especially livestock and fish) under intensive farming situations, which is inevitably leading to a greater spread of animal diseases and transmission to humans.

Specific review on zoonotic diseases has identified 1415 species of infectious organisms which are infective to man. Infectious organisms include virus and prions (like bovine spongiform encephalopathy and variant Creutzfeldt-Jacob disease), bacteria and rickettsia, fungi, protozoa and helminths.

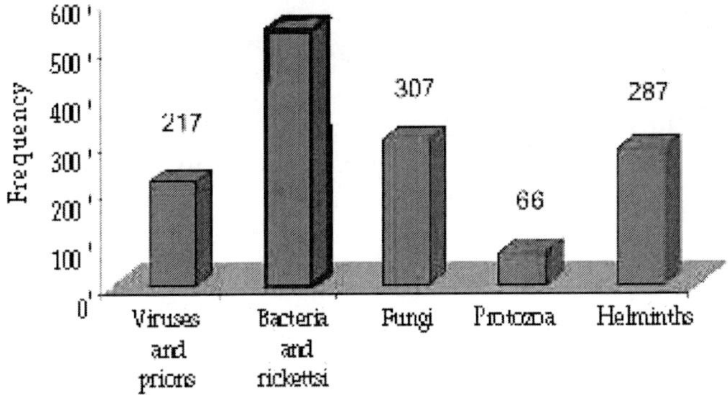

Fig. 16.1 : Frequency distribution of different types of infectious organisms

Some zoonotic pathogens are confined to animal reservoirs. Human beings serve as dead end host. Few important examples are anthrax, rabies, West Nile and Nipha/Hendra viruses. Some pathogens are well-established both in animals and man *viz.* bovine tuberculosis, salmonellosis. Some zoonotic diseases represent an intermediate situation with animals as the main hosts with occasional outbreaks occurring in humans *viz.* monkey pox, Hanta, Lassa and Ebola viruses. There are some diseases which are adapted to human-human transmission and are readily transmissible to humans (human tuberculosis). Subsequently, some pathogens of animal origin that suddenly appear in human populations *viz.* human immunodeficiency virus (HIV), influenza type A and probably severe acute respiratory syndrome (SARS).

Spread of zoonotic diseases occurs mainly due to ingestion of infective stages of the organism and approximately half of the world's population is affected by water-borne and food-borne infections. This is needless to say that, environmental changes, human and animal demography, pathogen changes and changes in farming practice play an important role for spreading emerging zoonotic diseases. Social and cultural taboos are also important aspects to be considered. Causes for emergence of zoonotic diseases are complex and multifactorial as well. Some factors also involve the changes at the molecular level like genetic shift and drift as occur in avian influenza virus. Modification of immune response of individuals also plays an important role. Social and ecological conditions influencing population growth and movement, food habits and the environment play more important role than changes at the molecular level. The different factors for spreading emerging zoonoses are :

1. Recreation
2. Companion animals
3. Consumption of bush meat
4. Globalization and Livestock movement
5. Tourism
6. Changed land use and urbanization

1. Recreation : Some sporting activities expose humans to zoonotic infections like hunting wild life and water sport which are responsible for spreading brucellosis, tularaemia and *Leptospira* spp.

2. Companion Animals : Are also responsible for spreading diseases.

Table 16.1 : Pet Animals Responsible for Transmission of Zoonotic Diseases

Pet Animal	*Disease/Aetiological Agent*
Cat	*Toxoplasma*, *Bartonella henselae*, cow pox virus, *Pasteurella multocida*, *Rickettsia felis*
Dog	*Toxocara*, leishmaniasis, methicillin-resistant *Staphylococcus aureus*, *Echinococcus granulosus*
Pet rat	*Leptospira icterrohemoragiae*, *Chlamydophila psittaci*
Pet reptiles	Exotic *Salmonella* spp.

3. Consumption of Bush Meat : Zoonotic pathogens can infect human being after consumption of bush meat. Specifically RNA viruses are transmitted due to high mutational rate.

Footnote : Neolithic transition : The capture and controlled breeding of major animal domesticates was part of a suite of transformations in human society known as the Neolithic transition.

Crowd Diseases – are small pox, measles, rubella and pertussis which emerged following advent of agriculture and associated settlement of major livestock species (species in temporal order are goat, sheep, pigs and cattle).

4. Globalisation and Livestock Movement : Transport of animals can result in mingling of different species in stressful and crowded condition. This type of mingling suppresses immune response to persistent of infections and increase pathogen shedding.

5. Tourism : More than one million international journeys are made each day and approximately 700 million tourists travel throughout globe on annual basis are act as potential carrier for different zoonotic diseases like rickettsial fevers, brucellosis, melioidosis, genotype I hepatitis E, tick borne encephalitis and schistosomiasis.

6. Changed Land Use and Urbanization : This leads to more incidences of Lyme borreliosis, ehrlichiosis, spotted fevers and anaplasmosis.

Classification of zoonoses is based mainly on (*i*) type of life cycle and (*ii*) type of aetiological agents.

TYPE OF LIFE CYCLE

(*a*) Direct Zoonoses : Infections are transmitted from the infected vertebrate host to susceptible vertebrate host either by direct contact, contact with fomite or mechanical vector. During transmission the agent undergoes no developmental and little or no propagative changes *viz.* Rabies, Brucellosis, and Trichinosis.

(*b*) Cyclo-Zoonoses : Infection requires more than one vertebrate host species in order to complete the life cycle of causative agent *viz.* Echinococosis, Taeniasis, and Pentastome infection.

(c) Meta-Zoonoses : Infection is transmitted biologically by invertebrate vector where the causative agents multiply or develop or do both in the invertebrate host and they essentially show extrinsic incubation before being transmitted to a suitable vertebrate host *viz.* Leishmaniasis, Plague and Schistosomiasis.

(d) Sapro-Zoonoses : Infection is transmitted from the inanimate developmental sites or reservoirs *viz.* larva migrans and some mycotic diseases.

(e) Anthroponoses/Zooanthroponoses : Infection transmitted from the lower vertebrate is called anthroponoses and vice versa mode of transmission is called zooanthroponoses.

TYPE OF AETIOLOGICAL AGENTS

The aetiologic agents involved in zoonoses are virus, bacteria, *Rickettsia,* parasite and fungus. Some important zoonotic diseases have been listed in Table 16.2.

Table 16.2 : Important Zoonotic Diseases and Mode of Transmission

Type	*Disease*	*Mode of transmission*
Bacterial	Anthrax (*Bacillus anthracis*)	Spore inhalation and ingestion
	Tuberculosis (*Mycobacterium bovis*)	Inhalation, ingestion and through break in skin
	Glanders (*urkholderias mallei*)	Contact with infected horses
	Brucellosis (*Brucella* sp.)	Milk and carcass of infected animals
	Salmonellosis (*Salmonella* spp of non-typhoidal)	Ingestion food of animal origin
	Plague (*Yersinia pestis*)	Rat flea bite
	Rabies (Rabies virus)	Infected dogs, and other mammal bite
Viral	Vesicular stomatitis virus	Insect or contact
	Japnese B encephalitis	Mosquitoes
	Rift valley fever	Mosquitoes
	Eastern, Western, Venezuelan encephalitis	Mosquitoes
	Bovine pustular stomatitis virus orf, contagious ecthyma	Handling of diseased animals

Contd...

Type	Disease	Mode of transmission
Parasitic	*Toxoplasma gondii*	Ingestion of oocysts of cat faces
	Dipylidium canium	Faeco-oral
	Dirofilaria immitis, D. tenuis	Mosquitoes
	Echinococcus granulosus	Ingestion
	Leishmania sp.	Sand fly
	Fasciola hepatica	Ingestion of snail
Rickettsial	*Rickettsia rickettsii*	Tick bite
	Ehrlichia canis	Tick bite
Fungal	*Sporothrix schenckii*	Cutaneous lesion infected with spore
	Microsporum spp.	Carrier animal direct contact and infected inanimate object
	Trichophyton spp.	Carrier animal direct contact and infected inanimate object

Important zoonotic helminth infections are caused by nematodes, trematode and cestode. In this chapter we have highlighted some important issues related to the helminth parasites.

ZOONOTIC NEMATODE INFECTIONS

Trichinellosis

This disease has been considered as truly emerging disease (or re-emerging) owing to increased infection rates as a direct result of changing human dietary trends and the breakdown of veterinary management practices in several developing countries. Uniqueness of the organism is related with lifecycle of the parasite. Since developing stage of the worm occupies both intracellular and extracellular niches. Human acquires the infection after ingestion of raw or uncooked meat containing encysted *Trichinella* larvae. Symptoms are non specific and disease is treated using combination of benzimidazole compound and corticosteroid. Diagnosis is done by conventional microscopy (biopsy of muscle), ELISA (using E/S product) and by nucleic acid detection. Treatment of the disease is done with anthelmintics and glucocorticoids.

Anisakiasis

This disease is caused by larval stages of nematodes (*Anisakis simplex* and *Pseudoterranova decipiens*). The infection is cosmopolitan in distribution and rate of infection is more where fishes are eaten in raw, smoked or undercooked condition. Majority of infected individual shows gastric disorder because nematode larvae reside in gastric mucosa. Main characteristic feature of this organism is expression of heat stable allergen. Therefore, detection of IgE isotype happens to be one of the test of choice to detect the infection. Conventional method (endoscopy) helps to detect the growing stage of the organism. Patient with intestinal obstruction are provided with nasogastric suction, followed by anthelmintic treatment. If suction fails, the worms are removed surgically to prevent intestinal rupture or blockage.

Hook Worms of Dogs and Cats

Hook worms of dogs and cats are responsible for cutaneous larval migrans (CLM). The common hook worms of dogs are: *Ancylostoma caninum, A. braziliense, A. ceylanicum* and *Uncinaria stenocephala*. In cats the species are *A. tubaeforme, A. braziliense, A. ceylanicum* and *U. stenocephala*. The geographical distribution of these parasites is imperfectly known because ranges overlap, hosts can harbour several species simultaneously. The geographical distribution of the parasites has been mentioned.

The worms produce cutaneous lesion which is characterised by erythematous papular or vesicular rash. Besides penetration, the larval stage may also cause follicuitis, myositis and eosinophilic enteritis. Systematic signs include peripheral eosinophilia (Loeffler syndrome), migratory pulmonary infiltrate and increased IgE levels. Diagnosis is done on the basis of cutaneous lesion, demonstration of organism from skin biopsy and presence of above mentioned systematic signs. Although CLM is a self limiting infection, antiparasitic and symptomatic treatment is often sought because of the associated discomfort and chances of secondary bacterial infection with this disease. Albendazole or ivermectin are the treatment of choice. Elevated doses of ivermectin kill the larvae in the muscle tissues. Attempts to freeze or surgically remove cutaneously migrated larvae are ineffective and can result tissue injury.

Table 16.3 : Geographical Distribution of Hook Worms of Dogs and Cats

Sl. No.	*Name of the species*	*Distribution*	*Remarks*
1.	*U. stenocephala*	North America, South America, Europe, Asia, Australia, New Zealand	Infection is prevalent in colder climate
2.	*A. caninum, A. tubaeforme*	—	Infection is prevalent in warmer climate
3.	*A. ceylanicum*	India, Taiwan, Malaysia, Borneo, Indonesia, Australia, South America (Surinam)	—
4.	*A. braziliense*	South-eastern Atlantic coast of North America, the gulf of Mexico and the Caribbean Sea, down to Uruguay in South America, in Africa, Australia and Asia	—

Visceral Larval Migrans (VLM)

Toxocariasis is a clinical term applied to infection in the human host with either *Toxocara canis* or *T. cati*. Infection of human host is acquired after ingestion of *viable* eggs. Infected patients present high circulating eosinophilia and suffer from long term multisystem diseases. Detection of infection is done by demonstration of organism by biopsy and serological test using excretory-secretory products of the parasite. Therapy in patients with VLM is aimed at relieving symptoms and is intended to diminish the host inflammatory response to the parasite. Corticosteroids and antihistamines are often used for the purpose. Antiparasitic agents, such as mebendazole, may help to reduce symptoms. However, systematic treatment with anthelmintics can result into hypersensitivity reactions and clinical trials have raised questions about their efficacy as well.

Heart Worm Infection

Heart worms (*Dirofilaria immitis*) are mosquito-borne filarial nematodes. In man the dead worms are arrested in pulmonary arteries and induce granuloma. Thereby the organism is responsible for producing "coin lesions" which could be detected through chest radiography. Extrapulmonary dirofilariasis has also been reported and is associated with lesions in brain, eyes and testicles. For diagnosis video-assisted thoracoscopic biopsy with histologic examination is the least invasive diagnostic method. Serological detection is possible using antigen of *Wolbachia* (a bacterial endosymbiont of *D. immitis*) and IgG isotype response is recorded using primary binding assay. Human infection does not require any treatment. Only surgical removal of parasite induced lesion is curative.

ZOONOTIC CESTODE INFECTIONS

Cysticercosis

The major cause of human cysticercosis is caused by bladder worm stage of *Taenia solium* and *T. saginata*. Human infection is acquired after ingestion of raw or undercooked meat of infected animals containing cysticerci.

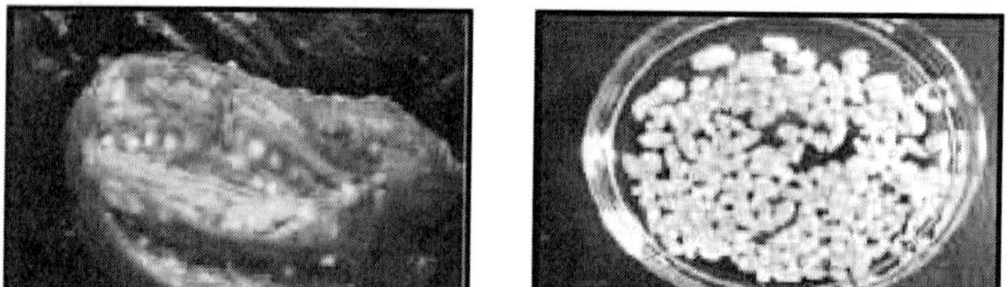

Fig. 16.2 : Isolated *Cysticercus Cellulosae* from Skeletal Muscle of Pig Slaughtered in Tangra Slaughter house of Kolkata.

Infection with adult tapeworm remains unnoticed but larval stage is involved with neurocysticercosis. A recent field study has suggested that, neurocysticercosis is responsible for around one-third of all cases of epilepsy in India and conservative figures suggest that, at least 50,000 people die each year as a result of this disease. Diagnosis of the disease is done by coproantigen test and serum antibody detection. The tests are done using purified antigen. Serological tests are further supported by magnetic resonance imaging (MRI) or computed tomography (CT). The drug of choice for human *Taenia* infections is praziquantel although niclosamide is also recommended. While these drugs offer a highly effective treatment for the disease, but reports of praziquantel and niclosamide-resistant populations are emerging. Hence, the use of both drugs has been tightly regulated.

Cystic Echinococcosis

The disease is caused by larval stage of tape worm, *Echinococcus granulosus*. Infection of the parasite is established in the suitable intermediate host (ungulates and human) after ingestion of eggs.

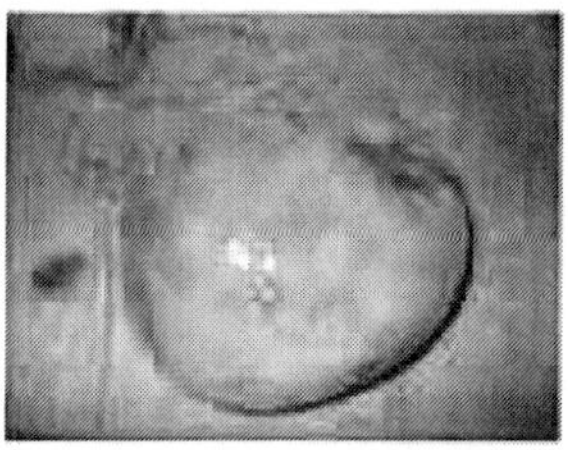

A. An Intact Pulmonary Cyst

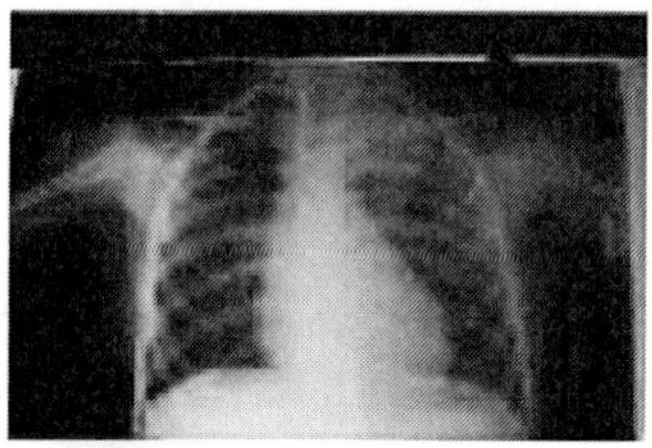

B. Radiographic

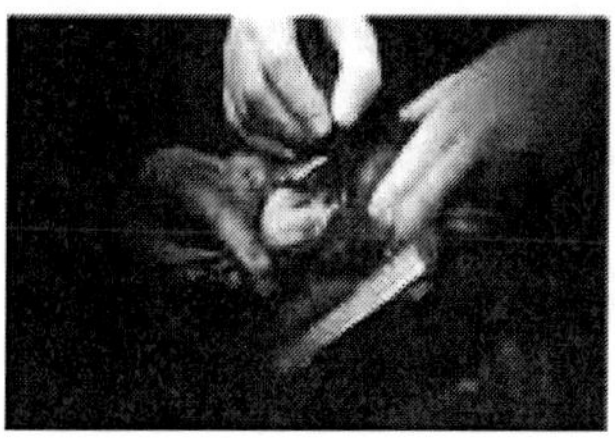

C. Surgical Approach to Operate Out the Cyst

Fig. 16.3 : Image of SOL caused by hydatid cyst.

The infection is common in poor pastoral communities where livestock are slaughtered in open areas with little or no veterinary management. In cystic echinococcosis, the fluid filled hydatid cysts take considerable time to develop. The infection is mostly seen in liver and lungs (90% of cases). Diagnosis of hydatid cysts in man is done by imaging techniques and serological test (using native and recombinant antigen). Detection of infection in canine is done by coproantigen ELISA and PCR based assay. The former test has been recommended by *Office des International Epizooties* (OIE). Coproantigen ELISA can detect the infection during incubation period of the organism. However, sensitivity of test is dependant on biomass of the parasite. Surgical removal of larval cyst is the preferred treatment; however, albendazole is also effective with or without surgery.

ZOONOTIC TREMATODE INFECTIONS

Fasciolosis

Fasciola hepatica and *F. gigantica* are the major causative agents of liver fluke disease with temperate and tropical climates, respectively. Although traditionally regarded as a disease of livestock, but now-a-days the disease has been regarded as emerging zoonotic disease. Prior to 1992, the total number of human cases of fasciolosis was estimated to be less than 3000. More recent figures suggest that between 2.4 and 17 million people are currently infected with this organism and 91.1 million people are at risk.

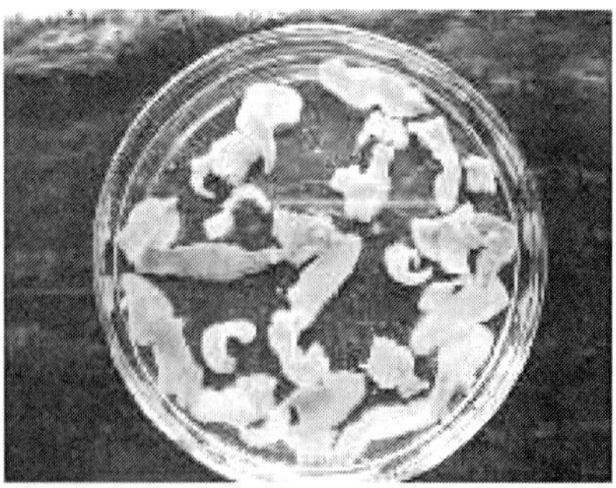

Fig. 16.4 : Isolated adult *Fasciola gigantica* from buffalo slaughtered at Tangra slaughter house, Kolkata

So far the clinical symptoms are concerned the disease undergoes two distinct clinical phases: acute fasciolosis corresponds to the migratory stages of the life cycle, whereas chronic fasciolosis is due to the presence of the mature adult flukes in the bile ducts. Most symptoms (including fever, abdominal pain, hepatomegaly and a range of gastrointestinal disturbances) result from the destruction of liver tissue by the migrating immature flukes and can lead to abnormal liver function tests. Eosinophilia and mild or moderate anaemia are also common features of acute infection. Chronic infection is often sub-clinical or shows symptoms that are indistinguishable from other hepatic disorders like cholangitis, cholecystitis and cholelithiasis. Definitive diagnosis of human infection is done by Kato-Katz method and popularly used for epidemiological survey. However, the result of the test may not be always reliable as eggs are passed sporadically with bile juices and low levels of infection are not often detected. Some progress has been made on PCR based detection of *F. gigantica* and *F. hepatica*. Treatment of fasciolosis is done by triclabendazole (TCBZ). This compound shows high efficacy (99%) against both immature and mature stages of the parasite.

Schistosomiasis

Schistosomiasis (bilharzias) is a tropical disease caused by digenean treamatodes of the genus *Schistosoma*. The impact of the disease on the human population is vast as it is endemic in 70 countries and more than 207 million people are believed to be affected and 779 million people are living at risk of infection. Transmission of the disease occurs through free swimming cercaria, released from fresh water snails that act as intermediate host. Adult worms reside in the mesenteric blood vessels and lay eggs. Eggs make their way through the intestine or bladder wall and are passed in faeces or urine. Many eggs are carried to the liver and induce T cell response that lead to development of granuloma. Granuloma further destroys the liver tissue and eventually causes hepatomegaly and splenomegaly. The gold standard for diagnosis of human schistosomiasis is microscopic examination of eggs in stool samples. Kato-Katz or thick smear method is used under field condition both for qualitative and quantitative evaluation. Quantitative evaluation gives idea about worm burden and morbidity. Serological tests are also used but the test can not distinguish present and past infection. Recently PCR based method has been standardised for detection of *S. japonicum*. This approach is particularly useful in cases with low level of infection. With the current absence of reliable and effective alternatives to praziquantel, the future control of human schistosomiasis relies on development of a vaccine. A number of anti-schistosme vaccine candidates that induce significant levels of protection in animals are currently under scanning. The majority are parasite membrane proteins or enzymes and include glutathione S–transferases, paramyosin, very low density lipoprotein-binding protein, serine protease inhibitors, fatty acid-binding protein, triose-phosphate isomerase and a 23 kDa integral membrane protein.

Fish-Borne Treamatodiases

Fish-borne treamatodiases is caused by liver flukes (*Clonorchis sinensis* and *Opisthorchis westermanii*) and lung flukes (*Paragonimus* spp.). The infection is a major public health issue and mostly prevalent in Southeast Asia. Infection in human being is transmitted either by fish or crustaceans. Diagnosis of fish-borne treamatodiases is done by coprological examination of human samples but this approach requires training and experience. Recombinant antigen based ELISA (lyophosphatidic acid phosphatase) has been found useful for detection of *C. sinensis*. Medical imaging techniques are also useful to detect clonorchiasis. These approaches are valuable alternative to conventional diagnostic methods. The drug of choice for fish-borne trematode infections is praziquantel. At present, praziquantel-resistant fluke populations are not thought to be wide spread.

This will be injustice for this chapter if we do not mention about commercial kits available in the market for diagnosis of several zoonotic diseases. ID VET innovative diagnostics, France has been marketed one diagnostic kit (ID screen Ò *Trichinella* Indirect ELISA kit) for detection of *Trichinella* infection. The test is based on the principle of indirect ELISA. E/S product of *T. spiralis* is used as test antigen. Equine and swine sera (pig and wild boar) and meat juices are also tested for specific antibody. Bordier Affinity Products, Switzerland has developed kit for detection of visceral larva migrance (VLM), cystic echinococcosis and schistosomiasis. E/S product of *Toxocara canis* (causative agent of (VLM) is used as test antigen and supplied precoated in ELISA plate. Sensitivity of the kit is more than 90 per cent. For detection of *E. granulosus*, hydatid fluid is used as antigen. Sensitivity and specificity of the kit is 96 per cent and 97 per cent, respectively. Soluble antigens of *S. mansoni* is used as test antigen for detection of specific IgG response. Sensitivity of the test kit is 94 per cent. Specificity of the test has been recorded as 99 per cent.

Canine heart worm kit is marketed by Synbiotics Corporation, USA and available literature suggests that, this kit is useful to determine low level of infection.

Despite advances in our understanding of the biology of helminth parasites, zoonotic helminth infections remain endemic in many parts of the world. The following measures may be taken to tackle the situation to save human health:

1. Good farm management.
2. Personal hygiene.
3. Proper food preparation practices.
4. Large-scale drug treatment of infected humans and animals.
5. Public awareness programme.

Above all there is always need for basic laboratory research. Extensive research is necessary on excretory-secretory (E/S) product which plays a crucial role to establish parasitism. Because E/S products are associated with immune evasion, detoxifying mechanism and having xenobiotic effect. These proteins are often used as immunodiagnostic and immunoprophylactic antigen as well as drug target. These proteins are often difficult to identify because parasites are difficult to be maintained by *in vitro* culture. However, with the increased knowledge on proteomics and genomics these difficulties have been tackled and we should be optimistic regarding the control of zoonotic helminth infections in future.

REFERENCES

Bowman DD, Montgomery SP, Zajac AM, Eberhard ML, Kazacos KR. (2010). Hookworms of dogs and cats as agents of cutaneous larva migrans. *Trends Parasitol.* **26** : 162-7.

Dorny P, Praet N, Deckers N, Gabriel S. (2009). Emerging food-borne parasites. *Vet Parasitol.* 7; **163** : 196-206.

Krueger A, Fischer P, Morales-Hojas R. (2007). Molecular phylogeny of the filarial genus *Onchocerca* with special emphasis on Afrotropical human and bovine parasites. *Acta Trop.* **101** : 1-14.

Kutz SJ, Jenkins EJ, Veitch AM, Ducrocq J, Polley L, Elkin B, Lair S. (2009). The Arctic as a model for anticipating, preventing, and mitigating climate change impacts on host-parasite interactions. *Vet Parasitol.* **163** : 217-28.

Lee AC, Montgomery SP, Theis JH, Blagburn BL, Eberhard ML. (2010). Public health issues concerning the widespread distribution of canine heartworm disease. *Trends Parasitol.* **26** : 168-73.

Macpherson CN. (2005). Human behaviour and the epidemiology of parasitic zoonoses. *Int J Parasitol.* **35** : 1319-31.

Mas-Coma S, Valero MA, Bargues MD. (2009). Climate change effects on trematodiases, with emphasis on zoonotic fascioliasis and schistosomiasis. *Vet Parasitol.* **163** : 264-80.

Mera y Sierra R, Artigas P, Cuervo P, Deis E, Sidoti L, Mas-Coma S, Bargues MD. (2009). Fascioliasis transmission by *Lymnaea neotropica* confirmed by nuclear rDNA and mtDNA sequencing in Argentina. *Vet Parasitol.* **166** : 73-9.

Periago MV, Valero MA, Panova M, Mas-Coma S. (2006). Phenotypic comparison of allopatric populations of *Fasciola hepatica* and *Fasciola gigantica* from European and African bovines using a computer image analysis system (CIAS). *Parasitol Res.* **99** : 368-78.

Robinson MW, Dalton JP. (2009). Zoonotic helminth infections with particular emphasis on fasciolosis and other trematodiases. *Philos Trans R Soc Lond B Biol Sci.* **364** : 2763-76.

Slingenbergh JI, Gilbert M, de Balogh KI, Wint W. (2004). Ecological sources of zoonotic diseases. *Rev Sci Tech.* **23** : 467-84.

Torgerson PR, Deplazes P. (2009). Echinococcosis: diagnosis and diagnostic interpretation in population studies. *Trends Parasitol.* **25** : 164-70.

Valero MA, Ubeira FM, Khoubbane M, Artigas P, Muino L, Mezo M, Pérez-Crespo I, Periago MV, Mas-Coma S. (2009). MM3-ELISA evaluation of coproantigen release and serum antibody production in sheep experimentally infected with *Fasciola hepatica* and *F. gigantica. Vet Parasitol.* **159** : 77-81.

Wilson M, Lountzis N, Ferringer T. (2009). Zoonoses of dermatologic interest. *Dermatol Ther.* **22** : 367-78.

17

CYSTICERCOSIS IN INDIA : AN OVERVIEW

Ashwani Kumar and Vijay J. Jadhav

Cysticercosis in cattle and pigs is an infection by the larvae of the human intestinal cestodes, *Taenia saginata* and *Taenia solium* respectively. These parasites have great zoonotic potential, which means that the parasitic worms or their developmental stages can be transmitted from animals to human beings and vice versa. Consumption of foods of animal origin, like meat, milk and their products, is the most common source of transmission of such infection from animals to man. In the developing world including India, neurocysticercosis (NCC) is the most common infestation of the central nervous system by this parasite in human. Keeping in view the public health significance of this infection, literature search was done for this chapter with special emphasis on Indian studies on cysticercosis in bovines and swines.

HISTORICAL PERSPECTIVE

Cysticercosis was first described in pigs by Aristophanes and Aristotle in 3rd century BC. Later it was noticed in human by Parunoli in 1550 (Prasad *et al.*, 2008). Vogt (1854) reported the first experimental infection in man. Kuchenmeister (1855) and Lockhart (1855) demonstrated that the bladder worm in the tissues of pig was the infective larval stage for man. *Taenia saginata* and *Taenia solium* were first distinguished in 1602 but the life cycles were worked out during the middle of 19th century (Sehgal and Bhatia, 1981).

BOVINE CYSTICERCOSIS

Taenia saginata is the adult worm which lives in small intestine of man and is white and semi-transparent; measuring 5-12 meters in length but it may be up to 24 meters. Many cases of taeniasis in man are asymptomatic, except for some anal pruritis due to emerging tapeworm segments but with severe infections human beings may experience loss of weight, anorexia, abdominal discomfort and digestive upset. Larval stage of this parasite is called *Cysticercus bovis* which mainly occurs in cattle, although other ruminants such as deer, reindeer, llama, buffalo, giraffe and antelope may harbour cysts. These cysts are round or oval in shape and when fully developed consist of a scolex invaginated into a small fluid-filled vesicle. The cystic stage is infective in about 10 weeks post-infection and can remain viable for up to 9 months. Degenerative changes in cysts often occur and such changes may not take place until 7 months. Degenerated cyst appears as oval with a thick connective-tissue capsule and is difficult to separate from the surrounding tissue and contains a yellowish-green caseous material. A dead cysticercus, usually with scolex evaginated may be found in this material. Cysts in bovine muscle may remain viable for up to 14 days after the death of the host.

In general, *C. bovis* cysts are usually encountered singly or in small numbers at meat inspection and are most commonly found in the muscles of mastication, especially the masseter muscles, the heart, tongue, diaphragm, esophagus, shoulder and occasionally in fatty tissues, lungs, liver and lymph nodes. To be infective, the cyst must be viable that can be ascertained by placing the cysts in normal saline solution with 30% ox-bile or 5% sodium taurocholate and incubating at 37°C. Evagination of the unarmed scolex in viable cysts normally takes place within 1-2 h. Microscopic examination of the viable cyst show a thin bladder wall and the scolex with four suckers but no rostellum or hooks (Gracey *et al.* 1999).

The incidence of *Cysticercus bovis* in cattle and buffaloes is reported mainly from Southern and North-Eastern parts of India. Krishana and Ranganathan, (1972), Sreemannarayana and

O, Christopher, (1977), Prabhakaran *et al.*, (1980), Thirumalaikplundusubramaniam *et al.*, (1983); Krishnan *et al*, (1984); Deka *et al.*, (1985) and Roy and Tandan (1989) have reported cysticercosis in cattle and buffalo from Madras, Andhra Pradesh, Trichur, Adhartal, Madurai, Madras, north eastern region, Mizoram and Nagaland respectively. Kolte *et al.*, (1981), Pramanik *et al.*, (1985) and Tamuli *et al.*, (2005) have also reported the prevalence of bovine cysticercosis from India. As per these studies the prevalence rates of *Cysticercus bovis* in cattle and buffalo were 1.73%-13.6% and 0.75%-2.3% respectively. Various sites on bovine carcasses found positive for *Cysticercus bovis* were heart, diaphragm, masseter muscles, tongue, esophagus, muscles of forelimbs and thigh, liver and peritoneal cavity.

SWINE CYSTICERCOSIS

Cysticercus cellulosae is the larval stage of *Taenia solium* which occurs most commonly in the musculature of the pig. It is of great public health and economic importance, the later occasioned by the condemnation of pig carcasses. Predilection sites of these cysts are heart, diaphragm and internal masseters, tongue, neck, shoulder, intercostals and abdominal muscles. The liver, lungs kidney, eye and brain are less often affected (Gracey *et al.*, 1999). Many reports of this infection in pigs are available in Indian literature. Pathak and Gaur (1989), Verma and Ahluwalia (1989), Rao and Paliwal (1996) and Deka and Gaur, (1990, 1993) reported infection of *Cysticercus cellulosae* in pigs from Uttar Pradesh at a rate of 1.91%-15.5% while Sharma *et al.*,(2004) reported it to be 6.35% from Ludhiana, Punjab. Various reports of this infection in pig carcasses are available from Southern (D'Souja, 1998; D'Souja and Hafeez, 1998; Hafeez *et al.*, 2004) Eastern (Pramanik *et al*, 1985) and North-Eastern(Deka *et al.*, 1985; Roy and Tandon, 1989) States of India and the incidence reported are 3.25%-6.35%, 1.79%-4.24%, 7.01%-20.8% respectively. The sites of the cysts in pig carcasses were muscles of neck, shoulder, hind limbs, thigh, masseter and gluteal muscles, tongue, heart diaphragm, liver, brain, spleen, kidney, eye, mesentery and omental fat. In some of the reports, cysts of *C. cellulosae* were mainly found in liver and mesentery and omental fat which are not the primary sites for such infection (Deka and Gaur, 1993).

HUMAN CYSTICERCOSIS

Cysticercosis (*i.e.*, tapeworm infection) is an increasingly common medical problem throughout the world where large populations migrated from endemic areas and among populations that often travel to these areas. Cysticercosis is caused by the metacestode, or larval, stage of *Taenia solium*, the pork tapeworm. The clinical syndromes caused by *T solium* are categorized as either neurocysticercosis (NCC) or extraneural cysticercosis (intestinal tapeworm infection). Neurocysticercosis refers to CNS infection with *T solium* and is probably the most common parasitic infestation of the CNS which has gained increased recognition in the last two decades because of the development of MRI and CT scanning. Neurocysticercosis is further divided into parenchymal and extraparenchymal disease. Parenchymal disease is characterized by infection with cysticerci within the brain parenchyma. Extraparenchymal disease develops when cysticerci migrate to the CSF of the ventricles, cisterns, and subarachnoid space or within the eyes or spinal cord. An estimated 50-100 million people are infected with cysticercosis worldwide. Areas of endemic disease include Central and South America, India, China, Southeast Asia, and sub-Saharan Africa. Studies in Latin America and India have noted adult-onset seizures in approximately 2% of the population, with as many as half due to neurocysticercosis. In India, the first report of the incidence of Taenia infection in humans was studied by Mhaskar (1917-1919) in certain areas of Tamil Nadu. Later on Chandler (1926-28), Maplestone and Bhaduri (1937), Salunkhe (1966), Mitra (1970), Ratnam and Khanna (1975, 1980), Sarma and Raychowdhari (1977), Veliath *et al.*, 1985, Pathak and Gaur (1989), Verma and Ahluwalia, 1989, Couta *et al.*, (1995), Parija and Sahu, 2003 reported this infection from Northern Bengal, Calcutta, Pune, Sikkim, Gauhati, Uttar Pradesh, western and central Uttar Pradesh, Goa, areas of South India around Pondicherry respectively.

DIAGNOSIS

Routine Inspection Procedures

Postmortem inspection is the most common method adopted to detect cysticercosis in carcass. Throughout the world the inspection techniques adopted and the final judgements exercised vary greatly. Gracey *et al.*, (1999) have described the procedures followed by member countries of the European Union, Canada, USA, South Africa and Australia. Routine inspection procedure includes incision (two incisions parallel to the mandible) and observation of lateral and medial masticatory muscles (cheeks) after tongue dropping; palpation of tongue; incision of heart from base to apex or vice versa through interventricular septum and observation of cut and inner surfaces; observation of oesophagus and cut surfaces of muscles and pillars of diaphragm. When *C. bovis* is detected during the routine examination, detailed examination is recommended. It includes thorough incision and examination of external and internal muscles of mastication, the heart and the muscular portion of the diaphragm including its pillars, the tongue, muscles of oesophagus and all the cut muscular surfaces of the split carcass. Developed countries like Canada and USA are stricter than South Africa and developing countries in putting the judgement for bovine cysticercosis. The former recommended total condemnation of carcass if the infestation is extensive (cysts are found in at least two of the sites *viz.* heart, tongue, muscles of mastication, diaphragm and its pillars, oesophagus and musculature that is exposed during dressing operations and in at least two of the sites exposed by incision into the rounds and forelimbs) during routine primary inspection while slightly infested carcass (infestation lesser than extensive infestation) may be passed for human food after removal and condemnation of the lesions with surrounding tissues. From less infested carcasses, the cysts and surrounding tissues shall be removed and condemned while the carcass or the meat derived there from shall be held in a freezer under inspectional control at a temperature not exceeding –10°C for not less than 10 days; or the meat is heated throughout, under inspectional control, to a temperature of at least 60°C. Edible viscera and offal shall be disposed off in the same manner as the rest of the carcass from which they were derived, unless any lesion of *C. bovis* is found in these by-products, in which case they shall be condemned.

Other Methods of Diagnosis

The diagnosis of cysticercosis in cattle and swine is based on the inspection of meat. However, a substantial number of infected carcasses are not detected by the present meat inspection techniques because incisions in the so called sites of predilection cannot be many due to economical reasons. A number of other diagnostic tests have, therefore, been tried to diagnose cysticercosis. These include intradermal test (Kumar *et al.*, 1989); western blot assay (Pathak *et al.*, 1994);Indirect fluorescent antibody test (Kumar *et al.*, 1987); double immune-diffusion test (DID)(Kumar and Gaur, 1989); immuno-electrophoresis test (Deka and Gaur, 1993); counter-immuno-electrophoresis (D'Souza, 1998, Sharma *et al.*, 2005, Hafeez *et al.*, 2004); latex agglutination test (Prasanna *et al.*, 2001); co-agglutination test (Selvam *et al.*, 2002); passive haemagglutination test (Tailliez *et al.*, 1976, Geerts *et al.*, 1977, Ratnam and Khanna, 1983, Kumar and Gaur, 1989, Parija and Sahu 2003); Enzyme-linked-immunosorbent assay (ELISA) (Pathak *et al.*, 1984, 1994; Kumar and Gaur, 1987, 1989; Deka and Gaur, 1993; D'Souza, 1998, 1999; Sreenivasamurthy *et al.*, 1999; Hafeez *et al.*, 2004; Dhanalakshmi *et al.*, 2006; Wanzala *et al.*, 2002, 2007; Monteiro *et al.*, 2006, 2007), Enzyme linked immune-electron transfer blot (EITB) (Sreenivasamurthy *et al.*, 1999); Polymerase chain reaction assay (Hiroshi *et al.*, 2004) . Prasanna *et al.*, 2001, Selvam *et al.*, 2002, Sharma *et al.*, 2005, Hafeez *et al.*, 2004 and Selvam *et al.*, 2004 compared routine meat inspection with latex agglutination test, co-agglutination test, counter-immune-electrophoresis (CIEP), ELISA and indirect haemagglutination test respectively and reported the superiority of these tests to diagnose cysticercosis.

PREVENTION AND CONTROL

Suitable control measures are chemotherapy, meat inspection, sewage treatement and disposal, stall feeding of animals and health education. Praziquantal at a single dose rate (50-100mg per kg body weight) is effective against larval stage of *T. saginata* in cattle. Benzimidazole derivative (albendazole) at a rate of 50 mg per kg of body weight was shown to have effect against *C. bovis* in cattle.These compounds may be tried for swine cysticercosis. In many countries, *T. solium* has been controlled by meat inspection, by improvement of living conditions, especially sanitation, and by the proper housing of pigs. In the case of *T. saginata*, however, meat inspection has not been so successful because of the difficulty of detecting all lightly infected carcasses. Refrigeration of meat at a temperature of 5°C or lower for not less than 21 days or thorough cooking (66°C is lethal for cysticercosis) of meat make it fit for human consumption.

There is strong evidence that mass travel, the migration of workers, problems of sewage disposal etc. have led to an increase in the prevalence of *T. saginata*. In defined foci of infection, mass treatment of humans may control infection, but in endemic areas, combined approaches are necessary. Cysticercosis is a zoonosis which especially requires the collaboration of and liasion between public health and veterinary officials.

REFERENCES

Couto, F., Nadkarni, N.S. and Menezes, S. (1995). *Cysticercus cellulosae* in Goa- a clinicopathological study. *J. Parasitic Dis.* **19** : 79-80.

D'Souza, P.E. (1998). Studies on porcine cysticercosis with special reference to serodiagnosis. *J. Vet. Parasitol.* **12** : 64.

D'Souza, P.E. and Hafeez, M. (1998). Studies on Cysticercus cellulosae in pigs in an organized abattoir in Andra Pradesh, *Indian J.Vet. Parasitol.* **12** : 33-35.

Deka, D.K. and Gaur, S.N. (1993). Epidemiological study on Taenia hydatigena cysticercosis in certain domestic animals of Uttar Pradesh. *J.Vet. Parasitol.* **7** : 29-34.

Deka, D.K. and Gaur, S. N. (1993). Immunoelectrophoresis test against porcine cysticercosis. *J. Vet. Parasitol.* **7** : 35-43.

Deka, D.K. and Gaur, S.N. (1993). Serodiagnosis of *Taenia solium* cysticercosis in naturally infected pigs by ELISA. *J.Vet. Parasitol.* **7** : 86-92.

Deka, D.K. and Gaur, S.N. (1990). *Taenia solium* cysticercosis in pigs in western parts of Uttar Pradesh. *J. Vet. Parasitol.* **4** : 59-63.

Deka, D.K., Borkakoty, M.R. and Lahkar, B.C. (1985). Cysticercosis in domestic animals in north eastern region of India. *Indian J. Parasitol.* **9** : 83-85.

Dhanlaxmi, H., Jagannath, M.S., Isloor, S. and D'Souza, P.E. (2006). Protein-A Elisa in the serodiagnosis of porcine cysticercosis. Journal of Veterinary Parasitology, **20** : 33-35.

Geerts, S., Kumar, V. and Vercruysse, J. Jr. (1977). In-vivo diagnosis of bovine cysticercosis. *Vet. Bulletin.* **47** : 653-664.

Gracey, J.F., Collins, D.S. and Huey, R.J. (1999). Meat Hygiene, 10th edition, W.B. Saunders Company Ltd., London.

Hafeez, M., Reddy, C.V.S., Ramesh, B., Devi, D.A. and Chandra, M.S. (2004). Prevalence of porcine cysticercosis in south India. *J. Parasitic Dis.* **28** : 118-120.

Hiroshi, Yamasaki., James, C. Allan., Marcello Otake Sato, Minoru Nakao, Yasuhito Sako, Kazuhiro Nakaya, Dongchuan Qiu, Wulamu Mamuti, Philip S. Craig, and Akira Ito (2004). DNA Differential Diagnosis of Taeniasis and Cysticercosis by Multiplex PCR. *J. Clinic Microbiol.* **42** : 548-553.

Kolte, G. N., Vegad, J. L. and Awadhiya, R P. (1981). Note on an unusual case of cysticercosis (Cysticercus bovis) in a Gir cow. *Indian J. Anim Sci.* **51** : 370-372.

Krishnan, K. R., Ranganathan, M. (1972). A survey on the incidence of Cysticercus bovis in bovines slaughtered at the Madras corporation slaughterhouse. *Indian Vet. J.* **49** : 1182-1184.

Krishnan, K.R., Ranganathan, M. and Ramamurthi, R. (1984). Occurrence of visible Cysticercus bovis in cattle and buffaloes. *Cheiron,* **13** : 109-111.

Kuchenmeister (1855). Cited by Sehgal and Bhatia (1981).

Kumar, D. and Gaur, S.N.S. (1989). Comparative evaluation of various immunodiagnosis tests for the diagnosis of Taenia solium cysticercosis in pigs, using fractioned antigens. *J. Helminthol.* **63** : 13-17.

Kumar, D. and Gaur, S.N.S. (1987). Serodiagnosis of porcine cysticercosis by enzyme-linked immunosorbent assay (ELISA) using fractionated antigens. *Vet. Parasitol.* **24** : 195-202.

Kumar, D., Gaur, S. N.S. and Varshney, K.C. (1987). Indirect fluorescent antibody test in the diagnosis of porcine cysticercosis. *Indian J. Anim. Sci.* **57** : 1204-1206.

Kumar, D., Gaur, S.N., Varshney, K.C. and Pathak, K.M. (1989). Intradermal test in the diagnosis of Taenia solium cysticercosis in pigs. *Ind. J. Anim. Sci.* **59** : 500-505.

Lockhart (1855). Cited by Sehgal and Bhatia (1981).

Maplestone, P.A. and Bhaduri, N.V. (1937). *Ind. J. Med. Res.* **25** : 155 (Cited by Sehgal and Bhatia (1981)).

Mhasker (1917-1919). Cited by Sehgal and Bhatia (1981).

Mitra, S.K. (1970). *Ind. J. Med. Res.* **58** : 6796 (Cited by Sehgal and Bhatia (1981).

Monteiro, L.L., Pinto, P.S.A. and Dias, F.S. (2006). Evaluation of the ELISA test for the antibody detection in cattle naturally and experimentally infected with Cysticercus bovis. *Vet. Parasitol.* **141** : 260-263.

Monteiro, L.L., Pinto, P.S.A., Salcedo, J.H.P., Araujo, J.V., Santos, W.L.M. and Cecon, P.R. (2007). Taenia solium metacestode antigens in ELISA for the diagnosis of bovine cysticercosis. Arquivo Brasileiro de Medicina Veterinaria e Zootecnia. **59** : 21-25.

Parija, S.C. and Sahu, P.S. (2003). A serological study of human cysticercosis in Pondicherry, South India. *J. Communicable Dis.* **35** : 283-289.

Pathak, K. M and Gaur, S. N. (1989). Prevalence and economic implications of Taenia solium taeniasis and cysticercosis in Uttar Pradesh State of India. *Acta Leiden.* **57** : 197-200.

Pathak, K.M. and Gaur, S.N. (1987). Serodiagnosis of porcine cysticercosis by enzyme linked immunosorbent assay (ELISA) using fractioned antigens. *Vet. Parasitol.* **24** : 195-202.

Pathak, K.M.L., Gaur, S.N.S. and Garg, S.K. (1984). Diagnosis of porcine cysticercosis by immunoelectrophoresis. *Indian J. Parasitol.* **8** : 79-80.

Pathak, K.M., Allan, J.C., Ersfeld, K. and Craig, P.S. (1994). A western blot and ELISA assay for the diagnosis of Taenia solium infection in pigs. *Vet Parasitol.* **53** : 209-217.

Pathak, K.M., Gaur, S.N. and Garg, S.K. (1984). Counter current immunoelectrophoresis, a new technique for the rapid serodiagnosis of porcine cysticercosis. *J. Helminthology* **58** : 321-324.

Prabhakaran, P., Soman, M., Iyer, R. P. and Abraham, J. (1980). Common disease conditions among cattle slaughtered in Trichur Muncipal slaughterhouse-a preliminary study. Kerala *J. Vet. Sci.* **11** : 159-163.

Pramanik, A.K., Bhattacharya, H.M. and Sengupta, D.N. (1985). Occurrence of Cysticercus cellulosae in slaughtered pigs in Calcutta and its public health significance. *Indian J. Anim. Hlth.* **24** : 143-146.

Pramanik, A.K., Bhattacharya, H.M. and Sengupta, D.N. (1985). Occurrence of Cysticercus bovis in slaughtered cattle and buffaloes in Culcutta and its public health significance. *Indian J. Anim. Hlth.* **23** : 141-145.

Prasad K.N., Prasad. A., Verma A and Singh A.K. (2008). Human cysticercosis and Indian scenario: a review; *J. Biosci.* **33** : 571–582.

Prasanna, K.M., Jagannath, M.S. and S'Souza, P.E. (2001). Diagnosis of *Taenia solium* cysticercosis in pigs by latex agglutination test. *J. Vet. Parasitol.* **15** : 47-49.

Rao, A. N. and Paliwal, O. P. (1996). Pathology of parasitic conditions affecting swine liver. *Indian J. Vet. Pathol.* **20** : 136-139.

Ratnam, S. and Khanna, P. N. (1975). MVPH Thesis Calcutta University (Cited by Sehgal and Bhatia (1981)).

Ratnam, S. and Khanna, P.N. (1980). Studies on the incidence of cysticercosis in animals and taeniasis in man in Calcutta, India. World Congress for Foodborne Infections and Intoxications, Berlin, West. 29th July to 3rd July 1980, pp 119.

Ratnam, S. and Khanna, P. N. (1983). Indirect haemagglutination test in the diagnosis of cysticercosis. *Cherion,* **12** : 173-175.

Roy, B. and Tandon, V. (1989). Metacestoidiasis in north east India: a study on the prevalence of hydatidosis and cysticercosis in Mizoram, Nagaland and Assam. *Indian J. Anim. Hlth.* **28** : 5-10.

Salunkhe, D.S. (1966). *J. Trop. Med. Hyg.* 69: 165. (Cited by Sehgal and Bhatia (1981)).

Sarma, G.C. and Roychowdhary (1977). MVPH Thesis, Calcutta University (Cited by Sehgal and Bhatia (1981)).

Sehgal, S and Bhatia, R. (1981). Manual on Zoonoses. National Institute of Communicable Diseases, Delhi, India.

Selvam, P., D'Souza, P.E. and Jagannath, M.S. (2004). Serodiagnosis of *Taenia solium* cysticercosis in pigs by indirect haemagglutination test. Veterinarski Archiv, **74** : 453-458.

Selvam, S. P., D'Souza. P.E. and Jagannath, M.S. (2002). Detection of circulating antigens of the bladderworm of *Taenia solium* in pigs by co-agglutination test. *Indian Vet. J.* **79** : 1012-1016.

Sharma, R., Sharma, D.K., Juyal, P.D. and Sharma, J.K. (2004). Epidemiology of *Taenia solium* cysticercosis in pigs of Northern Punjab, India. *J. Parasitic Dis.* **28** : 124-126.

Sharma, R., Sharma, D. K., Juyal, P.D., Asha Rani and Sharma, J.K. (2005) Seroprevalence of pig cysticercosis in Ludhiana. *J. Vet. Parasitol.* **19** : 143-145.

Sharma, R., Sharma, D.K., Juyal, P.D., Asha-Rani and Sharma, J.K. (2005). Comparative evaluation of counter immune electrophoresis and routine meat inspection for the diagnosis of swine cysticercosis. *Indian J. Anim. Sci.* **75** : 792-793.

Sreemannarayana, O. and Christopher, K. J. (1977). A case of combined infection of cysticercosis and sarcosporidiasis in bullock. *Indian J. Anim. Hlth.* **16** : 188.

Sreenivasmurthy, G.S., D'Souza, P.E. and Jagannath, M.S. (1999). Enzyme linked immunoelectro transfer blot in the diagnosis of *Taenia solium* cysticercosis in pigs. *J. Parasitic Dis.* **23** : 85-88.

Talliez, R., Biguet, J. and Doby, J. M. (1976). Attempts to diagnose bovine cysticercosis by passive haemagglutination. *Revue de Medicine Veterinarie.* **127** : 653-668.

Tamuli, S.M., Chakraborti, A. and Jamir, K.L. (2005). Cysticercosis in heart muscle of a heifer. *J. Vet. Parasitol.* **19** : 55-56.

Thirumalaikolundusubramanian, P., Thangam, T. and Mathuram, G. (1983). Cysticercosis in Madurai. *Indian J. Pathol. Microbiol.* **26** : 181-183.

Varma, T.K. and Ahluwalia, S.S. (1989). Incidence of Cysticercus cellulosae in slaughtered pigs and human taeniasis in western and central Uttar Pradesh. *Indian Vet. J.* **66** : 673-674.

Veliath, A.J., Ratnakar, C. and Thakur, L.C. (1985). Cysticercosis in South India. *J. Trop. Med. Hyg.* **88** : 25-9.

Vogt (1854). Cited by Sehgal and Bhatia (1981).

Wanzala, W., Kyule, N.M., Zessin, K.H., Onyango-Abuje, A. J. Kang'ethe, K.E., Ochanda, H. and Harrison, J.S.L. (2007). Evaluation of an antigen ELISA in the diagnosis of bovine cysticercosis in Kenyan cattle. *Parasitol. Res.* **100** : 539-548.

Wanzala, W., Onyango-Abuje, A.J. Kang'ethe, K.E., Ochanda, H. and Harrison, J.S.L. (2002). Serodiagnosis of bovine cysticercosis by detecting live *Taenia saginata* cysts using a monoclonal antibody – based antingen- ELISA. *J. South African Vet. Assoc.* **73** : 201-206.

18

PLASMID PROFILING AS AN EPIDEMIOLOGICAL TOOL FOR SURVEILLANCE OF PATHOGENS OF PUBLIC HEALTH SIGNIFICANCE

A.G. Karpe and R.P. Kolhe

Plasmids are covalently closed circular double stranded DNA which are present in many of the bacterial species. The role of bacterial plasmids and its association with development of multiple drug resistant strains is well known. It is an extra-chromosomal DNA molecule, separate from the chromosomal DNA and is capable of replicating independently of the chromosomal DNA. It is circular but may be linear in some of the species viz. *Borrelia burgdorferii.* They naturally occur in bacteria, but are sometimes also found in eukaryotic organisms like *Saccharomyces cerevisiae*. The number of identical plasmids within a single cell can range from one to even thousands under some circumstances. Plasmids are responsible for mechanism of horizontal gene transfer known as conjugation and they have very special importance in biotechnology. Unlike viruses, plasmids are 'naked' DNA and do not encode genes necessary to encase the genetic material for transfer to a new host. Plasmids may carry genes that provide resistance to naturally occurring antibiotics in a competitive environmental niche, or alternatively the proteins produced may act as toxins under similar circumstances. Host-to-host transfer of plasmid requires direct, mechanical transfer by 'conjugation' or changes in host gene expression allowing the intentional uptake of the genetic element by 'transformation'.

Plasmids are grouped depending on their ability of conjugation or based on various functions. *Conjugative* plasmids contain so-called *tragenes*, which perform the complex process of *conjugation i.e.* transfer of plasmids from one bacterial species to another bacterium in simulated environment. *Non-conjugative* plasmids are not capable of conjugation and can only be transferred with the assistance of conjugative plasmids by accident. An intermediate class of plasmids that are *mobilizable*, and carry only a subset of the genes required for transfer. They can 'parasitize' a conjugative plasmid, transferring at high frequency only in its presence.

Based on the various functions performed, they are classified into five main classes. *Fertility (F) plasmids*, contain tragenes and are capable of conjugation. *Resistance (R) plasmids*, contain genes responsible for development of resistance against bacteria. *Col-plasmids* contain genes that *code for* production of bacteriocins, the proteins that can kill other bacteria. *Degradative plasmids* enable the digestion of unusual substances, e.g., toluene or salicylic acid and *Virulence plasmids* which are responsible for development of virulence and pathogenicity of bacterial species. Plasmids are now being used to manipulate DNA and may possibly be a tool for curing many diseases. Plasmids serve as important tools in genetics and biotechnology labs, where they are commonly used to multiply or *express* particular genes.

HISTORY

The term *plasmid* was first introduced by Joshua Lederberg in 1952. A index case of gentamicin-resistant *Klebsiella pneumoniae* (R) plasmid was recorded in 1975 from an outbreak at Minneapolis. Plasmids with similar antimicrobial susceptibility patterns were isolated and characterized. An unusual antimicrobial susceptibility pattern, first seen in *K. pneumoniae* and then in other species, was the initial indication of epidemic due to single plasmid. Plasmid profile characterization by agarose gel electrophoresis was reported by Meyers *et al.* (1976) who also examined clinical isolates of *E. coli* from a study of traveller's diarrhoea in Mexico. Several other species were surveyed, including *K. pneumoniae, Citrobacter freundii, Shigella dysenteriae, Enterobacter cloacae, Salmonella serotypes, Haemophilus influenzae, Neisseria gonorrhoeae, Bacteroides fragilis,* and *Streptococcus faecalis*. The method was simple, relatively inexpensive, and applicable to many bacterial species. There are several reports on plasmid profiling studies of public health pathogens *viz. E. coli, Salmonella, Staphylococcus aureus* etc. in recent years.

ROLE IN EPIDEMIOLOGICAL STUDIES

Understanding the changing molecular epidemiology of pathogens and tracing their clonal origin is done by many molecular typing methods *viz.* ribotyping, phage typing, molecular fingerprinting by RFLP, PFGE, RT-PCR etc. Some of the earliest typing methods for bacterial isolates include serotyping, biochemical typing, auxotyping, isoenzyme typing, antimicrobial susceptibility testing, bacteriophage typing, bacteriocin typing, and plasmid profiles. All of these typing systems have been helpful in understanding the natural history of bacterial diseases with some advantages and disadvantages. Plasmid profiling of bacterial pathogens may be used as an epidemiological tool in epidemiological surveillance of bacterial pathogens. Plasmid sizes are denoted in terms of megadaltons (MD) and kilobases (kb). The conversion factor is 1 megadalton = 1.51 kb. An average-sized gene is about 1 kb and encodes a protein of 35,000 daltons. Plasmids are infectious and can be transferred between bacteria of the same genus or different genera. Usually all functions required for plasmid transfer, including synthesis of pili, are coded for by genes on the plasmids. Thus, after transfer to a second host, these genes may enable a newly formed trans-conjugant to become a donor in another round of conjugation. This process may be repeated several times. Plasmids can carry genes that code for functions other than transfer and replication, such as antibiotic resistance and toxin, adhesin, metabolic enzyme, and bacteriocin production.

PRINCIPLES

It gives best results when used in combination with other typing methods. The approach for using plasmid profiles as an epidemiological typing system is similar to that of other typing schemes. All the outbreak associated strains may have the same plasmid profile and are similar by any other typing system used in ideal case. There are many examples in which most of the isolates of a bacterial species from one geographic area are identical. While doing plasmid profiles, control isolates must always be matched with case isolates for accuracy. Plasmid profiling studies have many advantages over several other typing systems. A single set of reagents and equipment is applicable to many species of bacteria. Phage typing requires a battery of phage and indicator. Serotyping also requires a battery of antisera, which may be difficult and expensive to prepare and standardize. Antimicrobial susceptibility testing can be correlated to the plasmid content because of the wide variety of resistance genes that are plasmid encoded.

For any typing system to be effective, it must differentiate the case from non case isolates. Plasmid profiles offer a higher level of sensitivity in distinguishing between antibiotic resistance patterns. When plasmid profiles of groups of isolates are compared, there must be sufficient differences in the patterns to allow them to be readily separated. In some bacterial genera, such as Salmonella or Shigella, plasmids occur so frequently that multiple isolates of a plasmid-free strain from an outbreak setting would be an epidemiologically significant finding. The lack of plasmid itself may be used as a marker for some isolates in some situations.

HOST RANGE

Transfer of plasmids is very common between enteric and other gram-negative bacteria. The plasmid transfer between *K. pneumoniae, Enterobacter cloacae* and staphylococci are very common. Plasmid-mediated beta-lactamase production and aminoglycoside resistance have been reported in *Streptococcus faecalis* and other group D enterococci. Transfer of resistance determinants from gram-positive to gram-negative organisms and *Mycoplasma* spp. has also been recorded. Transposons carrying antibiotic resistance genes can also be inserted into a number of different replicons. A 92-kb conjugative plasmid with several antibiotic resistance genes was first observed in a *K. pneumoniae.*

The plasmid content of most bacterial strains is usually a stable feature but it may be lost during subculture in some of the cases. The genes carrying plasmid can be maintained with addition of antibiotics in the media. Change in plasmid may occur *in vivo* and *in vitro*. Plasmid profiles are relatively easy and inexpensive to perform as compared to other typing methods. Alkaline lysis and denaturation of nucleic acid forms the basis of plasmid isolation. Plasmids of identical size but different sequence and functions can exist in many bacteria. When only a single plasmid is present, restriction endonucleases must be used for knowing similarities and differences between strains.

EXAMPLES

Some of the examples of plasmid profile analysis used in understanding the epidemiology of outbreaks are summarized here.

Salmonella spp.

Plasmid profiling is useful tool in investigation of *Salmonella* outbreaks due to, the ability to find a previously unrecognized association between isolates from outbreak-related and sporadic cases, and documentation of the appearance and persistence of antibiotic-resistant strains that represent a serious public health threat. Combination of plasmid profile and antibiograms of *Salmonella* serotype Typhimurium and *Salmonella* serotype *Enteritidis* allowed the differentiation of thirteen and eight clones respectively from acute cases of food poisoning.

E. coli

Infections due to enterotoxigenic and enterohaemorrhagic *Escherichia coli* are very common in developing as well as developed nations. Toxin and adhesion factors are found to be plasmid coded with antibiotic resistance determinants. The toxins show some relationship to the animal species from which the organism was isolated. For example, the fimbrial adhesin K88 is associated with porcine disease, K99 is associated with disease in calves or lambs, and human enterotoxigenic *E. coli* strains usually express colonization factor antigen I or II. Considering this variety of plasmid-encoded virulence factors, plasmid profiles are used as markers for specific disease isolates. The plasmid from *E. coli* found to be transferred to *Shigella, Salmonella, Klebsiella, Enterobacter, Citrobacter, Edwardsiella, Serratia,* and *Proteus* species.

Shigella spp.

In addition to *R. plasmids,* a number of small cryptic plasmids were observed in *Shigella dysenteriae, Shigella flexneri,* and *Shigella sonnei.* Along with cryptic and *R. plasmids,* large plasmids in *Shigella flexneri* and *Shigella sonnei* have been shown to encode factors associated with invasiveness.

Legionella spp.

Plasmids of different size of 30 and 188 kb were observed in theses bacteria. A nosocomial outbreak of *Legionella pneumophila* was investigated, using isoenzyme typing, monoclonal antibody typing, and plasmid profiles. A high degree of correlation was recorded in comparisons of typing methods.

K. Pneumoniae

Multiple antibiotic resistances in several serotypes were recorded in neonatal outbreaks which revealed that a conjugative *R. plasmid* of about 106 kb was present in all of the isolates. Transfer of the plasmid into sensitive recipients suggested that all resistance determinants were carried on this plasmid.

Mycobacterium spp.

Plasmid profiles were used to compare human isolates with environmental isolates of *Mycobacterium avium, M.*

intracellulare, and *M. scrofulaceum*. This study showed that aerosol isolates most closely resembled human isolates, supporting the hypothesis that aerosols are major source of transmission of mycobacteria.

CONCLUSION

Various reports worldwide suggested the utility of plasmid profile as an epidemiological tool in investigation of clonal origin of drug resistant pathogens. It verifies the identity of bacterial isolates. It could be revealed from several studies that in some cases plasmid profile analysis is most accurate and important tool for typing and in other cases it has no value. The results of plasmid profiling study should always be compared with other typing methods for accurate analysis *viz.* restriction endonuclease digestion, phase typing, antimicrobial susceptibility testing, and PAGE. Such combinations with plasmid DNA analysis will provide precise knowledge on the origins and degree of relatedness of the strains isolated from different sources.

REFERENCES

Halawani, E and Shohaveb, M (2008). Epidemiological Typing of *Salmonellla enterica* Isolates Causing Acute Food Poisoning in Saudi Arabia Based on Plasmid Profiles and Antibiograms. American-Eurasian Journal of Scientific Research **3 (2)** : 178-187.

Meyers, J.A., Sanchez, D., Elwell, L.P. and Falkow, S. (1976). Simple agarose gel electrophoretic method for the identification and characterization of plasmid deoxyribonucleic acid. J. Bacteriol. 127:1529-1537.

Mayer, L.W. (1988). Use of Plasmid Profiles in Epidemiologic Surveillance of Disease Outbreaks and in Tracing the Transmission of Antibiotic Resistance. Clin. Microbiol. Rev. **1 (2)** : 228-243.

Milleman, Y., Lesage, M., Elizabeth, C and Lafont, J (1995). Value of Plasmid Profiling, Ribotyping, and Detection of IS*200* for Tracing Avian Isolates of *Salmonella typhimurium* and *S. enteritidis*. J. Clin.Microbiol. **33 (1)** : 173–179.

19

PESTICIDE RESIDUES IN FOODS OF ANIMAL ORIGIN IN INDIA AND THEIR MOLECULAR DETECTION AND CONTROL MEASURES

R.J. Zende and A.M. Paturkar

India's economic development during fourth to sixth five year plan is identified predominantly as the Green Revolution. Intensive agriculture with judicious use of inputs like water, fertilizers, new seed varieties etc. was successful in meeting the goals of self-sufficiency in food-grain production and adequate buffer stocks with imports being negligible. Indian farmers are adopting various newer technologies to achieve higher and economical production of crops and to continually improve quality of produce and their profitability.

Intensive agricultural production, however, is insufficient to fulfill the requirement for the ever growing population of India since large quantities of food produced are wasted during growing, harvesting and storage. Nearly 60,000 species of invertebrate pests and plant diseases in the agriculture field and storage, and 8000 species of weeds compete with man to incur a loss of 40 per cent of the production. Although several eco-friendly technologies such as integrated pest management system, use of neem based insecticides and other bio-pesticides are available for pest management, farmers rely mostly on the chemical pesticides because of their easy availability, immediate and spectacular effect. Synthetic pyrethroids have been used to control wide range of ectoparasites in cattle since 1970s, of which deltamethrin appears to the most potent, photostable, persistent, and effective at very low dosage and is used for control of tsetse flies as dipping or pour-on method in cattle. Fenvaterate is very effective in control of northern fowl mites and reduces population of face fly, horn fly and ticks in cattle. Lindane is also used in India for the treatment of maggot infestation and follicular mange in veterinary practice in the form of cream containing 0.1% w/w Gamma Benzene Hexachloride. These chemicals have contributed a lot to the betterment of human health too through the control of vectors of dreaded diseases like malaria, typhus etc. Pesticides are introduced in India in 1947 when 250 tonnes of DDT was imported for malaria eradication and now India ranks 10th in the world in pesticide consumption covering about 25% of total cultivated area.

Pesticides used in the agriculture activities can be classified into four major groups as organochlorines, organophosphates, carbamates and synthetic pyrethroids. Organochlorine pesticides (OCPs) have been used extensively world wide since it is effective against wide variety of pests, have low volatility and extreme stability which leads to their high persistence both in environment after application and in organisms after exposure. Despite a ban imposed by the WHO on use of certain OCPs, some of these pesticides are still used in limited quantity in many developing countries, including India for agricultural and public health programmes especially malaria control. During last decades much attention has been given to this group of substances at the International level after it became apparent that they are carried to an environment through "Global Distillation" and critical concentrations have been observed in some areas even in places where they have never been used or produced. Recently, nine OCPs have been targeted for global elimination under the signed Stockholm Convention on Persistent Organic Pollutants (POPs).

Organophosphate pesticides (OPPs), less persistent than OCPs, are frequently preferred choice of treatment because they are efficacious, biodegradable and cost effective in control of wide range of pests. However, they are generally more toxic than OCPs as potent cholinesterage inhibitors or carbamate compounds.

Synthetic pyrethroids are synthesized derivatives of naturally occurring pyrethrins and their insecticidal properties are derived from ketoalchoholic esters of chrysanthemic and pyrethroic acids which are strongly lipophillic and rapidly penetrate many insects and paralyze their nervous system. Pyrethroids are used to control horn flies, tsetse flies, mosquitoes and house flies in the form of shampoo or spray. In recent years pyrethroids have become popular because of their efficacy against wide range of insects including resistant strains and also due to their relatively faster biodegradability and low mammalian toxicity.

Modern agricultural production, though, involves the use of many pesticides to control pest and diseases of plants and also to increase crop production; it has also left an indelible and adverse impact on the environment. The extensive application of pesticides has lead to a human health hazard as well as deterioration in environmental quality. The principal sources of pesticides in crops, food animals, soil, water and almost all food commodities include carry-over from insecticide application to soil or to growing crops, leaching of pesticides (herbicides) or insecticides into ground water, drift of the pesticides from adjacent field, translocation of soil applied pesticide into growing crops, disposal of pesticides in streams, rivers and lakes, and disposal of effluents of pesticide industry in rivers and streams, and into soil which may be translocated in crops. No segment of the population is completely protected against exposure to pesticides and the potentially serious health effects leading to pesticide poisoning in about 1 million cases per year (Anonymous, 1999), though a disproportionate burden is shouldered by the people of developing countries and by high risk groups in each country.

Pesticides are known of inducing or aggravating certain health problems in humans such as endocrine disruption by mimicking or antagonising natural hormones in the body, immunosuppression, diminished intelligence, reproductive abnormalities and cancer. Although it is believed that adipose tissue acts as a protective reservoir, Dale *et al.* (1962) reported that *p,p'*-DDT residues in the adipose tissue can be mobilized during starvation, reach tissues such as brain and produce symptoms of neurotoxicity. Some products of pesticide metabolism are more toxic than the parent compound and are responsible for many of the undesirable toxic effects, both chronic and acute.

Although majority of the pesticides used for agricultural and domestic pest control purpose degrade rapidly in the environment, few find their way to animals through soil, contaminated water and plant tissues wherein they have specific affinity for adipose tissue and ultimately lead to contamination of the livestock products including milk, meat and organs . The livestock food constitutes significant part of human diet which leads to occurrence of high levels of these compounds in human adipose tissue and breast milk.

The increased global risk of adverse effects to human health and environment has led the international community to mandate the United Nations Environment Programme (UNEP) to convene an Intergovernmental Negotiating Committee for a Persistent Organic Pollutants (POPs) Convention to phase out production and use of certain long term persistent pesticides. As per the agreement in the convention, most of the countries including India have formed regulations to monitor the use of pesticides in agriculture. As on date, under section 9(3) of the Insecticide Act 1968, 171 pesticides have been registered for use in agriculture in the country, 29 pesticides have been banned to date, another 10 have been under restricted use and 25 pesticides are under review. Increased globalization has resulted in easy movement of agricultural products from one part of the world to another. Therefore, it is necessary to look into the diversity in rules and regulations across the different nations and harmonies different regulatory agencies globally to establish joint tolerances or maximum allowable residue limits (MRLs) and establish best/ uniform risk assessment guidelines.

Pesticide centric agriculture had taken centre stage in country's agricultural planning for protection of crop from pest attack and loss of valuable food production every year. Almost 67 per cent of the pesticides manufactured in India are used for two crops; namely rice and cotton, which are grown from July to November (Anonymous, 1996). Grazing animals may acquire these harmful pesticides through consumption of contaminated feed, water, direct skin absorption or inhalation which leads to contamination of their products such as milk, meat and tissues. The meat produced in India is very popular in most of the exported countries due to its most attractive unique characteristic of leanliness, competitive price, lack of animal origin feed ingredients in their diet as animals are grown by grazing. Indian meat production was 5,561 thousand tones in 2002. Of which 285 thousand tones was exported to various countries and rest 5,277 thousand tones was consumed locally. In the fiscal year 2005-2006 India has exported buffalo meat, sheep/goat meat and poultry products worth Rs. 2629.56, 80.37 and 167.58 crores, respectively.

Pesticide residues mean any specified substances in food, agricultural commodities, or animal feed resulting from use of pesticides. The term includes any derivatives of pesticides such as conversion products, metabolites, reaction products and impurities considered being of toxicological significance.

The levels of residues vary in different species of food animals and are proportional to the concentration of pesticides in their diet. The occurrence of pesticides or residues in edible food is a risk that has been main focus of public concern. It is reported that Indians take 75 and 91 per cent of HCH and DDT in their dietary intake through consumption of food of animal origin. On comparison of pesticide residues detected in food in India and world it was surprising to see that only 2.5% of food commodities in India are free of pesticide residues as compared to 80% at world level. The indiscriminate use of pesticides poses considerable risk due to presence of the residues in agricultural and animal husbandry practices. Therefore, the awareness and need for regular screening of various animal products such as milk and meat is imperative in the interest of trade and consumers society.

DETECTION METHODS OF PESTICIDE

The determination of pesticide residues is a requirement to support.

1. The enforcement of legislation.
2. Ensure trading compliance.
3. Conduct monitoring residue programmes in the dietary components and in the environmental samples.

Various analytical methods such as electrophoresis, enzyme linked immunosorbent assay, use of biosensors, chromatographic analysis using gas chromatography with array of detectors, high performance liquid chromatography and very recently gas chromatography with mass spectrometry have been developed in pesticide analysis. However, GC-ECD and GC-FTD are the most widely used analytical techniques employed for detection and quantitation of organochlorines & synthetic pyrethroids, and organophosphates, respectively since it provides high resolution of peaks, high sensitivity and specificity of detection of these pesticides by using capillary column which are able to detect multiclasses of these group of pesticides in single run. Many research workers also have recommended GC-MS as a confirmatory technique.

PESTICIDE CONTROL MEASURES

Thus, to avoid residues of pesticides in foods of animal origin following measures required to be implemented strictly:

1. The combined efforts of Departments of Agriculture and Animal Husbandry at state as well as National level, State Agricultural and Veterinary Universities, and various Governmental Regulatory Authorities to control residues in meat and poultry will be more effective in reducing the incidences of violative residues in meat and poultry products, and also in reducing potential risk to the consumers.
2. More incentives should be given to farmers for use of eco-friendly pesticides than chemical ones to avoid

accumulation and subsequent hazards to human health. Nationwide efforts are required to reduce/eliminate the use of chemical pesticides in agriculture.

3. Indian Regulatory Authorities should play even more effective role in preventing potentially harmful residues in animal origin foods including poultry products with improvement in technology for residue detection and control.

4. The regulatory authorities in India should encourage industry's participation in quality control programs for residue avoidance, strengthening the laboratories in India to a state-of-art-facility to undertake residue testing and regulatory programs and build up stronger link between detection and enforcement.

5. Producers having low regards for food safety must be persuaded through education, appropriate regulatory programs and enforcement actions to change their production and marketing practices.

REFERENCES

Aggarwal, A. (1996). Facing a silent spring. Down to Earth 5 : 27-37.

Agnihotri, N.P. (2000). Pesticide consumption in agriculture in India and update *Pesticide Research Journal*. 12 : 150-155.

Agmihotri, N.P. (1999). Pesticide safety evaluation and monitoring. All India Co-ordinated Research Project on pesticide residues. ICAR, New Delhi, 173 pp.

Anonymous (2006) Consumption of pesticides in various states during 2000-01 to 2005-06. http://cibrc.nic.in/pestconsum.htm.

Anupama Kumari, Sinha, R.K., Krishna, G.K. and Gopal, K. (2001). Quantitative estimation of DDT residues in some fresh water fish of river Ganga at Patna, Bihar. *Environmental and Ecology*. 19 : 396-399.

Au WW, Sierra, C.H., Cajas, S.N., Shipp B.K. and Legator M. (1999). Cytogenetic effects from exposure to mixed pesticides and the influence from genetic susceptibility. *Environ. Health Perspect.* 107 : 501-505.

Aulakh, R.S. (2002). Studies on insecticide residues in chicken and eggs and their public health significance. Ph.D. dissertation, PAU, Ludhiana, India

Battu R.S., Gupta, S.C., Chawla, R.P. and Kalra, R.L. (1984). Residues of DDT and BHC in market samples of meat of various animals. *Indian Journal Ecology* 11 (2) : 177-182.

Battu, R.S., Singh, B., Kang, B.K. and Chahal, K.K. (2001). Status of contamination of bovine milk with pesticide residues. Abst. PEF. Indian Agricultural Research Institute, Nov. 19-23, 2001.

Bedi. J.S., Gill, J.P.S., Aulakh, R.S., Joia B S and Sharma, J.K. (2004). Contamination levels of DDT and HCH residues in different goat tissues. *The Indian Journal of Animal Sciences* 74 (12) 11-13.

Bhinge, A.R. and Banerji, S.A. (1981). Estimation of Organochlorine pesticide residues in different organs of the Pomfert fish available in Bombay. *Scavanger* 11 : 25-30.

Chakravarty A. Pal S, Das, A.K. and Sukal, P. (1996). Monitoring of endosulfan residues in market fish samples. *Pesticide Research Journal* 8: 164-167.

Cheema, H.K. Kang, B.K. and Singh, B. (2005). Residues of chlorpyriphos in bovine milk in Punjab. Abst. 3rd Annual Conference of IAVPHS 9-10 Feb. PAU, Ludhiana.

Dinham B, Malik S. 2003 Pesticides and human rights. *Int J Occup Environ Health* 9 : 40–52.

Ekbom A., Wicklund, G.A. and Adami, H.O. (1996). DDT and testicular cancer. *Lancet* 347 : 553-554.

Fleming L., Monn, J.B., Briggle, T. and Sanchez Ramar, J.R. (1994). Parkinson's disease and brain levels of Organochlorine pesticides. *Ann. Neural* 36 : 100-103.

Gill, J.P.S. (2000). Studies on pesticide residues in milk and milk products and its public health significance. Ph.D. dissertation. PAU, Ludhiana, India.

Gill J.P.S., R.S. Aulakh, J.P.S. Mundi AND J.K. Sharma (2001) Pesticides residues in animal feed: a potential source of public health hazard. Paper in Post Conference proceeding of International Conference on Pesticides, Environment, Food Security from 19-23, November 2001 held at New Delhi.

Gill J.P.S., Aulakh R.S., Mundi J.P.S., Bedi J.S. and Sharma J.K. (2003) Pesticide residues in milk. Paper presented at Indian Dairy Industry Conference held at 5-7 March, 2003 at Chandigarh.

Gupta, R.C. and Gupta, P.K. (1979). Ecological impact of pesticideis. In Proc. Symp. Life and Toxic Environment pp 70-85. DAV College Muzaffarnagar.

Hassal, K.A. (1983). The Chemistry of Pesticides. Their metabolism, mode of action and uses in crop protection. The Mac Millan Press, London.

Jadhav, G.D. (1986) DDT and BHC residues in milk samples from Marathwada region. In: S.C. Goel (ed). Pesticide Residues and Environmental Pollution. Muzaffarnagar, India pp 72-85.

Jeyaratnam, J. 1990. Acute Pesticide Poisoning: A Major Global Health Problem. *World Health Statistics Quarterly* 43 : 139-144.

John, P.J. Bakore, N. and Bhatnagar, P. (2001). Assessment of Organochlorine pesticide residue levels in dairy milk and buffalo milk from Jaipur city, Rajasthan. *India. Environ. Int.* 126 (4) : 231-236.

Joia B.S. (2005). *Pesticide residues and the environment.* Third Annual Conference and National Symposium on New Approaches in Food Safety and Quality Control with Special Reference to Emerging Food Borne Diseases and Intoxications. pp 90-91.

Kalra, R.L. (2001). Implication of pesticide residues in human safety. Entended Abstracts: International Conference on Pesticides, Environment and Food safety. 19-23 Nov. 2001, pp.26.

Kalra, R.L. and Chawla, R.P. (1981). Monitoring of pesticide residues in the Indian Environment: In B.V. David (ed) Indian Pesticide Industry Facts & Figures. Vishvas Publications, Bombay, pp. 251-285.

Kalra, R.L. and Chawla, R.P. (1983) Studies on Pesticide Residues and Monitoring of Pesticidal Pollution. Final Technical Report. PL-480 Project, Punjab Agricultural University, Ludhiana.

Kalra, R.L. (1999). DDT and HCH residues in dairy milk samples collected from different geographical regions of India; a multicentric study. *Food contam. And Addit.* 16 : 411-417.

Kannan K, Tanabe S., Ramesh A, Subramanian A and Tatsukawa R (1992). Persistent Organochlorine residues in foodstuffs from India and their implication on human dietary exposure. *J. Agric. Food Chem.* 40 : 518-524.

Kannan K, Tanabe S, Giesy JP, Tastukawa R (1997). Organochlorine pesticides and polychlorinated biphenyis in foodstuffs from Asian and Oceanic countries. Rev. Environ. Contam. Toxicol. 152 : 1-55.

Kaphalia B.S. and Sethi, T.D. (1981). DDT and BHC residues in some body tissues of goats, buffalo and chickens, Lucknow. India. *Pestic. Monit. J.* 15 : 103-106.

Kathpal, T.S., Singh, G., Yadav, G.S., Dhankar, J.S. and Singh, A. (1992). Monitoring of milk and milk products for DDT and HCH contamination. *Pesticide Research Journal* 4 (2) : 123-131.

Lata, S., Siddiqui, M.K.J. and Seth, T.D. (1984). Chlorinated pesticides in desi ghee. *J.Fd. Sci. Technol*. 21 : 94-95.

Mahabir Singh (2002). Production and Utilization of pesticides in Asia and the pacific country. Report. India 190-202.

Manpreet, K. Gill, J.P.S., and Sharma, J.K. (2005). Presence of chlorinated insecticide residues in market fish samples. Abst. 3rd Annual Conference of IAVPHS 9-10 Feb. PAU, Ludhiana.

Mehrotra, K.N. (1985). Use of HCH and its environmental effects in India. *Proc. Indian Natu. Sci. Acad*. B51 : 581-595.

Mukherjee I. and Gopal M.(2003). Organochlorine pesticide residues in dairy milk in an around Delhi. Journal of AOAC International 76 : 283-286.

Narsimha Rao, B. Narsimha Reddy, K., Azam, S.M. and Prabhakara, R.K. (1989). HCH residues in milk and milk products. In: Abstr. Natn. Symp. Impact and Management of Pollutants on Crop Productivity : pp. 26-27, Haryana Agricultural University, Hissar.

Nath, B.S., Unnikrishnan, V., Usha, M.A., Sarwar: Organochlorine pesticide residues in milk from South India. Indian Journal of Dairy Science, 2005 (Vol. 58) (No. 4) 247-249.

Pandit, G.G., Rao A.M.M., Jha, S.K., Krishnamoorthy, T.M., Kale, S.P., Raghu K. and Murthy, N.B.K. (2001) : Monitoring of Organochlorine pesticide residues in the Indian marine environment. *Chemosphere* 44 : 301-305.

Pandit, G.G., Sharma, S., Srivastava, P.K. and Sahu, S.K. (2002). Persistent Organochlorine pesticide residues in milk and dairy products in India. *Food Addit. Contam*. 19 (2) : 153-157.

Regupathy A and Kuttalam S (1992). Monitoring of HCH and DDT residues in certain quail eggs in Tamil Nadu. *Pesticide Research Journal* 4 (2) : 149-153.

Sandhu, T.K. (1992). Pesticide in Food. *Proc. of 3rd World Congress on Food borne infections and intoxication*. June 2 : 710-714 held at Berlin.

Scheele, J., Teufel, M and Niessen., K.H. (1996). Chlorinated hydrocarbons in human bone marrow of healthy individuals and leukemia patients. *Arch Environ. Health* 51 : 22-25.

Shah. P.G., Patel, B.K. Raj, M.P. and Patanwala, R.D. (1992). Monitoring of HCH and DDT in ghee and butter samples in Gujarat. *Pesticide Research Journal*. 4 (2) : 117-121.

Sharma, N., Lakshmanan V. and Singh, M. (1984). Pesticide residues in livestock product with reference to meat. *Indian Food Industry* 3 : 52-56.

Sharma, R.C., Bhaskaran, M. and Bhinde, N.K. (1979). A simplified chemical method of DDT estimation in body fat. *Indian J. Exptl. Biol.* 17 : 1367-1370.

Sherman, J.D. (1996). Chlorpyrifos (Dursban) associated birth defects: report of four cases. *Arch. Environ Health* 51 : 5-8.

Singh Balwinder, Kang, B.K., Battu, R.S. (2004) Contamination of liquid milk and butter with pesticide residues in the Ludhiana district of Punjab state, India. Ecotoxicology and Environmental Safety, 2004 (Vol. 59) (No. 3) 324-331.

Straube E., Straube, W., Kruges, E., Bradatsch, M, Jacob, Meisel, M., Rose, H.J., Leng G and Hadnagy W (1999). Description of male sex hormones with regard to pesticides: pathophysiological and regulatory aspects. *Toxicol Lett* 107 : 275-231.

Tripathi, H.C. (1966). Organochlorine insecticide residues in agricultural and animal products in Tarai area. M.Sc. Thesis, Uttar Pardesh Agricultural University, Pantnagar, India.

WHO/UNEP Working Group. 1990. *Public Health Impact of Pesticides Used in agriculture.* World Health Organisation, Geneva, Switzerland.

Zaidi SSA (1987). Possible role of rat liver NADPH Cytochrome P-450 reductase in the detoxication of DDT to DDD. *Bull Environ. Contam. Toxicol* 39 : 327-333.

20

PESTICIDE RESIDUES IN FOODS OF ANIMAL ORIGIN : RESEARCH PRIORITIES

S.P. Singh and Rashmi Singh

A pesticide is a substance employed for preventing, destroying, attracting, repelling or controlling any pest during the production, storage, transport, distribution and processing of food, agricultural commodities or animal feeds. Use of pesticide dates back to more than 3,000 years as depicted in the writings of Greek, Roman and the Chinese civilizations. In the year 1939, Dr. Paul Muller, a Swiss entomologist discovered DDT which made the beginning of the wide use of pesticide for control of the pests. The DDT was considered a miracle substance for enhancing agricultural productivity and proved to be a boon during World War II when it saved lives of thousands of soldiers from threats of malaria and other vector born diseases.

There are a number of classes of pesticides as per their chemical structures and thousands of these formulations are available today in the market (Table 20.1). The major classes include organochlorines, organophosphates, carbamates and synthetic pyrethroids etc. Among these, organochlorines (OCS), organophosphates and carbamates display great persistence in the environment leading to the various health and safety problems.

Table 20.1 : Pesticides Registered for use in India Under Section 9(3) of Insecticides Act, 1968 (as on 7th March, 2005)

2,4-Dichlorophenoxy Acetic Acid	*Acephate*	*Acetamiprid*	*Alachlor*	*Allethrin*	*Alphacypermethrin*
Alphanaphthyl Acetic Acid	Aluminium Phosphide	Anilophos	Atrazine	Aureofungin	Azadirachtin (Neem Products)
Bacillus thuringiensis (B.t. & Bs.)	Barium Carbonate	Beauveria bassiana	Benomyl	Beta Cyfluthrin	Bifenthrin
Bitertanol	Bromadiolone	Butachlor	Benfuracarb	Captan	Carbaryl
Carbendazim Hydrochloride	Carbofuran	Carbosulfan	Carboxin	Cartap	Chlorofenvinphos
Chlorimuron ethyl	Chlormequat Chloride (CCC)	Chlorothalonil	Chlorpyriphos	Chlorpyriphos Methyl	Cinmethylene
Clodinafop-propinyl (Pyroxofop-propinyl)	Clomazone	Copper Hydroxide	Copper Oxychloride	Copper Sulphate	Coumachlor
Coumatetralyl	Cuprous Oxide	Cyfluthrin	Cyhalofop-butyl	Cymoxanil	Cypermethrin
Cyphenothrin	Dalapon	Dazomet	Deltamethrin (Decamethrin)	Diazinon	Dichloro Diphenyl Trichloroethane (DDT)
Dichloropropene and Dichloropropane mixure (DD mixure)	Diclorvos (DDVP)	Diclofop-Methyl	Dicofol	Difenocenazole	Difenthiuron
Diflubenzuron	Dimethoate	Dimethomorph	Dinocap	Dithianon	Diuron
Dodine	D-trans Allethrin	Edifenphos	Endosulfan	Ethephon	Ethion

Contd....

(Table 20.1 Contd....)

2,4-Dichlorophenoxy Acetic Acid	*Acephate*	*Acetamiprid*	*Alachlor*	*Allethrin*	*Alphacypermethrin*
Ethofenprox (Etofenprox)	Ethoxysulfuron	Ethylene Dibromide and Carbon Tetra-chloride mixture (EDCT Mixture 3:1)	Fenarimol	Fenazaquin	Fenitrothion
Fenobucarb (BPMC)	Fenoxaprop-p-Ethyl	Fenpropathrin	Fenthion	Fenvalerate	Ferbam
Fipronil	Fluchloralin	Flufenacet	Flufenoxyuron	Fluvalinate	Formothion
Fosetyl-Al	Gibberellic Acid	Glufosinate Ammonium	Glyphosate	Hexaconazole	Hydrogen Cyanamid
Imiprothrin	Imazethapyr	Imidacloprid	Iprobenfos (Kitazin)	Indoxacarb	Iprodione
Isoprothiolane	Isoproturon	Kasugamycin	Lambdacyhalothrin	Lime Sulphur	Lindane
Linuron	Mancozeb	Malathion	Mepiquate Chloride	Metalaxyl	Metaldehyde
Metasulfuron Methyl (MCPA)	Methabenzthiazuron	Methomyl	Methoxy Ethyl Mercury Chloride (MEMC)	Methyl Bromide	Methyl Chlorophenoxy Acetic Acid
Methyl Parathion	Metolachlor	Metoxuron	Metribuzin	Milbemectin	Monocrotophos
Myclobutanil	Nickel Chloride	Oxadiargyl	Oxadiazon	Oxycarboxin	Oxydemeton-Methyl
Oxyflurofen	Paclobutrazole	Paradichlorobenzene (PDCB)	Paraquat dichloride	Penconazole	Pendimethalin
Permethrin	Phenthoate	Phorate	Phosalone	Phosphamidon	Primiphos-methyl
Prallethrin	Pretilachlor	Profenophos	Propanil	Propergite	Propetamphos

Contd....

2,4-Dichlorophenoxy Acetic Acid	*Acephate*	*Acetamiprid*	*Alachlor*	*Allethrin*	*Alphacypermethrin*
Propiconazole	Propineb	Propoxur	Pyrethrins	Quinalphos (pyrethrum)	Quizalofop ethyl
S-bioallethrin	Simazine	Sirmate	Sodium Cyanide	Spinosad	Streptomycin + Tetracycline
Sulfosulfuron	sulphur	Tebuconazole	Temephos	Thiobencarb (Benthiocarb)	Thiodicarb
Thiomethoxain	Thiometon	Thiram	Thiophanate-Methyl	Transfluthrin	Triadimefon
Triallate	Triazophos	Trichlorofon	Trichoderma viride	Tricyclazole	Tridemorph
Trifluralin	Validamycin	Warfarin	Zinc Phosphide	Zineb	Ziram

Source : National Centre for Integrated Pest Management, Lal Bahadur Shastri Building, Pusa Campus, New Delhi 110 012. INDIA

In India, 40% of the food grain loss occurs either due to pests or other factors and, hence about Rs. 30 billion are spent on agrochemicals to reduce these losses. The Indian pesticide market is 12th largest in the world and since 1984 has grown by 13% per annum. India is the second largest manufacturer of technical grade agrochemicals in the south Asian countries after Japan. It stands 7th in the world in average consumption of pesticides per hectare.

Today, the usage of pesticides is highest in cotton (54%) followed by rice (17%), vegetables and fruits (13%), plantation crops (8%) and others (8%). About 81,000 mt of technical grade pesticides (80% in agriculture and 20% in public health) with more than 144 product registrations (Insecticides Act 1968 and Rules 1971) represent a huge quantity and diversification. Five major Indian states *viz.*; Andhra Pradesh, Karnataka, Gujarat, Punjab and Maharashtra contribute to more than half national consumption of the pesticides (especially insecticides).

Attempts have been made to reduce the pesticide use in India. Many hazardous pesticides have been either restricted or banned for the use (Table 20.2). DDT and BHC-Hexacholorocyclohexane (HCH/Gammaxane/Lindane) have been the major menace because of their wide spectrum of activity, easy availability and relatively low cost. However, their ban has a relief but the problem did not end there, since the residues are stably persistent in the environment.

Table 20.2 : Pesticides/Pesticides Formulations Banned in India

A. Pesticides banned for manufacture, import and use
1. Aldrin
2. Benzene Hexachloride
3. Calcium Cyanide
4. Chlordanepane
5. Copper Acetoarsenite
6. Chromochloropropane
7. Endrin
8. Ethyl Mercury Chloride
9. Ethyl Parathion

10. Heptachlor
11. Menazone
12. NitrofenNitrofenNitrofen
13. Paraquat Dimethyl Sulphate
14. Pentachloro Nitrobenzene
15. Pentachlorophenol
16. Sodium Methane Arsonate
17. Tetradifon
18. Toxafen
19. Aldicarb
20. Chlorobenzilate
21. Dieldrine
22. Maleic Hydrazide
23. Ethylene Dibromide
24. TCA (Trichloro acetic acid)

B. Pesticide/Pesticide formulations banned for use but their manufacture is allowed for export

1. Nicotin Sulfate
2. Phenyl Mercury Acetate
3. Captafol 80% Powder-(Use banned w.e.f. 17.7.2003)

C. Pesticide formulations banned for import, manufacture and use

1. Methomyl 24% L	2. Methomyl 12.5% L
3. Phosphamidon 85% SL	4. Carbofuron 50% SP

Source : DPPQ & S, Faridabad.

PESTICIDE RESIDUES IN FOODS OF ANIMAL ORIGIN

India is likely to cross one and a quarter billion mark by 2020 and to provide the livelihood to the fast growing population it would be inevitable to rely not only on agriculture production but also on foods of animal origin. Foods of animal origin such as meat, milk, eggs and their by products are consumed by the people world over. The pesticides are widely used to control pests and insects of crops, fruits and vegetables and in storage of seeds and grains in agriculture, various disease transmission vectors and external and internal parasites in animal husbandry and public health programmes.

Table 20.3 : Pesticides in Foods of Animal Origin

Commodity	*Pesticide*	*% samples positive*	*% of samples exceeding (MRLs)*	*States*	*Year*	*Investigator/reference*
Liquid Milk	DDT	82% of 2205	37% (0.05mg/kg)	12 states	1995-96	ICMR Bulletin 2001
	HCH	85%	42%	Ludhiana	2002	Pandit *et al.*
	DDT	6 of 92 or 7.4%	2 of 6			
	HCH	49 of 92 or 53.3%				
	Lindane	All 49	All (0.01mg/kg)		2004	Singh *et al.*
	Chlorpyriphos	All 20	11 (0.01mg/kg extraneous residue limit)		2005	Cheema *et al.*
Butter	HCH	56%			2000	Gill
	DDT	43%				
	Aldrin Dieldrin	1%				
	DDT	28 of 40			2004	Singh *et al.*
	HCH	8 of 40				
Ghee	DDT	All had less than MRL	(1.25ppm)		2000	Gill
	HCH	All had more than MRL	(0.2ppm)			

Contd....

Commodity	*Pesticide*	*% samples positive*	*% of samples exceeding (MRLs)*	*States*	*Year*	*Investigator/reference*
Fish	DDT	Organs of Pomfert 0.43-34.0 mg/kg		Bombay	1981	Bhinge & Banerjee
	DDT	50% of 14 had 0.02-3.02mg/kg	Ludhiana	1984	Battu *et al.*	
	HCH	0.03-1.12 mg/kg				
	Endosulfan	227 of 396	Kolkata and suburbs		(1988-93)	Ckakrabarty *et al.* 1996
	DDT	0.726-1.665 mg/kg	Fish from Ganga river in Patna	2001	Anupama *et al.*	
	DDT, HCH	0.18mg/kg and 0.004mg/kg respectively	Punjab market	2005	Manpreet *et al.*	
Meat	DDT		Tolerance limit 7 mg/kg	Reports from 1979 to 1986: levels of DDT and HCH in meat below the tolerance limit, except one sample from Lucknow 914.1mg/kg chicken meat.)		

DDT, HCH, endosulfan and heptachlor in chicken muscle; DDT, HCH, dieldrin, heptachlor, endosulfan detected in various tissues of goats.

(References cited by Gill, 2007)

The pesticide residues present in the foods of animal origin posses a great risk of health hazard to human consumers. The contaminated milk, meat and their products and drinking water with the pesticide residues becomes the cause of ill health in man. There is a growing awareness among the public with respect to the harmful effects of these dreaded agrochemicals. The increasing frequency of the presence of pesticide residues in different food products and the consequent safety concerns of these foods have been in the news. Table 20.3 enlists the presence of pesticides and their MRLs in different foods of animal origin.

The pesticides are used extensively and indiscriminately in agricultural, animal husbandry and public health operations and their residues tend to accumulate in vegetation and animal tissues and have great potential to cause health hazards to man and animals by disturbing the ecosystems of soil, water, air, phytoplanktons and zooplanktons. Pesticides after ingestion through contaminated feed and water or inhalation through lungs are absorbed, metabolized and excreted from animal body. Some of the residues are deposited in body tissue for longer duration particularly in adipose and nervous tissues and causes various neurobehavioral and other pathological changes in vital functions of the body including nervous, cardiopulmonary, hepatic, renal and immune system. Thus, there is a need to screen the feed, fodder and animal products for the presence of pesticide residues to prevent toxic hazards of pesticides.

Available data on the presence of pesticide residues in bovine milk in India indicate that majority of the samples tested, were found contaminated with DDT residues above the prescribed maximum residue limits (MRLs). The presence of HCH residues in dairy milk has also been recorded. Dieldrin residues in bovine milk have been found to the extent of 76 ppm (fat basis). Very high concentrations of DDT and BHC have been found in milk and milk products and their occurrence in dairy products has been shown in Table 20.4.

Meat samples collected from different meat animals from various parts of the country showed the occurrence of DDT

Table 20.4 : Pesticide Residue Levels in Milk and Milk Products in India

Product	*DDT (ppm fat basis)*	*BHC (ppm fat basis)*
Milk	0.01-55	0.02-61
Human Milk	1.4-102.2	1.25-27.52
Butter	1.6-11.36	0.55-1.51
Ghee	0.25-7.24	0.30-23.80
Infant milk	0.17-4.30	0.12-5.70
Skim milk powder	0.80-1.24	0.43-0.73

and HCH residues. The maximum levels of DDT residue reported were less than the prescribed limit (7 mg/kg). Residues of HCH were also detected in mutton, chevon, chicken and pork in different parts of the country. Residues of DDT and HCH were reported in various types of fish samples. Commonly consumed fish pomfert showed the presence of DDT.

In a study conducted at Pantnagar to detect the presence of pesticide (chlorpyrifos and endosulfan) residues in food of animal origin, a total of 2214 sample comprising of liver, kidney and muscle tissues from cattle (24), buffalo (71), goat (41), pig (302) and chicken (300) were analyzed. Of these, 18 of 72 (cattle), 14 of 213 (buffalo), 12 of 108 (goat), 78 of 906 (pig) and 46 of 900 (poultry) tissues samples were found to contain varying concentrations of endosulfan residues. However, only 1 of 72 (cattle), 40 of 906 (pig) and 7 of 900 (poultry) tissues were detected the presence of chlorpyrifos residues. (Project report 2003).

EFFECTS DUE TO PESTICIDES

Pesticides can have both acute and chronic health impacts depending on the extent of exposure. Acute effects may exhibit numerous symptoms including respiratory problems, nervous system disorders, and aggravation of pre-existing conditions such as asthma. Pesticides can cause irritation of the eyes, nose, and throat; burning, stinging, itches, rashes, and blistering of the skin; nausea, vomiting, and diarrhoea; and coughing, wheezing, headache, and general malaise. These effects can be delayed by up to four weeks and can include cramping in the lower limbs that leads to lack of coordination and paralysis. Very high doses may result in unconsciousness, convulsions and finally death.

In chronic poisoning, the person is repeatedly exposed to toxic agents over a long period, but only a low dose enters the body each time. Normally, no symptoms develop in relation to each exposure. Instead, victims gradually become ill over a period of months or years. This occurs when the toxic substance either accumulates in body tissues or causes minor irreversible damage at each exposure. After a long time, enough poison has been accumulated in the body to cause clinical symptoms. Chronic effects of long-term pesticide exposure include: impaired memory and concentration, disorientation, severe depressions, irritability, confusion, headache, speech difficulties, delayed reaction times, nightmares, sleepwalking, drowsiness and insomnia. Animal experiments indicate that exposure to cholinesterase-inhibiting chemicals can induce damage to the liver, kidneys and brain. Low doses of pesticides in animal and man can result in various pathological effects as given below.

Acquired Immunodeficiency

There is a marked immuno-suppressive effect by most of the commonly used pesticides. Organochlorines, organophosphates, carbamates and synthetic pyrethroids have been found to be immunotoxic at "no adverse effect dose" levels in poultry, sheep, and in bovine calves. The organochlorines are relatively much more harmful to immune system. It has also been reported that a state of immuno-suppression for a longer period may also lead to the development of neoplasm. Such animals also exhibit recurrent bacterial infections due to defective phagocytic machinery of the body.

Auto-Immunity

Pesticides are also known to initiate auto-immune response in body. Auto-immune glomerulonephritis or auto-immune hemolytic anemia or autoimmune rheumatoid arthritis is such manifestations in animals and man.

Hypersensitivity

Hypersensitive reactions are reported due to consumption of pesticide contaminated food stuffs. The dust of pesticides may cause allergic respiratory disorders like asthma. Cutaneous allergy has been known to occur due to contact of pesticide contaminated food items.

Carcinogenic Effect

Many pesticides have been implicated in causing or promoting cancers; leukemia, and non-Hodgkin's lymphoma, melanoma, multiple myeloma and soft tissue sarcoma. The most convincing evidence that pesticides are carcinogens comes from epidemiological studies. Cancers of the breast, testicles, ovary, lip, lung, prostate, bladder, cervix, and kidney, have also been frequently observed. Pesticides have been shown to induce brain tumor formation in animals. Some pesticides exert their carcinogenic effects either directly or indirectly through their metabolites.

Mutagenicity

Pesticides may cause alterations in structure or number of chromosomes resulting in trans-location, mutations and chromosomal breakage. The altered chromosomal number may become lethal during fetal stage. Several pesticides like DDT, Endrin, PCB and HCB are known to cause chromosomal aberrations. The mutagenic effect of pesticide poses a more serious threat to the future of human race.

Teratogenicity

The accumulation of pesticides in body tissue and congenital birth defects in young ones has not been well correlated so far. However, there are certain pesticides which cause teratogenic defects in animals. Carbaryl, thiram, propoxur, parathion, leptaphos, 2,4-D, lindane and diazinon are having teratogenic defects in animals. In mice cypermethrin, alphemethrin and malathian are found to exert birth defects in baby mice.

Neuropathy

Most of the organophosphates, organochlorines and carbamates may cause neuro-toxic effect in man and animals including increased irritation, loss of memory in coordination of movement, ataxia, delayed response, convulsions, spasms and paralysis. Pesticide residues are also responsible for marked behavioral changes in man and animals.

Nephropathy

Kidney, being an excretory organ, works continuously for the removal of waste and toxic substances from the body. The pesticide residues thus present in the food stuffs may enter the body system, a portion of it gets lodged in the tissues and remaining residues are eliminated through the excretory system. During the process of excretion, the kidney tissues get continuously exposed to this toxic substance resulting into kidney failure.

Hepatotoxicity

The pesticide residues in food may cause damage to the liver tissue as detoxification of the pesticides takes place in the liver. Continuous exposure of liver tissues with pesticides results into damage and death of the hepatic cells. There are instances of chronic liver disorders leading to cirrhosis. Certain pesticides are not so dangerous but their metabolites cause severe damage to hepatic parenchyma. The cirrhosis once starts; it never stops even after withdrawal of the primary cause.

Reproductive Disorders

It has been observed that the pesticides are lethal to dividing cells of genitalia. They may cause abnormalities in sperms leading to decrease their ability for fertilization. On the other hand, the ova become defective and not able to implant on the uterine surface leading to early abortion or miscarriage. The foods contaminated with pesticide residues may ultimately lead to sterility, early abortion, still births or repeat breeding. Various epidemiological studies on pesticide exposure has indicated increased risk of various types of congenital malformations mainly Cleft lip and palate, limb defects and cardiovascular malformations. Breast development occurs up to four years earlier among the young females. Chlorpyrifos has been linked to births of children with deformed heads, faces, eyes and genitals whereas; endosulphan has been linked to large numbers of serious birth defects in Keralites.

Respiratory Disorder

Pesticide applicators generally suffer from respiratory symptoms of wheezing due to paraquat, parathion, malathion, chlorpyrifos and thiocarbamate. Acute organophosphate or carbamate over-exposure is well known to cause broncho-constriction, increased airway secretions and respiratory distress.

Dermatological Disorder

Many pesticides can penetrate the skin and cause systemic exposure. Acute illness and death have been reported from per-cutaneous absorption of pesticides, particularly through damaged skin. Pesticides are reported to cause irritant dermatitis, allergic contact dermatitis.

REGULATORY CONCERNS REGARDING PESTICIDE RESIDUES

The persistent residues stay in food, biota and the environment for long time and impart potential threat to human health. In order to ensure the safety of food, the regulatory authorities have set Maximum Permissible Limits (MRLs) for the residues of these agrochemicals available in foods. Also the average daily intakes (ADI) have been worked out for many pesticides. Hence, adherence to the food safety norms rests with the national policies and the international trade of the food items. In India, steps should be initiated towards strict implementation of the recommendations made by different national as well as international bodies.

The nationwide network for monitoring pesticide residues in food ingredients is lacking. The statutory bodies such as ICAR (including State Agricultural Universities), ICMR, CSIR (Hyderabad, Pune, Jorhat, etc), NGOs, MNCs and other government and private (Rallis India, Bangalore and Jai Research Foundation, Vapi) institutions and agencies are involved in the residue research, development and the monitoring programmes. The Prevention of Food Adulteration Act (PFA)-1954 ensures the safety standards in food and the Insecticides Act-1968 emphasizes on the pesticide standard in India. Various test methods and specifications are provided by BIS apart from the MRL prescription by PFA-1954 for foods in general and foods of animal origin in particular. The Central Insecticides Laboratory (Faridabad) with its two regional and about 40 state pesticide testing laboratories, "BIS Mark Certification Scheme" and other private laboratories are involved in the quality assurance of the pesticides in the country.

In spite of all these, current monitoring systems to detect pesticide residue in milk, meat, and other food products (derived from animals) are inadequate. Therefore, more advanced screening and monitoring techniques should be deployed to protect consumers against the possible adverse effects of ingesting residues of drugs, some of which could be toxic or lead to diseases or allergic reactions. The accuracy of testing techniques should be improved to reduce the number of false-positive results and more resources are needed to develop testing methods for a wider range of drugs.

In United States, Department of Agriculture (USDA) which includes the Food Safety and Inspection Service (FSIS) and the Agricultural Marketing Service (AMS); the Food and Drug Administration (FDA); and the U.S. Environmental Protection Agency (EPA) are involved in regulation of drug residue analysis and food safety. FSIS is responsible for the wholesomeness and safety of fresh meat, poultry, and processed meat and poultry products intended for human consumption. It inspects slaughtering and processing establishments and samples and analyzes tissues derived from livestock and poultry at the time of or after slaughter. Inspection and analysis are intended to ensure, among other things, that meat and poultry do not contain residues of drugs, pesticides, or pathogens that cause them to be adulterated. AMS is responsible for the wholesomeness and safety of egg products. It conducts inspections and analyzes samples for chemical residues to ensure compliance with EPIA at plants that process egg products.

FDA enforces the federal Food, Drug, and Cosmetic Act (FDCA). FDA is directly responsible for ensuring the safety of milk and seafood for human consumption and that animal feeds are safe and contain no illegal residues of drugs, pesticides, or other environmental contaminants. FDA also approves drugs used for food-producing animals, establishes tolerance and safe levels for animal drugs and establishes action levels for unavoidable environmental contaminants that might adulterate food.

EPA is responsible for administering and enforcing the Federal Insecticide, Fungicide, and Rodenticide Act, which regulates the manufacture, sale, and use of pesticides. EPA also is responsible under FDCA for establishing tolerance levels and recommending action levels to FDA and FSIS for residues or pesticides in food. Under the Toxic Substances Control Act, EPA also regulates other chemical substances (such as industrial chemicals) that can adulterate food.

REFERENCES

CDS Tomlin (Ed).1997. The Pesticide Manual – A World Compendium, Eleventh edition, British Crop Protection Council, U.K.

European Council Directive (67/548/EEC), and subsequent amendments.

Karanth, N.G.K.. 2002. Challenges of Limiting Pesticide Residues in Fresh Vegetables: The Indian Experience. In: E. HANAK, E. BOUTRIF, P. FABRE, M. PINEIRO, (Scientific Editors), 2002. Food Safety Management in Developing Countries. Proceedings of the International Workshop, CIRAD-FAO, 11-13 December 2000, Montpellier, France, CIRAD-FAO. CIRAD CD-ROM, Montpellier, France.

Project Report. 2003. NATP on Quality assurance and monitoring of foods from livestock and poultry, ICAR, New Delhi.

Rotterdam Convention, 1998. UNEP/FAO, www.fao.org/pic.

Singh Mahabir. 2002. A chapter-India, in: report of the APO symposium on the production and utilization of pesticides in Asia and the pacific. Held in Tokyo from 9-15 Dec. 1998. Asian productivity organization. Tokyo.

UNEP Chemicals Newsletter 3(3), 1999.

WHO Recommended Classification of Pesticides by Hazard, and Guidelines to Classification 1998-1999, WHO/PCS/98.21, Geneva, 1998.

World Resources Institute, Intensification of Agriculture; www.igc.apc.org/wri/wri/wr-98-99/agrichem.htm#trends. www.fao.org/waicent/FAOINFO/economic/pesticid.htm.

21

MOLECULAR EPIDEMIOLOGY OF ANTIBIOTIC RESISTANCE

J.K. Sharma and Sandeep Ghatak

Emergence of resistance to antibiotic drugs is a recognized global problem in human and veterinary medicine. Resistance to antibiotic agents has been detected in a wide variety of pathogens and multiple drug resistance is increasingly becoming common. Far from just being a scientific curiosity, the development of multiresistant strains has required clinicians to shift empiric therapy regimens. This is true particularly for community-acquired organisms, such as pneumococci, for which high rates of penicillin resistance have necessitated the use of extended-spectrum cephalosporins in conjunction with vancomycin for empiric therapy of bacterial meningitis (Bradley and Scheld, 1997).

The evidence for widespread indirect dissemination of antibiotic resistance comes from varied sources, such as microbial population biology, microbial genetics, and clinical and epidemiological observations. Therefore studies in the molecular aspects of the emergence spread and detection of this menacing problem helps one understand the fundamental epidemiological features of the problem.

SOCIO-ECONOMIC COST OF ANTIBIOTIC RESISTANCE

Development and spread of antibiotic resistance has many direct and indirect implications. Among many these include higher treatment cost, increased laboratory testing, etc. It has been estimated that the national cost of direct impacts of antibiotic resistance in the United States was $4 billion per year in 1995 (Cosgrove. and Carmeli, 2003). Another estimate of hospital acquired infections by antibiotic resistant bacteria indicated an annual loss of $10 billion in USA, $ 450 million in Mexico and $ 40 million in Thailand (WHO, 2003). On the other hand other estimates indicate that in 1995 the cost of containing an outbreak of infection caused by methicillin-resistant *S. aureus* in a district general hospital in the United Kingdom was estimated to exceed US$ 560,000 (Cox *et al.*, 1995). AMR is the cause of professional, governmental, and public concern and has been classified as a national security risk in the USA (Neu, 1992, Tomasz, 1994, Fox, 1996 and Kaldec *et al.*, 1997).

MEDICAL COST OF ANTIBIOTIC RESISTANCE

The medical impact imparted by the phenomena of antibiotic resistances is complicated and includes increased morbidity and mortality in patients, longer hospital stay, lower treatment efficacy, etc. There is documented increase on the order of 1.3 – 2 fold in mortality, morbidity and cost for patients with resistant than susceptible infections. Moreover, due to increased resistance among common pathogens broader spectrum agents are now required for the empirical therapy of many common infections. These agents are usually more costly, exert more deleterious effects on protective normal microflora and at times are more toxic for the patients (Cosgrove and Carmeli, 2003, Tenovar, 2001).

There are at least five potential mechanisms by which antibiotic resistance can have adverse effects on human health. The first, relates to individuals who become infected only because they are taking an antibiotic to which the pathogen is resistant. The antibiotic, by suppressing their normal microbiota, renders them more vulnerable to infection. Second mechanism involves the linkage of virulence traits to resistance traits so that resistant organisms may be more virulent than susceptible organisms. A third mechanism is that treatment may be rendered ineffective by the choice of a drug to which the pathogens are resistant. Fourth mechanism is that the resistant pathogens from food animals may then be transmitted through the food chain to humans. Last, resistance traits can be acquired by the commensal flora of animals and from this reservoir, resistance traits could find their way through the food chain to commensals and pathogens of humans [Barza, 2002].

MOLECULAR GENETIC FACTORS IN EMERGENCE AND DISSEMINATION OF ANTIBIOTIC RESISTANCE

The emergence and spread of multiple resistant organisms represent the convergence of a variety of factors that include mutations in common resistance genes that extend their spectrum of activity; the exchange of genetic information among microorganisms in which resistance genes are transmitted to new hosts; the development of environmental conditions in hospitals and communities (selective pressures) that facilitate the development and spread of resistant organisms; the proliferation and spread, in some cases globally, of multiply resistant clones of bacteria; and the inability of some laboratory testing methods to detect emerging resistance phenotypes (Tenovar and Hughes, 1996., Doern *et al.*, 1998, Levin *et al.*, 1997).

ROLE OF MUTATIONS IN EMERGENCE OF ANTIBIOTIC RESISTANCE

In the early days of the "antibiotics," it was assumed that the development of resistance to antibiotics is a function of mutational events in the bacterial chromosome. However, when multidrug resistance first began to appear, particularly in gram-negative enteric bacilli, much of the resistance was plasmid mediated (Falkow, 1975). With the ensuing discovery of transposons and integrons, the role of mutations in the development of resistance in bacteria was often overlooked. However, for some organisms, such as *Mycobacterium tuberculosis*, mutations in genes that encode key metabolic pathways or housekeeping functions play a primary role in resistance to rifampin, streptomycin, ethambutol, and fluoroquinolones (Kapur *et al.*, 1995, Telenti *et al.*, 1997). Similarly, fluoroquinolone resistance in organisms, such as *Neisseria gonorrhoeae* (Deguchi *et al.*, 1995), *Streptococcus pneumoniae* (Jorgensen *et al.*, 1999), and *Salmonella* species (Griggs *et al.*, 1996), is often a result of mutations in the *gyrA*, *gyrB*, *parC*, and *par E.* loci. These types of mutations transform susceptible organisms into resistant ones. Some mutations in preexisting resistance genes, however, serve a different function by increasing the level of resistance to specific antibiotic or by expanding the spectrum of resistance [Tenovar, 2001].

In gram-negative bacilli, the progression of common α-lactamases that typically mediate resistance to ampicillin and narrow-spectrum cephalosporins into ESBLs—that is, enzymes that are capable of hydrolyzing extended-spectrum cephalosporins and monobactams—has become a classic example of mutation and selection of resistance determinants with an enhanced spectrum of activity. Mutations in 1 or more sites of the *bla*TEM or *bla*SHV genes, primarily in *K. pneumoniae*, *Klebsiella oxytoca*, and *E. coli*, lead to enhanced resistance. Such strains have been recognized throughout the world. At least 120 such ESBLs have been reported, and the list now includes enzymes of type *bla* OXA (Medeiros, 1997, Livermore, 1995, Jacoby and Bush).

ROLE OF GENETIC EXCHANGE

The ability of bacteria to exchange genetic information by a variety of mechanisms has been recognized for long time. The most commonly recognized modes of exchange are transformation and transduction (among Gram-positive organisms), and conjugation (among Gram-negative organisms). Among gram-negative organisms, plasmid transfer among a variety of enteric bacilli led to prolonged outbreaks of multiresistant organisms in hospitals (Tompkins *et al.*, 1980, Neuwirth *et al.*, 1996).

On the other hand, the ability of gram-positive organisms to exchange DNA via conjugation is often overlooked by microbiologists; however, it is a very effective means for transmitting antibiotic resistance genes among organisms. The sharing of aminoglycoside resistance genes among several species of staphylococci and enterococci is one example, of an active pathway. Genetic exchange pathways also exist between gram-positive and gram-negative organisms in which the transfer of kanamycin resistance genes has been observed (Clewell and Gawron, 1986, Trieu *et al.*, 1985).

Not all resistance genes that transfer among bacteria are expressed or even maintained; however, the limitations to expression are not well understood. Nonetheless, the ability of bacteria to acquire resistance genes from other organisms, including those that constitute the normal bacterial flora of humans, under the selective pressure of use of antibiotics should not be underestimated (Davies, 1994).

SELECTIVE PRESSURE

Selective pressure refers to the environmental conditions that enhance the ability of bacteria to develop resistance to antibiotics and to proliferate. This ability to survive may be the result of acquisition of new DNA (as is often the case with vancomycin resistant enterococci – VRE) or it may be due to spontaneous mutation, as is often the case for rifampin-resistant organisms. Expanded use of antibiotics in hospitals and in sites outside the hospital (*e.g.*, long-term care facilities, day care centers, animal feedlots, and other agricultural sites) increases the selective pressure for resistant organisms to emerge in these settings. The intensity of use of antibiotics appears to be proportional to the resistance levels in organisms in hospital settings (Nicolle *et al.*, 1996, Dupont and Steele, 1987).

MOLECULAR APPROACHES FOR STUDYING ANTIBIOTIC RESISTANCE

The determination of antimicrobial susceptibility of a clinical isolate is often crucial for the optimal antimicrobial therapy of infected patients. This need is only increasing with increasing resistance and the emergence of multidrug-resistant microorganisms. Testing is required not only for therapy but also to monitor the spread of resistant organisms or resistance genes throughout the hospital and community (Fluit *et al.*, 2000a, Fluit *et al.*, 2000b, Fluit *et al.*, 2001).

Nucleic acid-based detection systems offer rapid and sensitive methods to detect the presence of resistance genes and play a critical role in the elucidation of resistance mechanisms. During the last decade, nucleic acid-based detection systems have expanded tremendously and are becoming more accessible for clinical microbiology laboratories. This accessibility is not limited to the detection and identification of microorganisms but is extended to the detection of properties of these microorganisms, such as virulence factors and antimicrobial resistance. The application of nucleic acid-based technology is particularly useful for slow-growing or nonculturable microorganisms and for the detection of point mutations or certain genotypes (Fluit *et al.*, 2001).

For several reasons, molecular methods, compared to conventional susceptibility methods, have the potential to provide a more rapid and reliable assessment of antimicrobial resistance. (i) Molecular susceptibility testing methods can be performed directly with clinical specimens obviating the need for isolation of the organism by culture; (ii) these methods assess the genotype of the organism, whereas conventional susceptibility techniques asses the phenotype or expression of the genotype under artificial or laboratory conditions; (iii) in some cases, genotypes may be discerned long before phenotypes can be determined due to the slow growth of the organism; (iv) some organisms cannot be cultured or are not easily cultured and so only genotypes can be determined in these cases; (v) molecular methods may lessen the biohazard risk which may occur with the propagation by culture of a microorganism, a requirement for conventional test methods (Cockerill, 1999).

Most genotypic methods include an initial step where the "target" nucleic acid is amplified. This is usually accomplished by PCR. Other less frequently used methods which amplify either target nucleic acid or nucleic acid contained in probes annealed to target nucleic acid include self-sustaining sequence replication, strand displacement amplification, ligase chain reaction, and Qâ-replicase amplification. The signal generated from probes annealed to target nucleic acid can also be amplified *e.g.* branched DNA (bDNA) assay (discussed later).

The product of the PCR, referred to as an amplimer or amplicon, can be confirmed as the desired target nucleic acid (i.e., part or all of a resistance-associated genetic material) by electrophoretic mobility determinations, probe hybridization assays (Southern blotting of electrophoretic gels, slot, dot blot, enzyme-linked immunosorbent assay, or liquid hybridization formats), restriction fragment length polymorphism (RFLP) analysis, or DNA sequencing formats. Amplicons can also be assessed for specific mutations associated with antibiotic resistance by direct DNA sequencing methods and RFLP, single-strand conformation polymorphism (SSCP), dideoxy fingerprinting (ddF), Cleavase fragment polymorphism (CFLP), RNase cleavage, heteroduplex, line probe, molecular beacon, or microchip oligonucleotide array assays (Cockerill, 1999).

PCR

PCR technique involves exponential amplification of denatured target DNA molecule following hybridization with complementary sequence carrying oligonucleotides (called primers) in presence of a thermostable DNA polymerase (*Taq* polymerase in most cases) under a repetitive cycling with varying temperatures (e.g. 94°C – 60°C – 72°C) (Saiki *et al.*,1988). Amplified DNA fragments are then visualized usually under UV following agarose gel electrophoresis. Standard PCRs with amplicon sizing by gel electrophoresis are especially useful for identifying genes which encode antimicrobial resistance. These assays are highly specific, especially if there are no other nucleic sequences harbored by the organism which share significant homology with the target genetic material and large quantities of target nucleic acid are amplified. The latter condition exists when organisms are first propagated by culture and then isolated colonies are used for the PCR. Amplifying such large quantities of target nucleic acid reduces the sensitivity requirements for such assays, making it less likely that contamination with extraneous nucleic acid will be a significant problem. Therefore, provided that negative controls are used, specialized contained specimen processing areas and/or amplicon "sterilization" may be unnecessary. Amplicons can also be sterilized, that is, chemically or enzymatically modified, such that they cannot serve as a template for subsequent PCR assays which use the same oligonucleotide primers (Geha *et al.*, 1994, Wallet *et al.*, 1996).

bDNA ASSAY

The bDNA assay is a non-PCR-based signal amplification method that is commercially produced by Chiron Diagnostics (Norwood, Mass.) (Cockerill, 1999). It has been used to determine blood levels of viral loads HCV (Detmer *et al.*, 1996). The bDNA method depends on the amplification of a signal molecule and not the target nucleic acid. Signal generation is proportional to the amount of target gene sequences in the sample, which in turn is proportional to the number of organisms being analyzed. This assay have been reported to be able to detect the *mecA* gene directly from blood cultures containing staphylococci and was found to be as accurate as conventional PCR assays for detecting the *mecA* gene (Kolbert *et al.*, 1996). Upon automation the assay requires approximately 6 to 8 h to complete (Cockerill, 1999).

PCR-RFLP ANALYSIS

In RFLP analysis, the amplified DNA is digested (fragmented) with restriction enzymes. These endonucleases will only cleave DNA molecules at specific sites, i.e., unique short sequences of nucleic acid. Therefore, if the sequence of the target DNA is known, RFLP analysis can be used to confirm the target DNA in its amplified form.

Use of RFLP analysis to differentiate among genes encoding vancomycin resistance; have been reported (Patel *et al.*, 1997). Because of conserved DNA sequences which exist among vancomycin resistance genes, more than one vancomycin resistance gene may be amplified with the same PCR oligonucleotide primers. RFLP analysis then can be used to differentiate the vancomycin resistance gene amplicons, providing that sites for a restriction endonuclease are present in one but not another gene (Cockerill, 1999).

A potential advantage of the RFLP analysis is that PCR amplicons may be digested by a restriction enzyme to the extent that full-length amplicons are no longer available for subsequent PCR assays. Therefore, the amplicons are sterilized. The PCR-RFLP procedure can be performed in 6 to 8 h (Cockerill, 1999).

RFLP analysis is also useful for identifying mutations associated with antimicrobial resistance. It has been revealed through RFLP studies that point mutations in the catalase-peroxidase (*katG*) gene of *M. tuberculosis* are associated with isoniazid resistance (Brow *et al.*, 1996). RFLP analyses have also been demonstrated to be useful for identifying mutations associated with streptomycin resistance which occur in genes encoding 16S rRNA (*rrs*) and ribosomal protein S12 (*rspL*) in *M. tuberculosis* (Nachamkin *et al.*,1997), for classifying genes encoding TEM- (Cosgrove. and Carmeli, 2003) and SHV-type (Nuesch *et al.*,1996) extended-spectrum β-lactamases in gram-negative bacteria.

PCR-SSCP ANALYSIS

The technique of PCR-SSCP was first used to detect single nucleotide substitutions in human genes associated with hereditary disorders such as cystic fibrosis and phenylketonuria. The technique involves mobility shifts in high-resolution non-denaturing polyacrylamide gels are discernible for single-stranded mutated DNA versus wild-type DNA. After amplification of the target nucleic acid by PCR, it is denatured to a single strand and then electrophoresed. Mutations are inferred by the appearance of bands at positions different to those observed with the wild-type strain (Cockerill, 1999). Several investigators have reported on the utility of the PCR-SSCP method for identifying mutations in genes encoding SHV-type extended spectrum β-lactamases in the family

Enterobacteriaceae (Fatima *et al.*, 1996) and in several genes of *M. tuberculosis* associated with antibiotic resistance (Cockerill, 1999).

PCR-CFLP ANALYSIS

A genetically engineered structure-specific endonuclease, Cleavase I, has been used to detect mutations in the *katG* and *rpoB* genes of *M. tuberculosis* (Cockerill, 1999, Heisler *et al.*, 1996). The Cleavase I enzyme recognizes the folded structures which DNA strands form after denaturation and cleaves at the junction of the single-stranded and duplexed areas. After the fragments generated by Cleavase are separated by denaturing gel electrophoresis, unique polymorphisms occur with different mutations. So far, this method has had limited use (Cockerill, 1999).

PCR-RNA/RNA DUPLEX RNASE CLEAVAGE ASSAY

The method is based on the ability of RNase 1 and RNase T1 to cleave mismatches. Duplex RNA is transcribed from PCR products (test strain and wild-type strain) generated with primers containing opposing phage RNA polymerase promoters (T7/T7 or T7/Sp6). Following hybridization and RNase treatment, cleavage products of RNA/RNA duplexes occur due to mismatches. Mismatches are the result of mutation in the test strain compared with the wild-type strain. The assay has been successfully employed to detect mutations in the 23S rRNA gene of *Mycobacterium avium* complex which are associated with macrolide resistance (Nash and Inderlied, 1996). This method is commercialized and is available in kit form (Mutation Screener; Ambion, Inc.). It is relatively easy to perform but requires a longer time for completion than a PCR alone (Cockerill, 1999).

PCR-UNIVERSAL HETERODUPLEX GENERATOR ANALYSIS

DNA from a universal heteroduplex generator and the test strain are denatured simultaneously in the same reaction mixture and then allowed to reanneal. When separate strands of DNA from the heteroduplex generator and the test strain reanneal, four separate hybridizations can occur. Two of these hybridizations (heteroduplexes) will result in double-stranded DNA with a "bubble" occurring where no base-pair matches can hybridize. These hybrids will migrate as a single band when electrophoresed in a high-resolution gel. Two other bands will occur due to hybridization reactions (homoduplexes) which result in the formation of the double-stranded DNA of the heteroduplex generator and the test strain. If mutations are present in the test strain, the positions of the homoduplexes may vary compared to those of homoduplexes formed when no mutations are present. Williams and colleagues have used PCR-universal heteroduplex generator analysis to detect mutations in the *rpoB* genes of *M. tuberculosis* (Cockerill, 1999, Williams *et al.*, 1998).

PCR-LIPA

The PCR-line probe assay (LiPA) was first developed by Stuyer and colleagues to discriminate types and subtypes of HCV (Stuyver *et al.*, 1993). Biotinylated PCR fragments are hybridized to a selection of highly specific immobilized probes. The biotin group in the hybridization complex is then revealed by incubation with a streptavidin-alkaline phosphatase complex and the appropriate chromogen compounds. The assay has also been used to detect rifampin resistance-associated mutations in *M. tuberculosis* (Rossau *et al.*, 1997).

PCR-MOLECULAR BEACON SEQUENCE ANALYSIS

Molecular beacons are hairpin-shaped oligonucleotide probes that report the presence of specific nucleic acids in homogeneous solutions (Tyagi *et al.*, 1998). After these oligonucleotides anneal to their targets, they undergo a conformational change that restores the fluorescence of an internally quenched fluorophore. The assay has been used to detect mutations in the *rpoB* gene of *M. tuberculosis* associated with rifampin resistance (Piatek *et al.*, 1998).

DNA MICROARRAY

DNA microarray consists of orderly arranged single stranded DNA (ssDNA) from different known bacterial species on a solid surface (glass slide, silicon chip, nylon membrane, etc.). Unknown ssDNA from food samples are labeled with fluorescent dye and then hybridized on to the array. In the event of positive reaction or complementary binding between ssDNA on array and unknown target DNA, the particular spot(s) of the array fluoresce and emits signal. This signal is captured and analyzed to identify the unknown DNA and thereby the corresponding organism. Microarray technology holds immense potential due to their ability to identify multiple targets. Such matrix hybridization formats have great potential for rapid comprehensive detection of resistance genes or mutations associated with antimicrobial resistance. This is especially true if antimicrobial resistance in a specific organism can be due to multiple genes and/or multiple mutations. This technology also has the potential for significant automation and therefore should be easily adaptable to most clinical microbiology laboratories (Cockerill, 1999).

AUTOMATED DNA SEQUENCING

DNA sequencing remains the "gold standard" for identifying the products of amplification reactions. DNA sequencing of PCR products has become a much cheaper and faster method by virtue of automation (Cockerill, 1999). Instruments are now available for semi-automated running and analyzing of sequence gels. Therefore, any resistance gene or resistance mutation can be determined relatively easily and economically by direct DNA sequencing. Many researchers have reported successful use of automated DNA sequencing to determine antibiotic resistance-associated mutations for a variety of drugs and *M. tuberculosis* (Kapur *et al.*, 1994, Musser *et al.*, 1996).

EPILOGUE

Molecular analysis of antibiotic resistance has generated a wealth of information during the last decade. Applications of molecular techniques have aided our present understanding of the distribution and spread of antibiotic resistance among the species. Future challenges include the variety of point mutations or genes conferring resistance to pathogens and the repetitive nature of some of the current molecular methods. DNA microarray technology along with automated amplification-sequencing techniques has the potential to meet these challenges. Nonetheless, the conceptualizing, designing and fabricating of DNA arrays containing a wide range of resistance markers that are simultaneously applicable for many different species of pathogens presents a formidable challenge asking for a broader knowledge pool on antibiotic resistance markers.

REFERENCES

Barza, M. (2002). Potential mechanisms of increased disease in humans from antimicrobial resistance in food animals. *Clin. Infect. Dis.* **34** : S123–5.

Bradley, J.S., Scheld, W.M. (1997). The challenge of penicillin-resistant *Streptococcus pneumoniae* meningitis: current antibiotic therapy in 1990. *Clin. Infect. Dis.* **24** : S213–21.

Brow, M.A., Oldenburg M.C., Lyamichev, V., Heisler, L.M., Lyamichera, N., Hall, J.G., Eagen, N.J., Olive, D.M., Smith, L.M., Fors, L. and Dahlberg, J.E. (1996). Differentiation of bacterial 16S rRNA genes and intergenic regions and *Mycobacterium tuberculosis katG* genes by structure-specific endonuclease cleavage. *J. Clin. Microbiol.* **34**: 2139–3132.

Clewell, D.B. and Gawron-Burke, C. (1986). Conjugative transposons and dissemination of antibiotic resistance in streptococci. *Annu. Rev. Microbiol.* **40** : 635–9.

Cockerill, F.R. (1999). Genetic Methods for Assessing Antimicrobial Resistance. *Antimicrob. Agents Chemother.* **43** : 199–212.

Cosgrove, S. E. and Carmeli, Y. (2003). The impact of antimicrobial resistance on health and economic outcomes. *Clin. Infect. Dis.* **36** : 1433-7.

Cox, R., Conquest, C., Mallaghan, C. and Marples, R.R. (1995). A major outbreak of methicillin resistant *Staphylococcus aureus* caused by new phage-type (EMRSA-16). *J. Hospital Infect.* **29** : 87-106.

Davies, J. (1994). Inactivation of antibiotics and the dissemination of resistance genes. *Sci.* **264** : 375–82.

Deguchi, T., Yasuda, M., Asano, M. (1995). DNA gyrase mutations in quinolone-resistant clinical isolates of *Neisseria gonorrhoeae*. *Antimicrob Agents Chemother* **39** : 561–3.

Detmer, J., Lagier, R., Flynn, J., Zayati, C., Kolberg, J., Collins, M., Urdea, M. and Sanchez-Pescador. R. (1996). Accurate quantification of hepatitis C virus (HCV) RNA from all HCV genotypes by using branched-DNA technology. *J. Clin. Microbiol.* **34** : 901–907.

Doern, G.V., Brueggemann, A.B., Blocker, M. (1998). Clonal relationships among high-level penicillin-resistant *Streptococcus pneumoniae* in the United States. *Clin. Infect. Dis.* **27** : 757–61.

DuPont, H.L. and Steele, J.H. (1987). Use of antimicrobial agents in animal feeds: implications for human health. *Rev. Infect. Dis.* **9** : 447–60.

Falkow, S. (1975). Infectious multiple drug resistance. London : Pion Press.

Fatima-Hannachi, M., Gascoyne-Binzi, D.M., Heritage, J. and Hawkey, P.M. (1996). Detection of mutations conferring extended-spectrum activity on SHV β-lactamases using polymerase chain reaction single strand conformational polymorphism (PCR-SSCP). *J. Antimicrob. Chemother*. **37** : 797–802.

Fluit, A. C., M. E. Jones, F. J. Schmitz, J. Acar, R. Gupta, and J. Verhoef for the Sentry Participants Group. (2000a). Antimicrobial resistance among Urinary Tract Infection (UTI) isolates in Europe: results from the SENTRY Antimicrobial Surveillance Program 1997. Antonie Leeuwenhoek **77** : 147–152.

Fluit, A. C., M. E. Jones, F.-J. Schmitz, J. Acar, R. Gupta, and J. Verhoef for the SENTRY Participants Group. (2000b). Bacteremia in European hospitals, incidence and antimicrobial susceptibility. *Clin. Infect. Dis*. **30** : 454–460.

Fluit, A.C., Visser, M.R. and Schmitz, F.J. (2001). Molecular detection of antimicrobial resistance. *Clin. Microbiol. Rev*. **14** : 836- 71.

Fox, R. (1996). The post-antibiotic era beckons. *J. Res. Social Medi.* **89** : 602-603.

Geha, D.J., Uhl, J.R., Gustafero, C.A. and Persing, D.H. (1994). Multiplex PCR for identification of methicillin-resistant staphylococci in the clinical laboratory. *J. Clin. Microbiol.* **32** : 1768–1772.

Griggs, D.J., Gensberg, K., Piddock, L.J.V. (1996). Mutations in *gyrA* gene of quinolone-resistant *Salmonella* serotypes isolated from humans and animals. *Antimicrob Agents Chemother* **40** : 1009–13.

Heisler, L., Lyamicheva, N. and Olive, D.M. (1996). Detection of mutations related to rifampin resistance using Cleavase® fragment length polymorphism, abstr. U-95, p. 117. *In* Abstracts of the 96th General Meeting of the American Society for Microbiology.

Jacoby, G.H., Bush, K. Amino acid sequences for TEM, SHV, and OXA extended-spectrum and inhibitor-resistant β-lactamases. Available at http://www.lahey.org/studies/webt.htm.

Jorgensen, J.H., Weigel, L.M., Ferraro, M.J. (1999). Activities of newer fluoroquinolones against *Streptococcus pneumoniae* clinical isolates including those with mutations in *gyrA, parC,* and *parE* loci. *Antimicrob Agents Chemother* **43** : 329–34.

Kaldec, R., Zelicoff, A., Vrtis, A. (1997). Biological weapons control: prospects and implications for the future. *J. American Medical Assoc.* **278** : 351-6.

Kapur, V., Li L-L., Hamrick, M.R. (1995). Rapid *Mycobacterium* species assignment and unambiguous identification of mutations associated with antimicrobial resistance in *Mycobacterium tuberculosis* by automated DNA sequencing. *Arch. Pathol. Lab. Med.* **119** : 131–8.

Kapur, V., Li, L.L., Iordanescu, S., Hamrick, M.K., Wanger, A., Kreiswirth, B.N. and Musser. J.M. (1994). Characterization by automated DNA sequencing of mutations in the gene (*rpo*b encoding RNA polymerase b subunit in rifampin-resistant *Mycobacterium tuberculosis* strains from New York City and Texas. *J. Clin. Microbiol.* **32** : 1095–1098.

Kolbert, C.P., Varga-Delmore, P., Arruda, J., Zheng, X., Lewis, M. E., Kolberg, J. and Persing. D. (1998). A novel branched-DNA assay for detection of *mecA* gene in oxacillin-resistant and oxacillin-susceptible staphylococci. *J. Clin. Microbiol.* **36** : 2640–2644.

Levin, B.R., Lipsitch, M., Perrot, V. (1997). The population genetics of antibiotic resistance. *Clin. Infect. Dis.* **24** : S9–16.

Livermore, D.M. (1995). β-lactamases in the clinical laboratory and clinical resistance. *Clin. Microbiol. Rev.* **8** : 557–84.

Medeiros, A.A. (1997). Evolution and dissemination of β-lactamases accelerated by generations of β-lactam antibiotics. *Clin. Infect. Dis.* **24** : S19–45.

Musser, J.M., Kapur, V., Williams, D.L., Kreiswirth, B.N., van Soolingen, D. and Embden. J.D.A. (1996). Characterization of the catalase-peroxidase gene (*katG*) and *inhA* locus in isoniazid-resistant and susceptible strains of *Mycobacterium tuberculosis* by automated DNA sequencing: restricted array of mutations associated with drug resistance. *J. Infect. Dis.* **173** : 196–202.

Nachamkin, I., Kang, C. and Weinstein, M. P. (1997). Detection of resistance to isoniazid, rifampin, and streptomycin in clinical isolates of *Mycobacterium tuberculosis* by molecular methods. *Clin. Infect. Dis.* **24** : 894–900.

Nash, K.A. and Inderlied, C.B. (1996). Rapid detection of mutations associated with macrolide resistance in *Mycobacterium avium* complex. *Antimicrob. Agents Chemother.* **40** : 1748–1750.

Neu, H. (1992). The crisis in antibiotic resistance. *Sci.* **257** : 1064-73.

Neuwirth, C., Siebor, E., Lopez, J. (1996). Outbreak of TEM-24–producing *Enterobacter aerogenes* in an intensive care unit and dissemination of the extended-spectrum β-lactamase to other members of the family *Enterobacteriaceae. J. Clin. Microbiol.* **34** : 76–9.

Nicolle, L.E., Bentley, D., Garibaldi, R. (1996). Antimicrobial use in long term care facilities. *Infect. Control Hosp. Epidemiol.* **17** : 119–28.

Nüesch-Inderbinen, M.T., Hächer, H. and Kayser, F.H. (1996). Detection of genes coding for extended-spectrum SHV beta-lactamases in clinical isolates by a molecular genetic method, and comparison with the E-test. Eur. *J. Clin. Microbiol. Infect. Dis.* **15** : 398–402.

Patel, R., Uhl, J., Kohner, P., Hopkins, M.K. and Cockerill III F.R. (1997). Multiplex PCR detection of *vanA, vanB, vanC-1,* and *vanC-2/3* in enterococci. *J. Clin. Microbiol.* **35** : 703–707.

Piatek, A.S., Tyagi, S., Pol, A.C., Telenti, A., Miller, L.P., Kramer, F.R. and Alland, D. (1998). Molecular beacon sequence analysis for detecting drug resistance in *Mycobacterium tuberculosis*. *Nat. Biotech.* **16** : 359–363.

Rossau, R., Traore, H., De Beenouwer, H., Mijs, W., Jannes, G., DeRijk, P. and Portaels, F. (1997). Evaluation of the INNO-LiPA Rif. TB assay, a reverse hybridization assay for the simultaneous detection of *Mycobacterium tuberculosis* complex and its resistance to rifampin. Antimicrob. Agents Chemother. **41** : 2093–2098.

Saiki, R.K., Gelfand, D.H., Stoffel, S., Scharf, S.J., Higuchi, R., Horn, G.T., Mullis, K.B. and Erlich, H.A. (1988). Primer – directed enzymatic amplification of DNA with a thermostable DNA Polymerase. *Sci.* **239** : 487-491.

Stuyver, L., Rossau, R., Wyseur, A., Duhamel, M., Vanderborght, B., Heuverswyn, H. and Maertens, G. (1993). Typing of hepatitis C virus isolates and characterization of new subtypes using a line probe assay. *J. Gen. Virol.* **74** : 1093–1102.

Telenti, A., Honore, N., Bernasconi, C. (1997). Genotypic assessment of isoniazid and rifampin resistance in *Mycobacterium tuberculosis* : a blind study at reference laboratory level. *J. Clin. Microbiol.* **35** : 719–23.

Tenovar, F.C. (2001). Development and spread of bacterial resistance to antimicrobial agents: an overview. *Clin. Infect. Dis.* **33** : 5108-5115.

Tenover, F.C., Hughes, J.M. (1996). The challenges of emerging infectious diseases: development and spread of multiple resistant bacterial pathogens. *JAMA* **275** : 300–304.

Tomasz, A. (1994). Multiple-antibiotic resistant pathogenic bacteria. A report on the Rockefeller University workshop. *New England J. Med.* **330** : 1247-51.

Tompkins, L.S., Plorde, J.J., Falkow, S. (1980). Molecular analysis of R factors from multiresistant nosocomial isolates. *J. Infect. Dis.* **141** : 625–31.

Trieu-Cuot, P., Gerbaud, G., Lambert, T.(1985). In vivo transfer of genetic information between gram-negative and gram-positive bacteria. *EMBO J* **4** : 3583–3587.

Tyagi, S., Bratu, D.P. and Kramer, F.R. (1998). Multicolor beacons for allele discrimination. *Nat. Biotech.* **16** : 49–53.

Wallet, F., Roussel-Delvallez, M. and Courcol, R.J. (1996). Choice of a routine method for detecting methicillin resistance in staphylococci. *J. Antimicrob. Chemother.* **37** : *901–909.*

Williams, D.L., Spring, L., Gillis, T.P., Salfinger, M. and Persing, D.H. (1998). Evaluation of a Polymerase chain reaction-based universal heteroduplex generator assay for direct detection of rifampin susceptibility of *Mycobacterium tuberculosis* from sputum specimens. *Clin. Infect. Dis.* **26** : 446–450.

World Health Organization (2000). Overcoming antimicrobial resistance. Geneva. Switzerland 2000.

22

ANTIBIOTIC RESIDUES : DATA SHEET OF INDIA

A.M. Paturkar and R.J. Zende

Antimicrobial drugs are being used in veterinary medicine to treat or prevent diseases for more than five decades. Antibiotics are substances produced by microorganisms that are able to kill or inhibit the growth of other microorganisms. The term antimicrobials include both substances produced synthetically and by microorganisms. There are a range of antimicrobial drugs for different uses, for e.g. antibiotics to treat, prevent and control bacterial diseases, coccidiostats to control protozoal diseases particularly in poultry and anthelmintics to control internal parasites and to enhance animal growth and feed conversion efficiency. Currently, approximately 80% of all food-producing animals receive medication for part or most of their lives, 42% of all veterinary pharmaceuticals are used as feed additives, 19% are used to treat various ailments and 13% as parasiticides. The most commonly used antimicrobials in food animals can be grouped in six major classes' *viz.* α-lactams, tetracyclines, aminoglycosides, macrolides, quinolones and sulphonamides. Antimicrobials are administered to animals by injections (intravenously, intramuscularly, or subcutaneously), orally in feed or water, topically on the skin, by intramammary and intrauterine infusions and antimicrobial supplemented feeds. Theoretically, all these routes may lead to appearance of residues in foods of animal origin such as milk, meat and eggs. The withdrawal period is set out in the data sheet for the medicine and in the instructions for use which are part of the product packaging. The use of antimicrobial drugs and appearances of antimicrobial residues in foods are monitored by regulatory authorities at national or regional level with the help of government legislations to facilitate trade and for the protection of human and animal health. The datasheets for antimicrobial drug residues are generated in a structured approach through continuous monitoring and surveillance programmes at national or regional levels which reflects the trends and patterns of antimicrobial use in food animals and appearance of residues in animal origin foods.

ANTIMICROBIAL RESIDUES AND REASONS FOR ITS OCCURRENCE IN FOODS OF ANIMAL ORIGIN

Antibiotic residues are defined as "pharmacologically active substances (whether active principles, excipients or degradation products) and their metabolites which remain in foodstuffs obtained from animals to which the veterinary drug has been administered".

The question of biological significance of antimicrobial residues has been debated for over 20 years and remains the subject of considerable scientific and political activity. Before a medicine can be authorised for animals, it has to undergo rigorous and extensive testing. Even with rationalized use of antimicrobial preparations, their residues appear in the animal products. The residues can result from any of the following:

1. The most likely cause of violative drug residues is the failure to observe withdrawal periods. There is often a lack of veterinary advice regarding withdrawal periods and this may be compounded by illiteracy, making labeling and printed instructions for drugs of limited use.

2. Improper maintenance of treatment records or failure to identify treated animals adequately and traceability is often impossible which may lead to their occurrence.

3. Faecal recycling, where the drug excreted in faeces of treated animals contaminates the feed of untreated animals, can be the cause of residues of certain antimicrobial group.
4. For resource-poor farmers, the fear of economic loss may prompt the slaughter of casualty animals for food that received treatment and not recovered.
5. Violative drug residues can also occur as a result of improper use of a licensed product or through the illegal use of an unlicensed substance. Extra label dosages and use of drugs which have not been approved for the species in question by unqualified person or para-veterinary field staff may lead to violative residues.

MAXIMUM RESIDUE LIMIT (MRL)

The standards for antibiotic residues in food are known as Maximum Residue Limits (MRLs). It is the maximum concentration of residue following administration of a veterinary medicine which is legally permitted or acceptable in food under the laws. MRLs are established when an antibiotic is registered and approved for use in animals. MRLs will not be approved for any chemical where the residues could represent an unacceptable risk to public health and safety.

MRLs are adopted into central and state legislation and assist government health authorities in regulating the use of antibiotics. In addition, food legislation makes it illegal for food to be sold if it contains residues in excess of MRLs. The use of antibiotics and other pharmacologically active substances and their tolerance limits in foods are regulated by Prevention of Food Adulteration (PFA) Act (1954) and Rules (1955) in India.

STATUS OF ANTIBIOTIC RESIDUES IN FOODS OF ANIMAL ORIGIN IN INDIA

The Status of antibiotic residues in foods for a developing country is given in the form of data sheets. They contain authentic information regarding the trends in use of different antimicrobial drugs in food animals, their MRLs in foods, number of cases of recall or rejection of animal origin foods containing violative levels of drug residues, the type of foods involved, the levels of different antimicrobial drug residues detected and the economic losses due to recall or rejection of food lots in trade and the public health impact due to consumption of such foods which contain violative drug residues.

There is no national datasheet available for antibiotic residues in foods of animal origin in India. The reason for this is there is no continuous monitoring and surveillance program for veterinary drug residues at national and/or regional levels. Where as most of the developed countries have a continuous monitoring and surveillance program for veterinary drug residues at a national level and datasheets are available for antibiotic residues in foods of animal origin. In India, the detection and analysis of drug residues in foods is mainly restricted to export purpose and academic research. Implementation of national level residues monitoring and surveillance programme is the need of the hour and continued to be an important area in generating data sheet for the nation. Residue Monitoring Plans are implemented by the Export Inspection Agencies (EIAs) of Govt. of India in the dairy, poultry and egg sectors intended for export to European countries. During 2007-08, a total number of 618 samples were tested. During 2008-09, 1275 samples were tested for the entire range of residues from pesticides, antibiotics, heavy metals to other chemicals as required by the European Commission.

A survey on veterinary drug use and residues in milk was carried out by Sudershan, R.V. and Bhat, R.V. (1995) in Hyderabad (India) and surrounding suburban villages. Of 205 milk samples analysed, 9% of market samples and 73% of individual animal milk samples contained oxytetracycline residues. None of the government dairy samples contained oxytetracycline residues. D. Narahari and R. Amutha (2008) found that chloramphenicol was by far the most studied antibiotic as a residue in eggs. It could persist in yolk for up to

66 days, depending on the dosage. Sulphadimidine and arsanilic acid have been found as residues in egg albumen. Surveillance of muscle and organ samples of ovine and caprine for the presence of residues of gentamicin sulfate by HPLC was carried out by Barge *et al.* (2006) 5.56% samples showed violative amounts of gentamicin residues in muscle and organ samples of sheep and goat.

Processing of milk will help in inactivation of antibiotics like refrigeration causes disappearance of penicillin and in pasteurization most of antibiotics will loose their activity. Use of activated charcoal, resin and UV irradiation also help for antibiotic inactivation.

DEVELOPING A MONITORING AND SURVEILLANCE PROGRAMME FOR ANTIMICROBIAL DRUG RESIDUES IN ANIMAL ORIGIN FOODS IN INDIA

In recent years, the issue of veterinary drug residues in animal-derived foods has become increasingly important in many developing countries especially India. Concerns over veterinary drug usage and residues are primarily related to food safety and the possibility of the development of antibiotic resistant pathogens, but the main impetus behind the increased interest of government is the need to meet requirements for international trade. The ultimate outcome is an increase in foreign exchange and a contribution to the alleviation of poverty. The continuing development of international networks and collaboration between developed and developing countries must be actively promoted to progress towards the goal of a safe food supply.

PROBLEMS IN IMPLEMENTATION

Developing countries like India face many difficulties when planning to implement a residue control programme. However, with assistance from the developed world, the problems are not insurmountable. Several of the projects implemented by the FAO/IAEA have resulted in accredited (ISO/IEC 17025) screening laboratories and national plans being put in place, with a consequent positive impact on food quality and the ability to participate in international trade.

Infrastructure Limitations

With limited resources and personnel it is impossible for laboratories in many developing countries to meet the criteria set out for confirmatory analysis in EU Commission. The specific technical problems encountered in developing country laboratories are difficulties with supply of laboratory materials, analytical standards and reference materials, sourcing of analytical equipment and availability of local servicing and consumables. Scientific literature is not readily available and methodologies may not be available in the local language. Poor laboratory conditions such as high temperatures, unstable power supplies and inadequate safety facilities can adversely affect performance.

Training

It is difficult to recruit and retain specialised scientific staff in developing countries and there are few training opportunities. IAEA provides training through a number of mechanisms. Fellowships are arranged in established residues laboratories. Expert missions are also provided, the experts recruited being experienced scientists who can adapt the training to conditions in the counterpart laboratory and can provide a wider range of expertise if the need arises. Several international workshops and training programs have been organized. It is of key importance that the information flow is bilateral, so that the consultants from developed countries gain a better understanding of the problems and needs of the developing countries.

Guidelines

There is also confusion with respect to guidelines such as maximum residue limits (MRLs) and method validation. The EU sampling strategy and MRLs may differ from those set by Codex, which is intended to be used as a point of reference in trade disputes under the Sanitary and Phytosanitary Standards Agreement of the World Trade Organization (WTO). These differences can have a significant effect on developing country trade. For example, it is estimated that if Codex MRLs were adopted for tetracyclines, global trade in beef would increase by over $3.2 billion. It is usually difficult with the resources available to test for the complete range of compounds set out in European council directive. An approach must be defined to prioritise these substances in the development of a National Plan. One possibility is that the focus should be on compounds that have caused most disruption in international trade, for example prohibited compounds such as nitrofuran metabolites and chloramphenicol.

There is an urgent need to establish accredited laboratories for conducting continuous antibiotic residues screening tests and confirmatory analysis at different levels of food supply chain at regional levels. These laboratories can be coordinated through a national network to generate a national datasheet for veterinary drug residues in foods of animal origin in India which would help policy makers in formulating national guidelines/acts and implementing suitable control measures to prevent their occurrence in foods. This project can be undertaken in a manner similar to that of Pesticide residues monitoring programme at a national level which is in progress.

DIFFERENT TESTS USED FOR DETECTION AND QUANTITATION OF ANTIMICROBIAL RESIDUES

There are two main categories of analytical methods for antimicrobial residues. They are screening test methods and confirmatory test methods. Screening tests are generally qualitative and some are semi quantitative. They are designed to give a positive or negative result to indicate whether antibiotic residues are present or not in the foods. These methods neither identify the specific antibiotic residues present nor indicate antibiotic residues at a level above MRL. They are easy to perform, more rapid and relatively inexpensive. Confirmatory tests are performed for detection and quantitation of the drug residues accurately and used for comparing with MRLs and certification in international trade. Well trained scientific staffs in the area of drug residue analysis and highly sophisticated laboratories with modern analytical instruments and chemicals are required to perform these tests. High cost is involved in performing such tests. Screening test methods are of different types :

Tests Based on Acid Production

One of the earliest methods for detection of antibiotic residues in milk based on acid production by employing different cultures like *Streptococcus agalactiae, Streptococcus lactis, Lactobacillus bulgaricus* and active starter cultures and incubated at 37 °C and checked for colour development thus, indicating presence or absence of antibiotic residues. These tests were used in 1950-60's.

Tests Based on Reduction of Dyes

These tests are based on the principle that the dye reducing bacteria like *S. thermophilus, B. thermophilus* and *B. stearothermophilus* in milk fail to do so in the presence of residual antibiotics. Different dyes like methylene blue, resazurin and 2, 3, 5 Triphenyl tetrazollum chloride (TTC) were used for this purpose.

MICROBIAL INHIBITION TESTS

Nowadays, these tests are commonly used for screening antibiotic residues in foods.

Disk Assay

A disk of absorbent paper impregnated with the sample is placed on the surface of an agar medium which is inoculated with *B. stearothermophilus* var. *culidolactis*. Sample is heated to 32 °C for 2 min in order to destroy the natural inhibitory substances present in the sample. After a period of incubation, the presence of inhibitory substances in the sample is indicated by a clear zone around the disk. The size of the clear zone depends on the concentration and type of inhibitory substances present in the milk. Bulk tank samples are considered positive if a zone of inhibition exceeds 16 mm.

Delvo Test P

This test measures the growth inhibition of *B. stearothermophilus* var. *culidolactis* in a solid medium. The contents of the test organism ampule are mixed with a nutrient tablet. An aliquot (0.1 ml) of the milk sample is then combined with the mixture. The mixture is incubated for two and half hours at 54 °C and a colour reaction occurs based on a pH change in the medium. A yellowish colour indicates a negative reaction and purple colour indicates a positive reaction in the test sample.

Charm Inhibitory Assay

In this test *B. stearothermophilus* and a specially formulated agar medium is used. The antimicrobial substance in the milk sample inhibits microbial sporulation and growth, which results in reduced acid production. The pH Indicator changes from blue to greenish yellow, if the milk does not contain any inhibitory substance and it remains blue if milk contains inhibitory substances.

Fast Antibiotic Screen Test (FAST)

This test is used by USDA-FSIS and provides results within 6 hours. FAST growth medium contains sugar and a purple colour dye. Bacterial metabolism of the sugar results in acid production and a lowering of pH that causes a colour change from purple to yellow.

Frontier Post Test (FPT)

Qualitative and semi quantitative studies of antibiotic residues in meat and eggs were conducted by using this test. Optimal temperature for FPT is 37 °C and the reaction time after loading samples is 16 hours. The results of residual antibiotics determined by FPT were found similar with HPLC method.

Premi Test

It is a broad spectrum antimicrobial screening test which gives a reliable results within 4 hours. It is based on the inhibition of growth of *B. stearothermophilus.* A standard number of spores are imbedded in an agar medium with selected nutrients. An indicator dye is incorporated to show the growth of bacteria and colour change from purple to yellow colour.

IMMUNOLOGICAL METHODS

This assay format uses the binding of an antibiotic (the antigen) by an antibody. The category of the test system measures competitive interaction between drugs and sample contents. Various tests include:

Radio Immuno Assay (RIA)

One commonly used immunological method is RIA. Typically this test system uses specific antiserum or monoclonal antibody which provides the binding sites and an antibiotics tracer. The drug in the sample competes with the tracer or binding sites. After removal of the free (unbound) trace, the antibody tracer complex is counted. The more antibody tracer bound, the less antibiotic present in the sample.

β-Lactam LacTek

This assay system is based on immuno binding principle of the ELISA system. It uses a α-lactam specific antibody. The concentration of antibiotic in the milk is determined by comparing the optical density of each sample tube with that of test kit standard. The results are positive for the presence of α-lactam if the colour reaction of the sample is less than that of the assay standard.

Charm II Receptor Assay

This reaction assay is based on the binding reaction between the antibiotic function groups and the receptor or binding on or with added microbial cells. Antibiotic tracers

(C_{14} or H_3) compete with the drug present in the sample for binding site. Binding is measured by scintillation counter and is compared with standard antibiotic present in milk. The greater the amount of antibiotic present in the sample, the lower the count detected by the equipment.

ENZYMATIC ASSAY

Penzyme Test

This assay format is based on the development of a reddish orange colour which is produced by reaction of streptomyces DD-carboxy peptidase with synthetic oligo peptide containing D-alanine. If the milk sample contains certain substances that interfere with this reaction, the development of reddish orange colour is inhibited and yellow indicates a positive assay results.

DIFFERENT CONFIRMATORY TESTS

The methods require costly equipments, trained manpower and for each group you have to standardize and validate the method separately.

High Performance Liquid Chromatography (HPLC)

HPLC methods can be used for detection of antimicrobials from meat, milk, egg and egg products and their byproducts.

Gas Chromatography (GC)

For GC, the mixtures should be in volatile state for the separation of the components within the operating range of temperature of the instrument. The separated components are classified according to their relation times or by chromatographing spiked samples.

Liquid Chromatography-Mass Spectrometry (LC-MS)

These employ liquid mobile phases, sometimes containing inorganic salts. Materials of high relative molecular mass are readily separated by liquid chromatography. The separated components of the analyte are transferred to the mass spectrometer without interference from the solvent by ionization methods that produce less fragmentation in the mass spectrometer. The interface between the liquid chromatograph and the mass spectrometer is most vital part of the combined instrument.

ACCREDITATION AND QUALITY ASSURANCE

It is becoming essential that laboratories undertaking such analytical work should be accredited to standards as ISO/IEC 17025 or EN 45001. This requires laboratories to submit to inspection by the National Accreditation Body (NABL in India), have the methodology and its performance agreed, and thereafter ensure that the standard laid down is maintained. This requires the formal noting of all essential data associated with analytical work, keeping of training records of staff and maintenance and standardization records for all equipments. All these information is subjected to internal and external audit several times a year. This is desirable to the laboratories taking part in performance assessment schemes wherever possible to ensure that their analytical capability can be measured against other laboratories when analyzing standard or reference material. In the veterinary drug field, the Food Analysis Performance Assessment Scheme (FAPAS) provides such material.

Export Inspection Council (EIC) of India is concentrating on strengthening the capabilities of its laboratories with new equipments including Atomic Absorption Spectrophotometer (AAS), High Performance Liquid Chromatography (HPLC), Inductively Coupled Plasma Mass Spectrometry (ICPMS), Gas Chromatography Mass Spectrometry (GCMS), Gas Chromatography High Resolution Mass Spectrometry (GCHRMS) etc. depending on the requirements. Laboratories of EIC at Chennai, Mumbai, Kochi and Kolkata have implemented system of ISO 17025 and have been accredited by National Accreditation Board for Testing and Calibration Laboratories (NABL).

FUTURE PERSPECTIVES

The transmission of veterinary drug residues through foods of animal origin is in alarming rate but it has not been given necessary coverage primarily due to lack of infrastructure in detection of harmful residues as well as lack of monitoring and periodic surveillance system. So establishment of NABL accredited laboratories in each state for testing drug residues and a national level drug residues monitoring and surveillance programme should be the first priority.

This has necessitated the development of simple and economic field test to identify drug residue in edible animal products at the slaughter house level and prohibition of food containing antibiotics more than MRL. For this, the screening tests should be sufficiently sensitive to monitor the MRL and produce low incidence of results and almost zero false negative results while the confirmatory methods should be very sensitive and specific to measure very small amounts of residues.

The next most obvious development is that of multi residue detection methods. Presently, either single drug or single drug class are analyzed, but it is possible to develop methodology that will cope with multiple classes of drugs. At least, common extraction and clean up procedures should be first goal even if the final extracts are dealt with separately. This will reduce the time consuming aspect of the analytical methods.

Irrational use of antibiotics in field veterinary practices should be avoided. Ethno-veterinary practices may be promoted. Educational programmes and awareness campaigns targeted at farmers and para veterinary staff on the correct and appropriate use of veterinary drugs can help avoid many of these scenarios.

23

INDIAN MEAT INDUSTRY : CURRENT SCENARIO AND FUTURE POTENTIAL

B.D. Sharma

LIVESTOCK RESOURCE

India has the largest livestock population in the world. There are 176 million cattle, 98 million buffaloes, 64 million sheep, 125 million goats and 14 million pigs and 560 million chickens in the country (FAO, 2007). Livestock sector is an important contributor to the income and employment of large number of rural people of India. Presently, the share of livestock sector is as much as 25% of the total share of agricultural GDP, which is poised to increase further.

Our country shares about 56% of the buffaloes and nearly 15% each of cattle and goat population of the world. India ranks first in buffalo and third in sheep and goat population in the world. The contribution of livestock to the national economy is estimated to be over 11%. Livestock output as a percentage of agricultural output comes to around 26%. National sample survey has reported that in India livestock activities are carried out by over 90% of small cultivators and low wage earners to supplement their income. This is in contrast to the concept of large sized livestock farms in the developed countries. It is also noteworthy that 75% of our livestock population does not conform to the specific breed characteristics and has significantly reduced their production potential.

For a long time, meat industry has remained confined to a very small section of people in our country. These people had little knowledge of clean meat production and effective utilization of valued slaughterhouse byproducts. The scene is now changing. However, industry is still largely based on spent animals except for pig and farm poultry. Most animals are utilized for meat production after loosing their economic viability in the primary field. Cow (not bullock) slaughter is banned in India except in West Bengal and Kerala. The concept of meat type animals is yet to take roots in our country, although an awakening in this regard is discernible. Of late, particularly due to export potential, buffalo is emerging as a prospective meat animal. Meat industry provides direct and indirect employment to nearly 1.9 crore people at present and contributes to 16% of the income from entire livestock sector.

MEAT PRODUCTION

Meat is an important livestock product, which in its widest sense includes all those parts of the animals that are used as a food by man. Though meat has a very high biological value, its production and processing has always been the subject of social prejudice. This factor has adversely affected the growth of meat industry. In many cases, social resistance and ignorance have resulted in inordinate delay and deferment of abattoir modernization schemes. An important milestone in this area was the establishment of a modern abattoir at Bombay in 1973. Further, in the Fourth Five Year Plan, eight bacon factories were established with the foreign assistance. A few meat corporations were also formed to take up the development of slaughter houses.

Table 23.1 shows the population and meat production figures of our traditional million poultry are slaughtered annually yielding 6.3 million tonnes of meat. It may be noted that nearly 42.8% is contributed by the cattle and buffaloes in contrast to 12% by sheep and goats. Nearly, 99% pig population is slaughtered annually contributing 7.6% of the total meat production. Poultry with a population of 560 million contributes 2.2 million tonnes of meat (34 % of total meat production). There has been an impressive rise in the share of poultry meat during the last decade.

Table 23.1 : Livestock Population, Meat Production and Their Percentage Share in India

Species	*Population (Million)*	*Meat Production (Lakh Tonnes)*	*% Share*
Buffaloes	98.7	14.98	23.1
Cattle	176.5	12.82	19.7
Sheep	64.2	2.34	3.6
Goats	125.4	5.43	8.4
Pigs	14	4.97	7.6
Chicken	560	22.40	34.4

Source : FAO-2007

The traditional form of meat industry is characterized by unorganized sector in the hands of butcher-workers with very little knowledge of personnel hygiene. At present, there are 3600 licensed slaughter houses in the country. A large number of them are outdated and substandard according to the present production and processing technology specifications. These slaughter houses operate as service abattoirs where butchers slaughter the animals for a fee and both edible and non-edible parts of the carcasses are delivered to the butchers. Most of them need modernization with facilities for lairage, slaughter hall, chilling room, rendering plant etc; while it is imperative to have all these facilities in big cities, a semi-modern approach with mechanical hoist facility is the workable proposition for medium and small sized towns.

Eight new projects on modern mechanized abattoirs were initiated in 1990-91. In the Eighth Plan, five private sector export abattoirs became functional during the last decade, and ten modern abattoir complexes have come up in public sector. An equal number have come up in private sector also. The developmental activities are necessary to improve the image of the Indian meat sector.

WORLD SCENE

Although, the Indian meat industry is in developing phase, but it is the top food industry in the world. An analysis of world meat scenario reveals that Europe leads in production followed by Asia. Developed continents (N. America, Europe and Oceania) contribute about 60% to total meat production but they have a monopoly in meat exports as their share was as high as 84%. Nearly 55% of all world meat exports are being shared by European countries alone. The share of Asia in world meat export is very low (6.5%) but it is on the rise as evident in Table 23.2.

Table 23.2 : Producton of Meat in India and Share in World (2004)

Countries	*Production ('000 Tonnes)*		*Share in World (%)*	
	1999-2001	2004	1999-2001	2004
China	62833	74306	26.77	28.57
USA	37567	38891	16.01	14.95
Brazil	15332	19919	6.53	7.66
Germany	6377	6798	2.72	2.61
France	6538	6255	2.79	2.40
India	5272	6032	2.25	2.32
Australia	3743	3769	1.6	1.45
UK	3476	3270	1.48	1.26

India rank 6th in world meat production, but it is disheartening to note that India with a vast raw material base, contributes barely 2.3% to the world meat production. Our share in the export of meat is also of the same magnitude. The export of meat from India mainly comprises of fresh chilled meat, frozen meat and frozen meat products. A major chunk of meat exports amounting to Rs. 3213.74 crores is contributed by buffalo meat (2007). Vietnam, Malaysia, Bangladesh and UAE are the principal importers of buffalo meat from India. However, Indian exports of meat constitutes barely 2% of global export of this commodity. A great potential exists for exporting buffalo meat, beef and poultry in view of increased demand in gulf countries and higher cost of meat from developed countries. India has additional advantage of geographic proximity to gulf countries. There is an urgent need to tap the world meat export market by establishing modern and hygienic slaughter houses with chilling facilities solely for export purposes.

If the quality of Indian meat is strictly controlled, the country may boost its meat exports by selling to developing Asian, African and Latin American countries which is about 25% of the world meat exports. These measures will also help in fetching better prices for our produce which is nearly 30% lower than the average world meat export price.

PROCESSED MEAT INDUSTRY

Most of the meat produced in the country is sold by the retail butcher shops to the consumers as fresh hot meat (unchilled). This meat is then cooked in the households in many different ways depending on their taste and preferences. A very small proportion-less than 3% is sold as processed meat. The production of processed meat products in the organized sector got a fillip with the establishment of bacon factories in the Fourth Plan. These bacon factories stimulated the establishment of many processing units in those' areas. Nearly 220 licensed manufacturers under MFPO (1973) produce 22,000 tonnes of processed meat which comprises 50% cured products, 20% sausages and 20% canned products. Our production figures are in sharp contrast to developed countries where 65 to 80% of the total meat produced is sold in the processed form. Lately, Indian dynamics are changing in favour of processed meat products especially in big cities.

A look at the utilization pattern of meat in India will reveal that almost 90% of the meat is hot processed at home as per traditional methods. Nearly 8% of the production (mostly buffalo meat) is exported whereas only 2% is converted into value added meat products.

Table 23.3 : Export of meat from India (2006-2007)

	Quantity (Tonnes)	*Values (Rs. In Crores)*
Buffalo meat	494506.3	3213.74
Sheep/Goat meat	5777.53	65.87
Poultry Products	711245	318.17
Processed Meat	660.69	7.13
Total	1211290	3604.91

Major Export Destinations

Buffalo Meat : Malaysia,Vietnam, UAE, Quatar, Germany, Oman.

Sheep/Goat Meat : Saudi Arabia, UAE, Oman, Baharain and UK.

Processed Meat : Vietnam, Russia, Turkey, Scychelles, Ghana.

Poultry Products : Kuwait, UAE, Oman, Saudi Arabia, Japan, Denmark.

Several traditional meat products like *meat kabab, chicken biryani, tandoori chicken, meat curry* etc. are popular in the non-vegetarian population for a long time. Some other foods products adopted in meat like meat *samosa, meat tikka, meat kofta, meat pickle* etc. have been able to create an impact on the urban consumer. Various region-specific meat products like *Nihari* (Delhi), Goa sausage (Goa), Pork pickle (Himachal Pradesh), *Yakini and Gustaba* (Kashmir), *Rapka* (Arunachal Pradesh) etc. have good acceptability in their traditional consumers.

Western type meat products like cured ham, bacon, sausages, frankfurters, hot dog, meat patties, burgers, luncheon meat and loaves, liver paste etc. have good demand in cities. Eight bacon factories, five meat corporations and a fairly good number of MFPO licensees in private sector have taken up the production of a wide range of these products. They are catering to the requirements of defence, restaurants and household consumers. Canned meat products are relatively new entrants in the domestic market and are primarily being manufactured for defence supplies. The prices of canned meat is comparatively high rendering them beyond the reach of common consumers, although their presence can be noticed in the departmental stores in the metropolitan cities.

Animal protein consumption is lowest in India, even lower than the low income countries. This is mainly due to lower consumption of meat. National Institute of Nutrition has recommended per capita nutritional requirement of 12.4 kg meat per year, whereas the present per capita availability is only 5.5 kg meat. It points to the very high potential for growth of livestock and poultry sector in the country.

Processed meat products are poised for continuous growth in the country. In big cities, there is an ever increasing demand for 'heat and serve' and 'ready to eat' convenience or fast foods. These are delicious, nutritious and if required, easy to carry home. The growth of fast food parlours and restaurants is attributed to the rapid urbanization, changing life styles and upwards in the number of women entering the outdoor work force. It may be pointed out that increase in consumption of value added processed meat products are closely linked with increase in disposable income and growth of urbanization. Thus convenience type meat products are going to have spectacular growth in the coming years. Due to nutritional awareness and liberal food habits of the newer generation, the adoption of western type products with indigenous flavour profiles is bound to take place at a rapid rate.

ESTABLISHMENT OF NATIONAL MEAT AND POULTRY PROCESSING BOARD (NMPPB)

Meat and poultry processing industry has enormous economic potential and nutrition as well as employment significance. There is a considerable scope for increasing the production and export of meat and poultry products in our country. The issues of meat sectors were discussed at length with various stake holders and the need for setting up a professional and industry driven focal point organization was realized by the Ministry of Food Processing Industries in the 11th Five Year Plan. It was contemplated that National Meat and Poultry Processing Board would take an integrated approach to the development of meat sector and drive the sector forward in a professional manner. The Board will have sufficient autonomy, authority and empowerment to take the required actions to revitalize the meat sector in India. It will act as interface between industry and government.

NMPPB will be initially funded from the grant provided by MOFPI. For the first five years, the Board will work under the Chairmanship of Secretary, MOFPI.

MAIN OBJECTIVES

1. Helping the meat industry to establish viable new/ modern slaughter houses, slaughter house byproducts plants.
2. Set up Quality Control and analytical laboratories for meat and meat products.
3. Promoting GMP (Good Manufacturing Practices), HACCP (Hazard Analysis and Critical Control Points) and ISO-9001 in meat production to ensure food quality as well as safety and training all stakeholders.
4. Collaborating with other, like Ministries, Departments, NGO's and private sector for improving backward and forward linkages.
5. Work as a Central National hub to address all issues related to Meat and Poultry Sector.

CONCLUSION

Processed convenience and value added meat and poultry products sector has a very good potential in the country due to :

- Increase in double income families.
- Increase in disposable income.
- Less time availability for cooking.

At present India has a large population of over 250 million economically strong consumers having an adequate purchasing power for buying food, as a result of which the domestic demand for the livestock and poultry product is poised for rapid growth.

We must strive to export processed meat products rather than live animals and fresh meat. There is a need to study the consumption pattern of meat products in importing countries, so that we can tailor our products according to their requirements a shift from primary products to value added products besides fetching more profits will decrease the transportation cost and generate more employment. It will also encourage more efficient utilization of meat byproducts.

24

INDIAN DAIRY SCENARIO AND ITS IMPACT ON GLOBAL MARKETING

B.V. Venkateshaiah, G. Leena, H. Arunkumar, B. Sharanagouda and B.M Veeregowda

Agriculture is the backbone of Indian economy. Livestock and fishery are promising sub-sectors in the agricultural sector which have substantial growth prospects and presently accounting for 29.9 per cent of agricultural GDP and 6.29 per cent of total GDP of India as per the Government of India Report, 2005, besides, providing employment to around 19 million people. According to the 17th livestock census, crossbred cattle constituted 13.3 per cent of total cattle, of which, 86.7 per cent are indigenous cattle. India ranks first in the worlds milk production, the annual milk production in India is estimated about 108 million tons. This was achieved due largely to the bovine population of 283 million (185 millions cattle and 98 millions buffaloes) and its strong wide spread milk procurement system established by NDDB, through the operation flood programme, comprising of 15 state federations, 177 District unions and 1,28,799 village cooperative societies. Further, India is the second in goat and third in sheep population. It is one among the top five chicken-producing countries and among the top six egg-producing countries in the world.

In India's export earnings, livestock, poultry and related products amounts to Rs. 5120 crores, of which, Rs. 1720 crores emanated from meat and meat products. The demand for livestock products is increasing at a high rate in the domestic market. Simultaneously, the demand for value-added livestock products is also increasing in the international trade. In this context, analyzing the trends, opportunities and challenges of the marketing of livestock and livestock products in the domestic market as well as international market has a vital importance.

Besides this, the livestock sector also plays a significant role in the upliftment of rural people by means of additional income and employment. At times of crop failure or during drought situations, dairy offers an important and only viable livelihood option for the rural masses. The dairy sector alone engages nearly 70 million people, whereas nearly 5 million people are engaged in sheep and goat-rearing activities. The poultry sector, one of the important components of the livestock sector, contributes nearly Rs.260 billion to the national income of India by providing gainful employment to three million people.

The livestock sector can contribute a major share to the growing Indian economy and marketing has to play a vibrant and proactive role in exploring the potential of this sector. Domestic consumption of milk is estimated to grow to reach a level of 100 million tonnes in 2020, while during 2003-04, it amounted to only 88 million tonnes. Fourteen percent of total global milk production is accounted by India, while yield per animal is very low, due to inadequate nutrients. Seventy percent of dairy farm holding of 100 million in India is accounted for by small and marginal farmers. The contribution of Indian milk production can be increased by technological intervention, improved feed management and capacity building of the dairy farmers to make the dairy sector more lucrative.

Further, the combined effects of both domestic reforms and WTO commitments have transformed the Indian dairy industry from a predominantly sustenance-oriented economy to a market-oriented economy. India escapes the WTO provisions for domestic support or subsidies for the dairy sub-sector. The comparison of average Terms of Trade (ToT) values of dairy products shows that the price ratio (export price/import price) is higher in the pre-liberalization period than the post-liberalization period. There is a need to increase the processing efficiency of the Indian dairy industry to bring down the manufacturing cost of milk products.

LAUNCH OF NATIONAL MILK VISION

As envisaged in the India vision 2020, particularly for Milk, there is a need to launch a National Milk Vision, as a variant of White revolution. The implementation of this mission will empower the farmers and will certainly put India on the high yielding milk map, also brings sustainable development in the rural area enriching the agriculture, animal husbandry and food processing, creating value added employment opportunities to the 60 million families. The second green revolution can be hastened up by this National Milk Vision, because it will act as feeder channel and result into a economic multiplier for the nation especially during the recession. The 'National Milk Vision' is to be launched in an integrated manner to address the areas such as cattle breeding, feed and nutrition, cattle healthcare, farm management, milk procurement and transportation.

Cattle Breeding

It is essential to have a progressive national level breeding policy and make the consistent policies at the state level to enhance the input to output (feed to milk) ratio. The major technology implemented and tried so are cross-breeding through Artificial Insemination (AI), Embryo Transfer (ET) and development of transgenic animals. It is necessary to enhance and enrich the number of semen banks, properly trained manpower, infrastructure for monitoring blood levels of cross-breed cows and availability of good quality and proven bulls. There is also a need to add more than 30,000 AI centers before the 11th plan period. In order to active the progress, it may be established in Public Private Partnership mode to provide efficient door-step quality breeding services to farmers.

Feed and Nutrition

Feed accounts for almost 60 per cent of the cost inputs for milk production and has a direct bearing on the yield of cattle.

Presently the primary feed for cattle is crop residue and seasonal fodder because of which the yield, particularly of cross-bred animals, has been low in lean seasons. The area under cultivated fodder production is limited only to 4.60 per cent of the total cultivable land, it is essential to increase fodder production by increasing area under cultivation to 12 per cent of the total cultivable land. Also there is a need to carry out research for dry land fodder production techniques. According to International Dairy Federation (IDF), the farmers in India get paid lowest price for their produce in the world. A situation of crisis is already developing as dairy farmers find it more profitable to sell off buffaloes. Since export of meat is fetching good prices, due to the export imitations by the government. Thus, there is a dire need to formulate such policies which will provide feed and nutrition of cattle at an affordable price.

To increase India's share in the international trade, it is essential to concentrate on

1. Improving the quality of raw milk by 'Clean Milk Production Programmes'. Formulation and implementation of a quality assurance system for the export of dairy products through an independent agency. In order to increase our exports, we have to improve quality of our milk and in order to improve the quality of milk, we need to undertake; (*a*) training the farmers, (*b*) chilling of raw milk at collection point, (*c*) testing for adulterations and antibiotics, (*d*) checks for low SNF problems, (*e*) as many as 23 tests on every sample of milk received in the dairy to maintain the quality of raw milk. Further, to augment the export, the quality of raw milk should be such that it has less than one lakh SPC and not more than 0.5 ppb aflatoxin and nil pesticides. Dairy hygiene standards by HACCP programmes : The farmers should be trained and given the incentive to maintain high degree of hygiene from cattle, vessel, transportation, delivery and the right type of feed given to the cattle.
2. Maintaining the consistency of supplies.

3. Formulation of an export policy: We have to generate a consistent export policy with suitable incentives and long term market creation goal in view of the global competition.

4. Improving the dairy product packaging system: Formulation and implementation of product diversification strategy to cope with wide fluctuation in pricing of international milk products, particularly milk powder.

At the same time, activating the water bodies in the rural village should become corporate social responsibility of the industries and the enterprises in that region. However, at present, **India's Dairy Industry is at the crossroads.** In spite of having a huge livestock population and having a tremendous potential to produce and export livestock and its products in the present liberalized era. India plays an insignificant role in the world trade of livestock and its products. Globalization and liberalization have a multifaceted effect on the livestock economy of India. Although meat and meat preparation has shown a stable and promising performance on the export front, it has had an adverse effect on the dairy sector.

It is reported that India has now become third largest meat exporter in the world and trade has now touched one billion dollar mark. Unfortunately, government is encouraging such exports rather than imposing restrictions. In this way very good quality germplasm is being lost. The Government has reduced duty on butter oil from 15 per cent to 5 per cent and therefore butter oil is being imported in our country which would naturally affect prices of ghee in our country. IDA should demand that the government recommend milk industry as a priority sector. Very alarming situation is developing at the village level. The young generation is leaving villages and going to the cities or abroad. It is feared that the milk production will be severely affected if the present situation continues. To overcome this situation the following policies may be envisaged.

(*a*) Government should impose duty on import of SMP and butter oil in such a way that it discourages import of cheap and subsidized SMP and butter oil from New Zealand, Europe and America. If this is not done our local industry will get crashed.

(*b*) Government should discourage the export of oil cakes. If this is not done then the cost of production of milk will go high. Under the present situation of economic crisis, industry is not able to offer better prices to the farmers which will effect the milk production in our country.

(*c*) The government should strictly impose enforcement of laws pertaining to adulteration of milk which is reaching at an alarming level. We are finding contaminants such as maltose, chemicals, pesticides, in milk. Government should take this aspect very seriously, otherwise our dairy industry will not be able to export milk and milk products because the rules and regulations are very strict at international level. Further clean milk production and hygienic milk production practices are beneficial to our citizens also. The government should encourage the formation of consumer forums in order to pressurize the farmers and processors to produce good quality milk.

(*d*) The government should reduce VAT to the level of not more than 4 per cent in all the states. In this way milk will be available for children and poor people at affordable rate.

(*e*) The co-operative dairy industry works on the principle of no profit no loss. The surplus generated during the year is ploughed back to the user members in proportion to their business with co-operatives based on the quality of raw milk. Therefore, there is no justification of government imposing income tax on the entity which is essentially a non-profit organization. Therefore the present level of tax may be brought down.

(*f*) The NCDFI, NDDB and IDA should come together and represent to GOI on above issues and a delegation of farmers, co-operators and private industry should talk to the government to put forward their demands.

Dairy sector contribution is around 65-70 per cent to livestock sector. We have less than 1000 milk processing centers in India. The goals of the 11th five year plan for the livestock sector are expected to achieve an overall growth between 6 to 7 per cent per annum for the sector as a whole and the milk production growth is estimated to 4-5 per cent per annum from 100 million tonnes from 2008 to 126.42 million tonnes by 2011-12. The main priority of every nation is to ensure food security for its citizens. The best way to achieve this goal in a harmonious and sustainable manner is by ensuring economic well-being of the men and women who feed our nation. The giant strides that India has taken in terms of ensuring food security for its citizens during the last sixty years, may get compromised, if our policy makers do not take consistent and long term measures that sustain the momentum.

REFERENCES

Bhaskar Goswami. (2007). Can Indian Dairy Cooperatives Survive in the New Economic Order? WTO PUBLIC FORUM 2007, *How Can the WTO Help Harness Globalization?* 4-5 October, 2007, Geneva.

Karmakar, K.G and Banerjee, G.D. (2006). Opportunities and Challenges in the Indian *Dairy Industry* by Technical Digest, NABARD, **9**.

Manitra Rakotoarisoa and Ashok Gulati (2006). *Competitiveness and trade potential of India's Dairy Ind. Food Policy*. **31** : 216-227.

Milk and Dairy Products in India-Production, Consumption and Exports, Aug 2009 M2 Communication.

Vijay Paul Sharma (2002). Trade liberalization and Indian dairy industry by, Oxford & IBH Pub. Co. (New Delhi)

www.indiadairy.com

25

VETERINARIANS PREPAREDNESS FOR DISASTER RESPONSE

S.R. Garg and V.J. Jadhav

Disasters, whether natural or manmade, cause great distress and loss of life. India is particularly vulnerable to the impact of disasters because of dense human and livestock population, insufficient resources, illiteracy and poverty. Though the threat to human life is a prime concern in emergency situations, the consequences of disasters on animals can not be ignored. The mortality of livestock not only gives a severe financial blow to the farming community; the innumerable dead animals also pose a major threat to the environmental health of man and animals. Veterinarians can provide considerable relief in such situations by virtue of their specialized qualification and experience in emergency medicine. Their proximity to the rural folks makes their task easier. Veterinarians can be helpful in the rescue operations and crisis management as well as in mitigating the after effects of disasters. With their knowledge of epidemiology, hygiene, sanitation, water quality management, nutrition, livestock health and zoonotic diseases, they can contribute vastly in improving the quality of life of both humans as well as animals in the post-disaster scenario. The responsibilities of veterinarians should extend beyond the traditional animal health related functions to the general welfare of the society in the events of emergency. The potential of the veterinarians in such situations should be given due recognition.

Any occurrence that causes damage, economic destruction, loss of human life and deterioration in health and health services on a scale sufficient to warrant an extraordinary response from outside the affected community or area is considered as disaster. Millions of people are affected by natural catastrophe from floods, cyclones and tsunami, earthquakes, landslides and volcanic eruptions across the world. Apart from the loss of human life, disasters cause great loss to the economy. The countries worldwide are estimated to have lost an average of 2 to 5 per cent of their GDP from natural calamities in the recent past (Goel, 2007).

TYPES OF DISASTERS

Disasters are classified broadly as natural disasters, man-made disasters and other disasters. These may either be major disasters or minor disasters. Depending upon the cause, disasters may be grouped as given below :

1. Water and Climate Related Disasters : Floods and drainage management, cyclones, tornadoes and hurricanes, hailstorm, cloud burst, heat wave and cold wave, snow avalanches, droughts, sea erosion, thunder and lightning.

2. Geology Related Disasters : Landslides and mudflows, earthquakes, dam failures/bursts, mine fires.

3. Chemical, Industry and Nuclear Related Disasters : Chemical and industrial disasters, nuclear disasters.

4. Accident Related Disasters : Forest fires, urban fires, village fires, mine flooding, oil spill, major building collapse, bomb blasts, festival disasters and fires, electrical disasters and fires, and air, road, rail and waterway accidents.

5. Biology Related Disasters : Biological disasters and epidemics, pest attacks, cattle epidemics and food poisoning.

DISASTER POTENTIAL OF INDIA

Due to the unique geo-climatic conditions, India is quite vulnerable to natural disasters. Floods, droughts, cyclones, earthquakes and landslides have been recurrent phenomena in the country. According to the estimates, more than four thousand people lost their lives and about 30 million people were affected by disasters every year during the decade 1990-2000 (Anonymous, 2004). According to the international specialized database, about three thousand persons were reported killed while more than 12 million people were affected by disasters in India during the year 2008 (EM-DAT, 2008). The loss in terms of private, community and public assets has been astronomical. Some prominent disasters that occurred in India are listed in Table 25.1.

IMPACT OF DISASTERS

The direct devastating impact of disasters in terms of loss of human life, property and infrastructure is well known but this is not all. Disasters have long term impact and their effects can be detected for months and sometimes even years after the disaster. The after effects of a disaster are due to the loss of crops, unavailability of essential food, and diseases that may occur due to malnourishment, hunger, poor hygiene etc. Loss of farmland infrastructures, industrial setup, employment opportunities cause severe financial distress to the people.

Disasters affect animals as well. Traditionally animals are viewed as human property during emergency management. However, the disaster-hit animals may have serious public health consequences, such as threat to food supply, water contamination and transmission of zoonotic diseases. Emotional attachment of the animal owners with their animals affects people's mental health too (Sen and Chander, 2003).

Table 25.1 : Some Major Disasters in India

Disaster	*Year*	*Location*	*Damage*
Earthquake	1991	Uttarkashi	Death of 769 persons
	1993	Latur district of Maharashtra	9,484 persons killed and around 14,845 cattle head lost with infrastructure loss of about Rs. 250 million
	2001	Kutch region of Gujarat	13,805 human deaths with loss of assets to worth Rs. 28,423 crores
Cyclones	1977	Andhra Pradesh	Death of 8,547 persons
	1998	Kandla, Gujarat	1,680 persons died
	2000	Tamilnadu	Heavy loss of plantation, houses and crops
Flood	2004	Assam	All 27 districts of states affected causing death of 251 persons and crop area loss of around 12.58 lakh hectares
	2004	Bihar	20 districts affected causing loss of 683 human lives, 2497 livestock, 13.95 lakh hectares of crop area
Landslides	1994	Varundh ghat, Konkan coast, Maharashtra	20 persons killed, breaching of *ghat* road damaged to the extent of 1 km
	1995	Aizwal, Mizoram	25 persons killed, road severely damaged
	1998	Malpa, Kali river	210 persons killed, the village wiped out in the event
Snow avalanche	1979	Lahaul and Spiti, Himachal Pradesh	About 237 persons killed
	2005	Jammu and Kashmir	More than 200 persons died
Road accidents	2002	India	82,717 persons killed in 4, 02, 158 accidents
Rail accidents	1999	Gaisal, Bihar	286 persons killed involving Awadh-Assam Express and Brahmaputra mail
	2000	Punjab	46 persons killed as Howrah-Amritsar mail rammed into a derailed goods train
	2001	Kerala	40 persons killed when the Mangalore-Chennai mail tumbled into Kadalundi river

Source : Goel (2007)

MANAGEMENT OF DISASTERS

Disasters may be of different kinds but all of them have typical similarities regarding unpredictability, speed, urgency, uncertainty and threat. These features make the possibility of prevention of disasters very bleak. Therefore, problem of disasters is addressed through a management system that helps to cope up with the after effects and minimize the losses. Disaster management is a complex process that requires a system to be in place at the national, state, district and local level, comprising of different components and participating stakeholders, with most of the coordination being done by the disaster management department. It requires collective and participative action of many people from various government departments, NGOs, community based organizations, panchayats, paramilitary organizations, military services, media and even common people. Management system is in place in many countries including India.

There are four generally recognized phases of emergency management, namely, mitigation, preparedness, response, and recovery (FEMA, 1998). Mitigation phase involves preventing future emergencies or minimizing their effects. This includes any activities that prevent an emergency, reduce the chances of an emergency or reduce the damage due to unpreventable disasters. Mitigation activities take place before and after the emergency. Preparedness includes plans or preparation to handle an emergency and to save lives. Preparedness related activities take place before an emergency occurs and it helps in responding appropriately in emergency. The response phase includes the actions taken to save life and prevent further property damage in an emergency situation. It involves putting preparedness plans into action. The response activities take place during an emergency. The last phase *i.e.* recovery phase includes action taken for recovering from an emergency. It helps to return to a normal or an even safer situation following an emergency. Recovery activities take place after an emergency. The same phases also apply to the management of animals, both livestock and pets, during disasters (FEMA, 1998, Sen and Chander, 2003).

In India, the main responsibility for disaster relief lies with the state governments, while the Government of India supplements the efforts of the state governments by offering logistic and financial support. Various government agencies play different roles in disaster management as presented in Table 25.2

Table 22 : Agencies Associated with Disaster Mitigation in India

Disaster	*Agencies*
Earthquake	Indian Meteorological Department, State Earthquake Research Institute, Geological Society of India
Flood	Indian Meteorological Department, Irrigation Department
Cyclones	Indian Meteorological Department
Epidemics	Public Health Department
Industrial chemical accidents	Industry, Mutual Aid and Response Group, Departments of Industry, Police, Bhabha Atomic Research Centre
Drought	Indian Meteorological Department, Public Health Department

Source : Anonymous (2002).

The National Crisis Management Committee is headed by the Cabinet Secretary, who is the highest executive officer. Secretaries of all the concerned Ministries and Departments are the members of the Committee. The Crisis Management Group headed by the Central Relief Commissioner consists of senior officers (nodal officers) from different Ministries. The nodal officer is responsible for preparing Sectoral Action Plan/ Emergency Support Function Plan for managing disasters.

DISASTER RESPONSE OF VETERINARIANS

No doubt, the first priority of disaster relief is protecting and saving human lives. Protection of human property and animals is generally of secondary concern (Heath *et al.*, 1997a). In disaster management, the basic responsibility of the veterinarian is to protect the livestock and animal food products, thus, contributing to human health.

Veterinarians can play major role in promoting local pre-disaster planning at community level for timely and safe evacuation of livestock and pet animals (Heath, 2000a). This will facilitate the evacuation of people who otherwise may be reluctant to leave their animals behind. During relief efforts, veterinarians can play crucial role in increasing the survivability of animals that are victims, and of those that are deployed in relief operations. The contribution of veterinarians will be most effective if they integrate their expertise with other local, national and international groups and agencies involved in disaster management (Heath, 2000b).

Veterinarians should provide their inputs at the time of preparation of disaster management plan at state and local level. They should assist the planning committees in developing the animal evacuation and care plans during emergencies. They should help in the development of action plans concerning evacuation routes that do not conflict with human evacuation routes, safe destination sites and alternate shelters for the animals. As animal mortality is an expected sequel to disaster, veterinarians should prepare the carcass management and disposal strategies in advance to avoid environmental and public health crisis.

After disaster, the veterinarians should carry out search and rescue operation of all animals including domestic and stray animals. Rescued animals should be transported to safe places and should be treated. The surviving animal populations should be immunized against epidemic outbreaks. Veterinarians should also help in restoration of animals to the claimants.

Apart from these animal related relief measures, veterinarians can also contribute directly to public health through emergency care and treatment of humans, sanitary supervision, food inspection and prevention and control of diseases. Veterinarians are familiar with medical emergencies and they are professionally trained to respond in situations with limited resources (Heath *et al.*, 1997b). Their proximity to rural folks makes their task easier. With their knowledge of epidemiology, hygiene, sanitation, water quality management, nutrition, livestock health and zoonotic diseases, they can make significant contribution in improving the quality of life of both humans and animals in the post disaster scenario.

Specialized trainings in disaster management can further strengthen the capacity of veterinarians to function in the emergency situation. The Veterinary Council of India has already taken initiative in this direction.

REFERENCES

Anonymous (2002). Disastersin India:Riskandvulnerability.http://www.managedisasters.org/indiapaper00.asp

Anonymous (2004). Disaster Management in India-A status report. National Disaster Management Division, Ministry of Home Affairs, Government of India.

EM-DAT (2008). The OFDA/CRED International Disaster Database. Université Catholique de Louvain, Brussels. www.emdat.be accessed on 5th October 2009.

FEMA (1998). Animals in disaster (Module A) : Awareness and Preparedness. Federal Emergency Management Agency, Emergency Management Institute (EMI) Independent study course. EMI, Emmitsburg, Maryland.

Goel, S.L. (2007). Disaster administration and management. Deep and Deep Publications Pvt. Ltd, New Delhi, India.

Heath, S.E., Dorn, R., Linnabary, R.D., Hooks, J., Casper, J. and Marshall, K. (1997a). An overview of disaster preparedness for veterinarians. *JAVMA* **210** : 345-348.

Heath, S.E., Hooks, J., Marshall, K., Dorn, R., Linnabary, R.D. and Casper, J. (1997b). Participation of veterinarians in disaster management. *JAVMA* **210** : 325-328.

Heath, S.E. (2000a). The role of veterinarians in disasters. World Veterinary Association Press Release, Washington, DC. Cited from Sen and Chander (2003).

Heath S.E. (2000b). Building an animal disaster program. In: Proceedings of Outbreak Symposium at AVMA, Schaumburg, USA. Cited from Sen and Chander (2003).

Sen, A. and Chander, M. (2003). Disaster management in India: The case of livestock and poultry. *Rev. Sci. Tech. Off. Int. Epiz*. **22** : 915-930.

26

RODENT TRANSMITTED DISEASES OF MAN AND ANIMALS

Ashok Kumar, I. Shakuntala,
A. Deka and H. Rahman

Rodents are the groups of animals characterized by two continuously growing incisors in the upper and lower jaws. They are classified as:

Kingdom – Animalia,

Phylum – Chordata,

Class – Mammalia,

Order – Rodentia

The rodents exploit a wide variety of habitats and environment even those with extreme conditions throughout the world. Most of them live in wild areas having little interaction with human, however, some of them, especially mice and rats live in close proximity of human dwellings. They are generally harmful to mankind as they carry many diseases as well as cause extensive damage to food grains, feed stuffs and agricultural fields. There are more than 200 species of rodents in the world. Common rodents include mice, rats, hamster, gerbils, bandicoots, squirrels, gophers, beavers, voles, chipmunks, guinea pig and porcupines, etc. Around 99 species of rodents belonging to 43 genera and 4 families are found in India (Corbet and Hill, 1986). The common species found in

India are *Tatera indica, Bandicota bengalensis, B. bengalensis kok, B. indica, Nisokia indica, Millardia meltada, M. gleadowi, Mus booduga* and *Rattus rattus,* etc. Among the rodents, mice and rats, particularly House mice (*Mus musculus*), Roof rats (*Rattus rattus*) and Norway rats (*Rattus norvegicus*) are considered the most important carriers of diseases. In the North East region of India, bamboo flowering makes favourable conditions for explosion of rodent population, which ultimately lead to famines called *Mautam* and *Thingtam* in Mizoram due to heavy destruction of food grains (Pathak and Kumar, 2000).

EPIDEMIOLOGY AND TRANSMISSION OF DISEASES

The role of rodents in transmission of diseases was well known even during old times as reflected by mention "Desert your dwelling, if you see a dead rat" in Bhagwat Purans (Pathak and Kumar, 2000). Rodents are involved in direct or indirect transmission of many diseases including zoonotic infections. The ability of rodents to carry and transmit the diseases is encouraged by their habit and habitat and similar physiologies that rodents share with human. Besides eating foodstuff, they contaminate food with their droppings, urine, excreta, hair, etc. carrying the infectious agents. Thus rodents play a very important role in transmission of several dreadful diseases of man and animals. Some of these diseases can be transmitted through breathing of contaminated dust with rodent urine and droppings, contact with biting wound, conjunctiva, and abraded skin, eating or drinking contaminated food or water and handling of contaminated materials or infected animals. Some of these infections can also be indirectly transmitted by the bite of vectors like mosquitoes, flies, ticks, flea or mites. The diseases transmitted by rodents and their causative agents are summarized in Table 26.1.

Some of the important rodent-borne diseases, as the detail description of all of the diseases in the list is beyond the scope of this chapter; the features of some of the important diseases are discussed.

Table 26.1 : List of Zoonotic Diseases Transmitted by Rodents

Disease	*Causative Agent(s)*
Bacterial :	
Erysipelothrix infection	*Erysipelothrix insidiosa (rhusiopathiae)*
Leptospirosis	*Leptospira* species
Lyme disease	*Borrelia burgdorferi*
Melioidosis	*Burkholderia pseudomallei*
Plague	*Yersinia pestis*
Rat bite fever	*Spirillum minus*
	Streptobacillus moniliformis
Salmonellosis	*Salmonella* species
Tularaemia	*Fransilla tularensis*
Yersiniosis	*Yersinia pseudotuberculosis*
Viral :	
California encephalitis	California encephalitis virus (*Buniya virus*)
Colorado tick fever	Colorado tick fever virus (*Orbivirus*)
Eastern equine encephalitis	Eastern equine encephalitis virus (*Alpha virus*)
Hanta virus infection	*Hanta virus*
Korean haemorrhagic fever	*Unku virus*
Kyasanur forest disease	KFD virus (*Flavivirus*)
Lassa fever	*Arana virus*
Lymphocytic Choriomeningitis	*Arena virus*
Mayaro fever	*Mayaro virus* (*Alpha virus*)
Omsk haemorrhagic fever	*Flavi virus*
Rota virus gastroenteritis	*Rota virus*
Tick borne encephalitis	*Flavi virus*
Venezualan equine encephalitis	Venezualan equine encephalitis virus (*Alpha virus*)
Vesicular stomatitis	Vesicular stomatitis virus (*Vesiculo virus*)
Rickettsial :	
Indian tick typhus	*Rickettsia conorii*
Murine typhus	*Reckettsia typhi*
Q-fever	*Coxiella burnetii*

Contd...

Disease	Causative Agent(s)
Rickettsial pox	*Rickettsia akari*
Rocky mountain spotted fever	*Rickettsia rickettsii*
Scrub typhus	*Rickettsia tsutsugamushi*
Siberian tick typhus	*Rickettsia siberica*
Actinomycetic :	
Nocardiosis	*Nocardia* spp.
Mycotic :	
Coccidioidomycosis	*Coccidioides immitis*
Histoplasmosis	*Histoplasma capsulatum*
Ring worm	*Dermatophytes*
Protozoan :	
Amoebiosis	*Entamoeba histolytica*
Leishmaniasis	*Leishmania* spp.
Toxoplasmosis	*Toxoplasma gondii*
Trypanosomiasis	*Trypanosoma* spp.
Helminthic :	
Capillariasis	*Capillaria* spp.
Echinococcosis	*Echinococcus* spp.
Echinostomiasis	*Echinostoma* spp.
Gnathostomiasis	*Gnathostoma spinigerum*
Gongylonemiasis	*Gongylonema pulchrum*
Hymenolepiasis	*Hymenolepis nana*
Paragonimiasis	*Paragonimus westermani*
Rallietiniasis	*Rallietina celebensis*
Schistosomiasis	*Schistosoma* spp.
Sparganosis	*Spirometra* spp.
Trichinellosis	*Trichinella spiralis*
Ectoparasitic :	
Scabies	*Sarcoptes scabiei*

A. Bacterial Diseases

1. Leptospirosis (Weil's disease, Stuttgart's disease, 7 days fever, mud fever, swamp fever, cane cutter's disease, autumnal fever or swine herd's disease) :

Leptospirosis is caused by the organisms of genus *Leptospira* that consist of 8 pathogenic species, 23 serogroups and 280 serovars. These eight species are namely *Leptospira interrogans, L. borgpefersenii, L. inadai, L. meyeri, L. naguchii, L. santarosai, L. weilli, L. kirschneri* (WHO 2003). The disease may appear in acute or chronic form. The infection occurs approximately in 160 mammalian species (Alexander, 1991). The mouse, vole, rat, mongoose, shrew, jackal, dog, pig, cat and cattle are the important reservoirs.

Leptospirosis is world wide in distribution including India where the disease is more common in coastal areas. The Leptospirae can survive in moist warm environment but these are sensitive to desiccation, UV ray irradiation and more vulnerable at pH range of 6.2 – 8.0. Transmission occurs through contact with an environment contaminated by urine, aborted fetus and uterine discharge of reservoir host or other infected animals. The Leptospirae can colonize the kidney and may thus be excreted in urine of infected animal. *Leptospira* can also enter through abraded skin and mucous membrane during bathing or swimming in lake, river or canal polluted with the urine of infected animals. Venereal transmission also occurs in rodents. Man is considered as "dead end host" but transplacental transmission has been reported.

The incubation period in man is usually 8-12 days. The disease may manifest in human in two phases. 1st phase is septicaemic and 2nd phase is due to immune response. The disease may appear in 2 forms which are icteric and anicteric. The icteric form is characterized by impaired renal and hepatic function, vascular collapse and haemorrhages. The onset is sudden with chills, headache, conjunctival infection, myalgia, prostration, nausea, vomiting, photophobia and nuchal rigidity in anicteric form. Persistent headache may occur that is indicative of meningitis.

Among animals, cattle may suffer with acute and chronic infection. Fever, anorexia, flaccid mastitis, stiffness, abortion, haemataemia, haemoglobinaemia and death may occur. Pyrexia, anorexia, jaundice, haemorrhage, neurological signs, abortion and stillbirth are the important clinical signs in pig. Horses suffer from pyrexia, icterus, periodic opthalmia and abortion. Sheep suffer from abortion, fever, agalactia, dysponea, jaundice, haemataemia and sudden death. Jaundice, haemoglobinaemia and abortion have been reported in goat. Dogs suffer from fever, anorexia, listlessness, conjunctival infection, vomiting intussusceptions, haemorrhages, ulcerated gums, foul breath, uraemia and sudden death. Nephritis and icterus has been reported in cat and nephritis, hepatitis and abortion in deer. Poultry are resistant to leptospirosis.

Diagnosis of Leptospirosis can be made by observation of clinical symptoms supported by laboratory investigations. The leptospirae can be directly visualized under dark field microscope in clinical material *viz.*, urine, faetal tissues, blood etc. collected from the infected animals. The preparations can be stained employing silver impregnation technique of Fontana. Immunoperoxidase staining is done for demonstration of Leptospirae in tissues. The organisms can be isolated from clinical materials by using Ellinghausen-MacCullough-Johnson-Harris (EMJH) medium, Kurthoff's medium and Fletcher's medium. Organisms take 1 to 6 weeks to grow. Animal inoculation is done in guinea pig or hamster and can be re-isolated from urine serologically, Microscopic Agglutination Test (MAT) is the most widely used test for the diagnosis of Leptospirosis. Live leptospira cells are used as the antigen in this test and a titre of 1:100 or above indicates presence of past infection. Enzyme linked immunosorbant assay (ELISA) has also been recognized as a useful test for detecting *Leptospira* antibodies. It is preferred over MAT as it is more sensitive and does not require live antigens. Polymerase chain reaction (PCR) is used for selective amplification of target DNA sequence of *Leptospira* cells present in clinical samples even in small concentration. Nucleic Acid Hybridization is based on the detection of leptospiral DNA in infected tissues by hybridization with a radio or non-radio labeled single stranded nucleic acid probe, either whole or derived from cloned sequence.

Preventive measures include rodent control, disinfection of water and protective clothing by agricultural workers. Prophylactic vaccination of dogs, cattle and pig has been performed with little success. Treatment is relatively unsatisfactory even though penicillin, erythromycin, streptomycin, tetracycline are used in acute illness. Dihydro streptomycin is recommended for carriers.

2. Plague (Black Death, Pestilential fever, Mahamari (in Northern India), Pest or Mad rat disease): It is a highly fatal zoonotic disease caused by a Gram-negative bacillus, *Yersinia pestis*. The disease affects wide variety of species like man, camel, deer, dog, cat, donkey, antelope, rabbit, rat and squirrel. It was a pandemic disease with worldwide distribution but mostly prevalent in Europe, Middle East, China and India. Plague is a re-emerging disease as it may cause outbreak after a long gap of quiescence. There is a report of re-emergence of this disease in Algeria in 2003 after a gap of 50 years.

Several epidemics of plague have occurred in India causing the great losses to mankind. There were 12.5 million deaths in Agra epidemic during 1612. The epidemics were reported in Beed District of Maharashtra (bubonic plague) and in Surat District of Gujarat (pneumonic plague) in 1994. A total of 876 cases were presumptively diagnosed in both epidemics, out of which 54 cases were reported as dead. Recent outbreaks were reported in Shimla District of Himachal Pradesh in 2002 and Uttaranchal in 2004. These outbreaks were contained by appropriate actions including immediate surveillance, chemoprophylaxis and management.

Normally the transmission of the disease occurs through bite of rat flea, *Xenopsylla cheopis*. Commensal rat (*Rattus rattus*) may pick up plague bacilli from interactions with wild rodents or from their fleas and spread the disease in urban areas.

Clinically plague has three forms : (i) Bubonic plague that involves the legs and inguinal lymph nodes causing intense haemorrhagic inflammation of the lymph node; (ii) pneumonic plague which is now rare but highly fatal disease involving the lungs; and (iii) Septicemia plague that is the terminal stage of both bubonic and pneumonic plague. If bubonic plague is not properly treated then it may lead to meningitis (meningeal plague). The important symptoms are nausea, chill, fever, dysponea, chest pain, pneumonia, epistaxis, haematuria, diarrhoea, constipation, painful and oedematous buboes, cyanosis, staggering gait, delirium, prostration, coma and death.

In case of animals, the disease may be acute, chronic or inapparent. Animals exhibit the symptoms like pneumonia, fever and lymphadenitis. Haemorrhagic buboes and spleenomegaly is found in dead animals. Feline plague is characterized by abscess formation, lymphadenitis, lethargy and fever.

Tentative diagnosis of plague is based on the clinical signs like high fever, lymphadenitis, and appearance of buboes. The organisms can be demonstrated in aspirated fluid from lymph node employing Fluorescence Antibody Techniques (FAT). Smear of pus, cerebrospinal fluid (CSF), sputum, blood, throat swab and spleen tissue also contain the organisms. The bone marrow aspirate from femur of dead rodent and heart blood is used for screening. Cultural examination by growing the organisms in blood agar and MacConkey's agar and animal inoculation test are also performed to confirm the disease. ELISA is used to diagnose the disease serologically. PCR and gene sequencing are the recent aids to confirm the infection.

The basic measures to control the plague include (i) reduction of rodent population by rodenticide and eradication of rat flea using insecticide; (ii) using killed and live vaccines as prophylaxis. Tetracycline is the drug of choice for treatment of this disease. Chloramphenicol and streptomycin are also used.

3. Tularemia (Rabbit fever, Deer fly fever, Francis disease or Ohara's disease) : Tularemia is caused by a small, Gram-negative, non-motile, aerobic, capsulated, non-sporulating bacillus called *Francisella tularensis*. The organism has two biovars, viz: *F. tularensis* biovar *tularensis* (Jellison Type A) and *F. tularensis* biovar *palaearctica* (Jellison Type B), of which former is more virulent. The disease affects man, rabbit and rodent and reported through out the world. The rodents involved in transmission are musk rat, ground squirrel and beaver. The disease is transmitted among the rodent population by the bite of infected tick or deer fly. Transmission to human occurs through handling or eating infected animals or drinking contaminated water. Inhalation of contaminated dust may also transmit the disease to healthy one or by bite of *Chrysops discalis* tick.

The disease is manifested in human in three clinical forms: (*i*) Ulceroglandular form with presence of small, rugged ulcer at the entry point of organism, enlargement of local lymph nodes, which sometimes become suppurative and painful; (*ii*) Abdominal or typhoidal form with nausea, gastroenteritis and diarrhoea; and (*iii*) Pulmonary form which is associated with increased respiration, coughing, pneumonia and bronchopneumonia. Fever, rigid gait, diarrhoea, frequent urination and difficulty in respiration are the main symptoms observed in animals.

Provisional diagnosis can be made on the basis of clinical manifestations that can be confirmed by laboratory-based investigations. Detection of causative organism in pus samples from the local lesion or suppurative lymph node, blood, sputum is done by smear or cultural examinations in laboratory. Serodiagnosis is based on tube agglutination test and ELISA. Skin test in pig is performed with intradermal inoculation of tularin for detecting delayed type of hypersensitivity reaction.

A live vaccine from a virulent strain of *F. tularensis* has been used as prophylaxis in Russia. Control of tick is essential to break up the transmission process of infectious agent through tick bite. Streptomycin is the drug of choice. Gentamicin, chloramphenicol and tetracycline can also be used.

4. Lyme disease (Lyme borreliasis, Lyme arthritis or Erythema migrans).

It is a zoonotic disease caused by a spirochete, *Borrelia burgdorferi*. The disease is prevalent in United States, Europe, Australia, England and Asia including India. It affects cattle, sheep, horse, dog and human. Deer, mice, raccoon, squirrel and opossum are also affected. White footed mouse and tree squirrel are involved in maintenance and perpetuation of infectious agent and the ticks of these rodents belonging to genus *Ixodes* namely *I. ricinus, I. dammini, I. pacificus* and *I. pensulcatus* are the major vectors. The disease in human is manifested three stages: Stage-I is characterized by Erythema Chronicum Migrans (ECM) that develops within days or weeks after tick bites. The main symptoms in this stage are fatigue, fever, chills, headache, myalgia, migratory arthalgia, lymphadenopathy and stiff neck. Stage-II occurs within weeks or month and is characterized by cardiac and neurological disorders. Stage-III may occur at any time from months to year after bite of infected tick. It is characterized by swelling and pain of large joints, arthritis of several joints especially knee joints. Shoulder, ankle, elbow and jaw may also be affected with arthritis. Clinical manifestations in animals include fever, polyarthritis, encephalitis, hepatitis, photophobia, uveitis and lameness.

Diagnosis of the disease is made on the basis of clinical symptoms. Barbour, Stoener, Kelly (BSK)-11 and modified Kelly's media are used to grow the organisms for cultural examinations of clinical samples in laboratory. Microscopically, the organisms are examined under dark field illumination. ELISA, IFA and FA techniques are used for serodiagnosis. Molecular techniques like DNA hybridization, PCR and Restriction endonuclease analysis are used for detection and confirmation of the pathogen.

Preventive measures include the avoidance from tick bites and control of tick population by acaricidal drugs. A commercial adjuvant vaccine (Lymerix) is now available for dogs as prophylaxis. Procaine penicillin is the drug of choice. Other antibiotics used are oxytetracycline, ampicillin, doxycycline and erythromycin.

5. Melioidosis (Whitmore's disease, Pseudoglander or Rodent glander).

It is a direct bacterial zoonosis caused by *Burkholderia* (previously known as *Pseudomonas*) *pseudomallei*. It is primarily a disease of rodent with occasional cases in humans and farm animals. The infection has been reported from camel, cat, dog, goat, guinea pig, horse, pig, monkey, kangaroo, koala and wild animals. The disease has been reported from Malaysia, Indonesia, Thailand, Vietnam, Australia, Central and South America, Iran, New Guinea, France, Bangladesh, Pakistan and India. The infection may occur from faeces of infected animals, by ingestion of contaminated water, through abraded skin from contaminated soil and rarely through venereal transmission.

The disease in human is characterized with fever, chills, bronchitis, pneumonitis, productive cough, haemoptysis, septicaemia, gastroenteritis, insomnia, weight loss, pruritis, vesicles, pustules on hands and feet and abscesses. The clinical manifestations in animals are associated with respiratory problems, nervous disorders, abscess in joints, visceral organs and lymph nodes, prostration, fever, dysponea and arthritis.

Diagnosis is based on demonstration of the organism by isolation from clinical samples such as sputum, blood, urine and abscesses in MacConkey's agar added with gentamicin. Young hamster is used for animal inoculation test where development of abscess is observed in positive cases. Meliodin test, an allergic skin test is done in animals. Development of skin lesions indicates positive cases. False positive reaction in goat and false negative reaction in pig are observed. Serodiagnosis can be done by Complement Fixation test (CFT), Indirect Haemagglutination test (IHA) and Indirect Fluorescent Antibody (IFA) technique.

Elimination of infected animals and the disinfection of contaminated utensils is the way to control this disease. Treatment can be done with oxytetracycline, novobiocin, chloramphenicol, sulphadiazine, ceftazidime and cefotaxime against this disease.

6. Rat Bite Fever : The disease caused by *Spirillum minus* and *Streptobacillus moniliformis* comes under this group. The disease is worldwide in distribution. The susceptible host are man, rat and mice.

The infection caused by *S. moniliformis* is also known as Haverhill fever, epidemic arthritic erythema or Streptobacillary fever. The incubation period in this case ranges from 3 to 5 days, which may be up to 10 days. Infections occur due to ingestion of milk contaminated by faeces of rodent and through rat bite as the organism lodge in the nasopharynx of rat. It can also be transmitted through rat scratch. The disease is rare in man and occurs sporadically. It is characterized with fever, chill, headache, myalgia, maculopapular rash on the extremities and polyarthritis. Endocarditis, myocarditis, hepatitis and meningitis are some possible complications. Prognosis is good if treated properly. Polyarthritis and gangrene are noticed in rat. Regional lymph nodes are affected showing lymphadenitis with large abscess in guinea pig.

The infection caused by *S. minus* is called Sodoku or spirillary fever. The incubation period ranges from 2 to 3 weeks or may be up to 4 months. The disease is worldwide in distribution but mostly prevalent in Far East countries. Infection is transmitted through saliva of rodent during bite. In case of man, the arthritis is not so common but there will be maculopapular and urticarial rashes around the area of bite. Other symptoms exhibited are fever, chill, headache, malaise, vomiting, diarrhoea and neuralgia. In animals, the *S. minus* infection is asymptomatic but sometimes there may be conjunctivitis and staring coat.

Diagnosis is based on the clinical symptoms confirmed with laboratory tests. *S. minus* does not grow *in vitro* where as *S. moniliformis* can be isolated in laboratory media which can be seen in isolated form or in chain under microscope. *S. minus* can be isolated by animal inoculation in guinea pigs and mice where the organisms multiply in blood and can be detected in blood smear using Wright's stain. The organisms appear as spiral shaped with 2 or 3 twists.

Control of rat population, construction of rat proof dwellings and immediate attention to rat bite are the essential measures for prevention and control of this disease. Penicillin is the drug of choice. Streptomycin and tetracycline are other antibiotics used to treat the disease.

7. Relapsing Fever : It is a zoonotic disease caused by *Borrelia* species (*B. recurrentis, B. persica, B. hermsii, B. venezuelensis, B. mazzottii* and *B. hispanica*) and transmitted by tick and lice from natural reservoir wild rodents. The disease is widely spread in Asia, Africa and Europe.

Human suffer with sudden onset of fever with temperature up to 38.9-41°C that becomes normal after 3-7 days. Headache, body pain, nausea and vomiting are the main symptoms during the febrile period. There is spleenomegaly and hepatomegaly. Death is due to damage of liver, lobar pneumonia, subarachnoid haemorrhage or splenic rupture. Experimental infections can be produced in monkeys, guinea pig, mice and rats with relapsing course of illness resembling to man.

For diagnosis, organisms can be demonstrated in blood collected during pyrexial period. The actively motile Borreliae can be seen in unstained blood drop by phase contrast or dark field microscopy. Gram-negative spirochetes can be stained with Giemsa stain. Animal inoculation test is done in suckling mice.

Control of the disease includes early diagnosis and treatment of affected person or animal, use of acaricidal drugs, avoidance from tick and lice bites by protective clothing. Penicillin and tetracycline are commonly used for the treatment of this disease.

B. Viral Diseases

1. Kyasanur Forest Disease (KFD) : It is an Indian haemorrhagic disease caused by a RNA virus called KFD virus that belongs to genus *Flavivirus* of family *Flaviviridae*. The disease is named after the Kyasanur Forest of Karnataka State where the first case was diagnosed. Birds (jungle fowl) and small mammals are the reservoir of this virus and infection is transmitted by the bite of tick *Haemophysalis spinigera*. Transovarian transmission in tick is also possible. Langur (*Presbytis entellus*) and Bonnet monkey (*Macaca radiata*) play an important role in amplification of the virus. Man and cattle are accidental hosts. Deforestation and introduction of cattle have increased the exposure of population to tick vectors and thus the incidence of disease.

Incubation period in man is 3-7 days. Sudden onset of fever with headache, vomiting, myalgia, cephalgia, insomnia, bradycardia, haemorrhages on mucous membranes, encephalitis, leucopenia, neck stiffness, tremor and mental disorder are the main symptoms. Gastrointestinal and bronchial problems are common.

Intravenous inoculation with the virus in monkey develops diarrhoea, bradycardia and hypotension. Phagocytosis of erythrocytes and nuclear material was observed in peripheral blood. During epidemic haemorrhage and nonspecific degenerative changes in the parenchymatous viscera were observed. Sometimes, monkey may show encephalitis but the infection in other animals is of subclinical type.

Diagnosis is done by isolation of virus in mice and use of CFT, haemagglutination inhibition (HI), ELISA for serodiagnosis. Avoidance from tick infested area, use of chemical repellent or wearing protective clothes and use of acaricides for ticks are the preventive measures. Immunization with killed vaccine may be used for population at risk otherwise no satisfactory treatment is available.

2. Lassa Fever : It is a direct zoonosis involving man and rodents caused by Lassa virus that belongs to genus *Arenavirus* of Family *Arenaviridae*. It is a single stranded RNA virus. The disease occurs mainly in Central and Western Africa. Multimammate rat (*Mastomys natalensis*) is the main reservoir host. Infection is transmitted to man directly through contact with rodent's saliva and urine or contaminated food and water. Ingestion of raw meat of infected rodent also transmits the disease. The main symptoms of disease in man include fever, headache, myalgia, abdominal cramp, nausea, vomiting, diarrhoea, coughing, chest pain, tonsillitis, pharyngitis, oedema of face, capillary haemorrhages and shock. Death occurs due to cardiac failure. Clinical symptoms have not been reported in animals.

Diagnosis is done by isolation of virus in tissue culture from pharyngeal washings or swabs and blood. Serological diagnosis is done by CFT and indirect immunofluorescent technique. Isolation of the infected person and rodent control are essential measures to control the disease. There is no satisfactory treatment.

3. Lymphocytic choriomeningitis (LCM or Armstrong's disease) : It is caused by a single stranded RNA virus, *LCM virus* that belongs to genus *Arenavirus* of family *Arenaviridae*. The disease occurs in Argentina, Germany, Hungary and USA. *LCM virus* may affect mouse, monkey, man, dog and guinea pig. The house mouse, *Mus musculus* is mainly involved in transmission of disease. It is transmitted through contact with mice, may also spread through dust contaminated with urine or via skin abrasions. The laboratory borne infections also occur. The disease is more prevalent in the area densely inhabited by mice population. Person-to-person contact has also been reported.

The symptoms in man are mild. The disease starts with influenza like illness after an incubation period of 6-13 days. The patients show fever, malaise, coryza, myalgia and bronchitis. Meningitis is common but it is benign and recovers within few days. Chronic infections also occur with headache, paralysis, erythematous rash and mild pharyngitis. An early leucopenia followed by lymphocytosis is a common finding. Death may occur due to meningoencephalomyelitis. The animals do not usually present clinical symptoms.

Diagnosis is based on clinical symptoms. Laboratory confirmation of *LCM virus* is based on serological tests and isolation of the virus. The virus can be isolated from blood, CSF and brain tissues. Avoidance of contact and control of mice and proper precautions in the laboratory are the important measures for prevention of disease.

4. Colorado Tick Fever : It is caused by a double stranded RNA virus composed of 12 segments, Colorado tick fever virus that belongs to genus *Coltivirus* (previously *Orbivirus*) of family *Reoviridae*. It affects mainly man, rodents and squirrel. The disease is prevalent in USA and Canada. Deer mouse, bushy tailed wood rat, ground squirrel, porcupine and chipmunk are the rodents involved and the disease is transmitted by bite of rat tick, *Dermacenter andersoni*. Transmission through person to person contact and blood transfusion has also been reported.

The symptoms of disease in man are similar to that of dengue. The onset is sudden with fever which is biphasic in approximately 50% of patients, headache, myalgia, retro-orbital pain, lumber backache, nausea, vomiting, maculopapular rashes, encephalitis, aseptic meningitis, fever and leucopenia. It remains asymptomatic in animals.

Diagnosis is based on clinical signs supported by laboratory investigations. Hamster or suckling mice are used for isolation of the virus. Indirect fluorescent antibody test may be used for early serological diagnosis. Avoidance of tick bites and control of ticks are the preventive measures. There is no satisfactory treatment.

5. Mayaro Fever : It is caused by an RNA virus, *Mayaro virus* that belongs to genus *Alphavirus* of family *Togaviridae*. The disease is reported from South American countries. It affects man, rodent, migratory birds, howler monkey and marmoset and is transmitted by bites of mosquitoes infected with *Mayaro virus*.

The disease affects human as a benign febrile illness of brief duration for 2-6 days with fever, headache, conjunctivitis, prostration, joint pain, joint oedema, photophobia and rash. It remains asymptomatic in animals.

For diagnosis, the virus can be isolated from the blood of febrile patients at the beginning of the disease by inoculating newborn mice by intra cerebral route. CFT and HI tests are used to diagnose the disease serologically. Avoidance from mosquito bites and mosquito control are the measures for prevention. Laboratory personnel may be infected via air borne transmission and therefore should take precautions against exposure accordingly. There is no satisfactory treatment.

6. Hanta Virus Infection : The causative agent is RNA virus called *Hantavirus* or *Hantaanvirus* that belong to family *Bunyaviridae*. The virus was first reported from Korea in 1975 and was named after the river 'Hantaan'. It is worldwide in distribution including India. It causes two types of illness, *viz.* haemorrhagic fever with renal syndrome or HFRS (old world *Hantavirus* infection) and Hantavirus pulmonary syndrome or HPS (New world *Hantavirus* infection). The rodents involved are cotton rat (*Sigmodon hispidus*), rice rat (*Oryzomys palustris*), white-footed mouse (*Peromyscus leucopus*) and deer mouse (*Peromyscus maniculatus*) for different hantaviruses, later one being important reservoir. The virus is shed via saliva, urine and faeces of the reservoir rodents. The disease mainly affects the animal caretakers and laboratory workers. Transmission occurs through water contaminated with rodent excreta, urine, and saliva or through inhalation. It may also be transmitted through contact with abraded skin or conjunctiva.

In case of HFRS, severe malaise, loss of appetite, nausea, vomiting, conjunctivitis that later becomes haemorrhagic, erythema of face, neck and thorax followed by haematuria, proteinuria, oliguria, uraemia, epistaxis, intracerebral, gastrointestinal and urogenital bleeding are the main symptoms. Blood pressure is increased along with increased haemorrhagic diathesis. Renal functions become hampered and an irreversible shock occurs.

In case of HPS, high fever with rigor, malaise, nausea, vomiting, myalgia, diarrhoea, headache, retrosternal pain, respiratory distress, rhinitis, pharyngitis, pneumonia, hypoxia, alveolar edema and increasing respiratory insufficiency are the main symptoms.

Tentative diagnosis can be made on the basis of clinical manifestation. The isolation of Hantavirus is difficult. RT-PCR is done for detection of virus. Postmortem examination, especially examination of kidney specimens is useful for detection of the disease in dead cases.

Control of rodents and use of disinfectants in the infected areas are the important measures. Vaccine is not yet available.

Symptomatic treatment including dialysis, use of cardio tonic drugs and electrolyte therapy is useful. Ribavirin can improve the condition.

C. Rickettsial Diseases

1. Q-Fever : The disease is caused by *Coxiella burnetii*. It was first observed in Australia. But now it is worldwide in distribution. The organism is maintained by two interacting cycles, one in wild animals with their ticks and another in domestic animals. It affects cattle, camel, cat, goat, gerbil, hedgehog, pig, rabbit and sheep. It is an occupational disease affecting the abattoir workers and dairy farmers. The disease may be transmitted to human by inhalation of aerosols containing the *C. burnetii* or through consumption of contaminated milk.

After an incubation period of 14 to 26 days, the onset of disease in man is sudden with fever, shivering and shaking malaise, pain in the limb and joint, frontal headache that does not respond to ordinary analgesics, thrombophlebitis and pulmonary embolism. Endocarditis may occur in chronic cases. It causes bronchopneumonia and abortion in pregnant animals. Infected animals shed the organism in urine, faeces, milk and foetal fluid.

It is difficult to diagnose the disease on the basis of only clinical signs. The history of exposure to livestock, isolation of organism from clinical samples preferably in embryonated chicken eggs by yolk sac route and confirmation by PCR based techniques are the methods for diagnosis. Serological tests used are ELISA, rickettsial agglutination test, CFT, capillary agglutination test and indirect immunofluorescence test. Breaking the infection cycle and pasteurization of milk are the measures for prevention. Inactivated Q fever vaccine has been used for prevention. Chlortetracycline, penicillin and chloramphenicol are used for treatment.

D. Actinomycetic Diseases

1. Nocardiosis : It is caused by *Nocardia asteroids*, *N. brasilliensis* and *N. otitidiscavianum* and affects a wide variety of species including rodents and sometimes affecting man. The disease is worldwide in distribution including India. Infection mainly comes from contaminated soil. Infection to man occurs through inhalation of organisms and introduction of infectious agent through skin of hand and feet. Nosocomial transmission may also occur.

Development of localized subcutaneous abscesses that are invasive and destructive to soft tissues and the underlying bone (mycetoma) along with lymphangitis and lymphadenitis are the main symptoms in man. The discharge of pus, often containing yellow or black colored granules is observed. Among animals, cattle and dogs are mainly affected with fever, dysponia, coughing, convulsion, sub laryngeal swelling, subcutaneous mass draining sinus, corneal ulcer and pus formation with small granules. Granules disseminated through haematogenus or lymphatic route to other organs.

The provisional diagnosis can be made on the basis of clinical symptoms. Gram staining of the pus showing the filamentous branching bacteria and isolation using nutrient agar or blood agar is done for confirmation of the disease. Proper hygiene and sanitation measures reduce the frequency of disease. Disinfection of animal specifically lower limbs, proper udder hygiene should be done before and after milking to prevent the disease in animals. Drainage of abscess and treatment with penicillin and nalidixic acid are effective.

E. Protozoan Disease

1. Toxoplasmosis : The disease is caused by Toxoplasma gondii and affects all warm blooded animals like cattle, buffalo, sheep, goat, pig, horse, camel, dog, cat, monkey, rodent and man. The disease is worldwide in distribution but more prevalent in warm, moist climate than cold and dry climate. The principal host is cat in which the organism reproduces sexually and the cysts are shed in faeces of cat and spread the disease to other animals and man. The disease may be transmitted through contaminated food, undercooked meat and meat products, milk, water, inhalation, through semen and by transplacental routes.

Congenital as well as acquired infection occurs in man. There may be abortion, premature birth, hydrocephaly, microcephaly, hepatomegaly, spleenomegaly, fever, icterus, blindness, epileptic convulsion, cerebral calcification and mental retardation in congenital infection. In case of acquired infection, there may be pyrexia, lymphadenopathy, headache, stiff neck, pain in joints and maculopapular rash. The disease is more important in immunocompromised persons as the dormant cyst in the body of such individuals can alive again, may show cerebral illness and ultimately death. Fever, dyspnea, pneumonia, diarrhoea, enteritis, ataxia, encephalitis, bilirubinaemia, abortion, still birth and death has been reported in animals.

The diagnosis is difficult on the basis of only clinical signs. The organism can be observed microscopically in CSF, body fluid and tissue with the help of Giemsa stain. Isolation of organism can be done in embryonated eggs, mice or in tissue culture. Sabin-Feldman dye test, indirect fluorescent antibody test, indirect haemagglutination test, CFT and intradermal skin test are employed for diagnosis of Toxoplasmosis.

Avoidance of cats, hygienic practices for drinking water and foods, proper cooking of meat and restriction on consumption of raw meat, and restriction of flies and cockroach to access foods are the important measures. SDDS (sulphadiamino diphenyl sulfone) is the most effective drug. Pyrimethamine, sulphonamides, spiramycin, barnerine, clindamycin are also tried but there is no satisfactory treatment against this disease with success.

It is mandatory to break the cycle of causative agent by interfering at reservoir level or its transmission to prevent and control any infectious disease. The same is true for rodent related diseases. The control of rodents has to be adopted by reducing their population and by avoiding the direct or indirect contact of rodents to human population, domestic animals and the materials used by them.

Control of Rodents

Different strategies have to be evolved for control of rodents depending upon agro climatic zones and physiographic conditions, type and density of rodents, type of operations at farm and residential area. The following measures in general have to be adopted for effective control of rodents:

Sanitation

Good sanitation is essential for not only the control of rodents but also the vectors transmitting infectious agents. Dirty and jungle areas are attractive habitats to rodents. Therefore, the weeds, bushes, jungles surrounding the residential area and livestock farms should be regularly cleaned. Elimination of nesting sites of rodents helps to reduce the population of rodent. There should not be any place where rodents could hide, nest or rest in and around human dwellings, animal farms, store houses and feed processing house particularly feed store houses. Feed should be always stored in containers wherever possible.

Rodent Proof Constructions

The rodent proof buildings should be constructed as far as possible. All the openings and holes in building should be sealed with durable materials. Steel wool can be used to seal the openings tightly. The edges should be covered with metal to prevent gnawing by rodents. A layer of heavy gravel can be constructed along the perimeter of buildings to discourage the burrowing of rodents. Rodents normally use the same pathways to move from place-to-place. So, these runways should be identified and broken and cleaned properly.

Reduction of Rodent Population

Population reduction becomes necessary in the area heavily populated by rodents. It can be done by trapping and poisoning. Trapping is one of the effective measures to reduce or control the rodent population. It is simple and inexpensive method but requires skill and labour. Traps are set along with bait of feed tied to the trigger close to walls behind feed stuff in dark corners and in places actively inhabited by rodents. Poisons along with bait are offered to rodents to kill them. The rodents get attracted to the bait, eat and die. Tracking powders are used specifically around the perimeter of the rodent nest and in buildings or structures. A very small amount of these poisons is required to cause lethality in rodents. Generally two types of rodenticides are used : (*i*) Single dose and (*ii*) Multiple doses.

Single dose poisons like barium carbonate, zinc phosphide, red squill, norbromide, sodium fluoroacetate, aluminium phosphide, fluoroacetamide, strychnine, arsenic trioxide, rodenticide phosphorus, thallium sulphate, etc cause acute poisoning. In India, mainly zinc phosphide, aluminium phosphide and barium carbonate are used; other acute rodenticides are not in much use because of their toxicity and efficacy problems (Parshad, 1999). Occasionally, a phosphorous based rodenticides 'Ratol' containing inorganic phosphorous is used in the fields. Zinc phosphide is effective against all species of rats and mice. It remains one of the most widely-used rodenticides due to its fairly good safety records, low cost and reasonably high effectiveness against rodents (Chow, 1971). It rapidly breaks down into less hazardous phosphine gas in the presence of acid in rodents' gut, unlikely to cause secondary poisoning because of its degradability (Solymar, 2001).

Multiple dose (cumulative) rodenticides poisons include anticoagulant compounds. These compounds must be fed repeatedly to become effective (4-6 days). Death from these compounds results from internal bleeding and can take from 1-10 days after the initial poisoning. They act by depressing the hepatic vitamin K dependant synthesis of substance, prothrombin, essential to blood clotting, which subsequently increases capillaries permeability leading to widespread internal hemorrhages. These compounds have been used widely and successfully for control of rodents. The degree of toxic hazards to animals and human is low. Many formulations of anticoagulants are available. The anticoagulant rodenticides-warfarin, diphacinone and chlorophacinone are slow acting and antidote, vitamin K1, is available. Newer anticoagulants, brodifacum and bromadiolone can cause death in a single feeding. In India, the first anticoagulants have long been available but have not gained popular acceptance because of its low toxicity and repeated feeding, however, among the newer anticoagulants, bromadiolone has been commercially available for the control of agricultural and commensal rodents (Parshad, 1999).

Fumigation

It is effective method to destroy both rodent and rodent fleas. A number of chemicals are used for fumigation. Those are calcium cyanide (also called as cyanogas or cymag), carbon disulphide, methyl bromide, sulphur dioxide etc. among these; cyanogas is extensively used that is pumped into the rat burrows by a special pump. Calcium cyanide releases hydrocyanic acid gas (HCN) when contact with air.

Chemosterilants

The chemicals are used to make the rodents sterile temporarily or permanently in either sex or both. A number of chemicals have been evaluated against several species of Indian rodents. Alpha-chlorohydrin was found to be most susceptible to *B. bengalensis*, the most predominant species of field rodents in India (Saini and Parshad, 1999).The synthetic steroids like ethinyl oestradiol, methyl testosterone or Org 5933 were evaluated as potential chemosterilants for rodent control and methyl testosterone was found to be more effective (Gao and Short, 1993).

Biological Control

Biological control involves the use of predators like cats, mangoose, varanid, weasel, owl, etc., parasites and pathogens. Use of parasites or pathogens as bio-control agents has been ignored because of possible potential health risk to livestock and humans. However, use of predators like barn owls has been reported in Bangladesh and India (Parshad, 1999).

Conclusion

Though the accurate figures for actual damage caused by rodents are not available, it is true that rodents damage and consume vast quantities of food in agriculture fields and storage houses. The losses have been reported up to 25% in some of the countries. The rodents act as reservoir to important infectious agents and contaminate the environment causing health hazards to human and animals. Strategic preventive and control measures are required to check these losses to mankind. The well established and organized surveillance system for rodent related diseases can be of immense help for timely warning. The rapid response teams should be set up at local, district, state and national levels along with motivation of people for properly managing outbreaks of such diseases and control of rodents. There should be long term and short term plans for control of rodent population in accordance to the ecological factors and occurrence of rodents in a particular area or region.

REFERENCES

Alexander A.D. 1991, Leptospira. In: Manual of clinical microbiology: Eds. Balows A, Hausler W.J., Hermann K.L., senberg H.D. and Shadomy H.J. 5th edition. Washington, D.C. American Society for Microbiology.

Chow C.Y. 1971. The Biology and Control of the Norway Rat, Roof Rat and House Mouse. World Health Organization, WPR/165/71, 1-22.

Corbet GB and Hill JE. 1986. A world list of mammalian species. London. (Cited from VC Agarwal and Ishwar Prakash 1992. Ecological distribution of Indian rodents. In Rodents in Indian Agriculture, Vol 1. Eds. Ishwar Prakash and PK Ghosh, Scientific Publishers, Jodhpur.

Gao Y and Short RV. 1993. Use of an oestrogen, androgen or gestagen as a potential chemosterilant for control of rat and mouse populations. J-Reprod-Fertil. 97 (1) : 39-49.

Parshad VR. 1999. Rodent control in India. Integrated Pest Management Reviews 4 : 97-126.

Pathak KA and Kumar DK. 2000. Bamboo flowering and rodent outbreak in north eastern hill region of India. Indian J Hill Farmg. 13 : 3-7.

Saini MS and Parshad VR. 1988. Evaluation of a toxicantsterilant; alpha-chlorohydrin, for the control of Indian mole rat *Bandicota bengalensis*. *Ann. Appl. Biol*. 113, 307–12.

Solymar B. 2001. Rodent management on farms and in new tree planting to prevent accidental poisonings of raptors and other non-target Wildlife. http://www. bsc-eoc.org/ download/Rodent.

WHO. 2003. Human leptospirosis: Guidance for diagnosis, surveillance and control. World Health Organization, Geneva.

27

GLOBAL PREVALENCE OF ROTAVIRUS AND NOROVIRUS AND THEIR GENOTYPIC DIVERSITY IN INDIA

Z.B. Dubal, K.N. Bhilegaonkar and Shriya Rawat

Diarrhoeal diseases are major cause of childhood morbidity and mortality all over the world. Many pathogenic bacteria like *E. coli, Salmonella, Shigella* etc. and enteric viruses like rotavirus, norovirus, astrovirus, enterovirus etc. are responsible for gastroenteritis. Of the enteric viruses, rotavirus and norovirus have been recognized as the most common cause of severe gastroenteritis in a wide variety of animal species worldwide. In low income countries, diarrhoea is the third most common cause of death with 17% deaths is under 5 yrs age group (WHO, 2004). In India, annually 18.6 million children under 5 yrs are affected with nearly 3,86,000 deaths. The two enteric viruses i.e. rotavirus and norovirus, though contributing a major chunk of these diarrhoeagenic agents, are neglected especially in India. Both are RNA viruses with rotavirus (family Reoviridae) possessing 11 segments of dsRNA, while norovirus (family Caliciviridae) has ssRNA as the genetic material. Rotavirus infection is mainly encountered in very young animals and children below five years of age, whereas norovirus affects all age groups and is usually associated with food-borne outbreaks in cafeterias, hospitals, ships etc.

ROTAVIRUS AND NOROVIRUS

Rotavirus has a distinct wheel like appearance by negative staining electron microscopy (EM) and thus the name *rota* which in Latin means "wheel". The virus particles are about 70 nm in diameter and posses icosahedral symmetry. They have triple layer capsid, the innermost layer of which, the core, contains the viral genome. This genome consisting of 11 segments of dsRNA that code for 6 structural proteins (VP1, VP2, VP3, VP4, VP6 and VP7), and 6 non-structural proteins (NSP1-NSP6). However, gene segment 11 encoding both NSP5 and NSP6 proteins. They are classified into seven different group (A-G) based on the antigenic specificity of the VP6 capsid proteins, as well as the pattern of the electrophoretic mobility of the 11 dsRNA segments of viral genome (Ramani and Kang, 2007) (Fig. 27.1). Of these seven groups, only group A, B and C are known to infect human and animals whereas, group D-G found only in animals (Broor *et al.*, 2003). Group A rotaviruses are consider as an important viral diarrhoeal agents in children and young animals worldwide which can be further typed based on the outer capsid proteins that elicit neutralizing antibodies-VP7 (G serotypes) and VP4 (P serotypes) or based on sequence comparison as G genotypes and P genotypes. Thus, because of two surface proteins which carry neutralizing specific antigens, a dual classification has been established. Group A rotaviruses have been characterized as possessing 15 G and 21 P genotypes (Das *et al.*, 2002). However, to date, 23 distinct G genotypes and 31 P genotypes have been identified (Mukherjee *et al.*, 2010). Genotype P[27] was recently identified from porcine origin (Khamrin *et al.*, 2008).

Norovirus (NoV) is non-enveloped, 27 to 40 nm in diameter with single-stranded, positive-sense, polyadenylated RNA virus (Fig. 27.2) with genome of 7.4 to 7.7 Kb and buoyant density of 1.33 to 1.41 g/cm^3. Noroviruses (NoVs) have been divided into seven genogroups (GI-GVII) based on genome sequence variability of their RNA dependent RNA polymerase (RdRp) and capsid protein of which, 5 genogroups (G) *viz.*, NoV GI, GII, GIV, GVI and GVII have been associated with human gastroenteritis (Phan *et al.*, 2007; Vinje *et al.*, 2004). To date, molecular characterization of NoVs has revealed 16 genotypes of GI, 23 genotypes of GII, 2 genotypes each of GIII and GVI, but only 1 genotype of GIV, GV, and GVII. The genome of NoVs comprises of 3 Outer Reading Frames (ORFs) *viz.* ORF1 encodes six nonstructural polyproteins [p48, NTPase, p22, VPg, 3CL and RdRp], ORF2 encodes the major capsid protein [VP1] and ORF3 encodes the minor structural protein [VP2] (Hardy, 2005, Glass *et al.*, 2000).

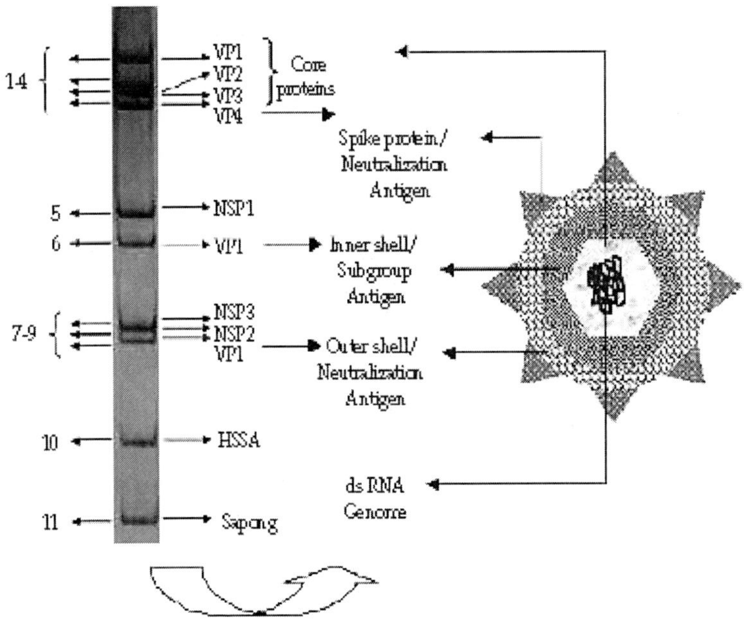

Fig. 27.1 : Structure of rotavirus coding 11 RNA segment (left) and schematic diagram of rotavirus (right).

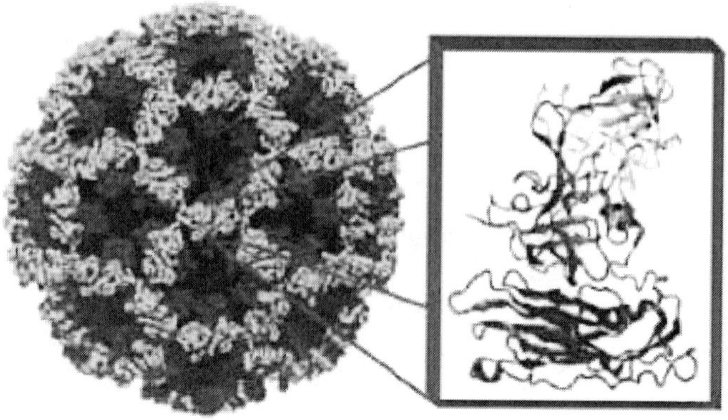

Fig. 27.2 : Structure of norovirus

PREVALENCE OF ROTAVIRUS AND NOROVIRUS IN HUMANS AND ANIMALS

Worldwide Prevalence

Of all rotavirus types, rotavirus A which is endemic worldwide, accounts for more than 90% of gastroenteritis in humans. In Asia, >55% of all rotavirus disease-associated deaths have been estimated to occur because of large population centres and some of the most populated countries of low socio economic status (Parashar *et al.*, 2003). Virtually every child experiences rotavirus gastroenteritis during the first few years of life. Boys are twice as likely to be admitted to hospital as girls. Overall, 95% of sick children were <2 years of age, of these 65% were boys and 35% were girls. The incidence of rotavirus was 56.8 and 151 cases/1000 childrens <5 yr of age in Republic of Korea and China, respectively (Kim *et al.*, 2005, Wang *et al.*, 2005). The incidence of rotavirus has also been reported from Japan, Thailand and other countries with varied prevalence rate. An outbreak caused by contaminated municipal water occurred in Colorado in 1981 (Hopkins *et al.*, 1984). During 2005, the largest recorded epidemic of diarrhoea occurred in Nicaragua. Similar large outbreak occurred in Brazil in 1977 (Linhare *et al.*, 1981). Rotavirus B, also called adult diarrhoea rotavirus or ADRV, has caused major epidemics of severe diarrhoea affecting thousands of people of all ages in China. These epidemics occurred as a result of sewage contamination of drinking water (Hung *et al.*, 1984).

Rotavirus has been shown to infect mammals (for example, apes, cattle, pigs, sheep, rats, cats and dogs, mice, rabbits) and birds (chickens and turkeys). There is evidence that animal rotaviruses can infect humans, either by direct transmission of the virus or by contributing one or several RNA segments to reassortants with human strains (Cook *et al.*, 20004, Muller *et al.*, 2007). Porcine rotaviruses have been detected by many countries with different prevalence rate. It is highly prevalent in Mexico, USA, Europe and Thailand. It is also reported from other countries like Australia, Quebec, Canada, India etc. (Ramani and Kang, 2007). Similarly bovine rotaviruses were also reported from many countries with varying prevalence rates.

NoV causes approximately 90% of epidemic non-bacterial outbreaks of gastroenteritis around the world(CDC, 2001), and responsible for 50% of all food-borne outbreaks of gastroenteritis in the US. In countries like Netherlands and England, NoVs have been reported to account for 5-17% of cases of diarrhoea. In a 5 year (1998-2002) study in Finland, norovirus was incriminated in 60.6% of viral gastroenteritis cases. NV has been shown to be a common cause of "traveler's diarrhoea". In an evaluation of 124 travelers to Mexico who had acute diarrhoea, NoV were the second most commonly identified pathogen in diarrhoeal stool samples (21/124, 17%), exceeded only by enterotoxigenic *Escherichia coli* (50/106, 47%) (Ko *et al.*, 2005). Norovirus infected cases were also reported from United Kingdom, Australia and France with varied prevalence rate (6.5-53%) (Kirkwood *et al.*, 2005). Malawi, China, Vietnam, Mongolia, and India have reported NoVs associated with 6-25% of acute gastroenteritis cases. GII-4 strains which are widely distributed in the world and have recently caused multiple outbreaks in Europe, Asia, and Australia (Bull *et al.*, 2006).

Bovine norovirus (BoNVs) genotype 1 and 2 have been identified in UK, Netherlands and the USA. In The Netherlands,

31.6% of pooled stool specimens from veal calf farms and 4.2% of individual stool specimens from dairy cattle were positive for NoVs related to the Newbury virus (Vander *et al.*, 2003). The variable faecal prevalence of 8-72% of BoNVs infection in diarrhoeic calves has been reported from UK, Ohio, USA and South Korea with the leading strain being GIII/2 BoNVs (Park *et al.*, 2007). The detection rate of swine NoVs in Japan was low (0.35%), and a similar low detection rate (2%) was reported in The Netherlands (Vander *et al.*, 2003). Porcine NoV detected in Japan, the Netherlands, and the United States is closely related to the human NoV. Furthermore, human NoV can replicate and induce an immune response in gnotobiotic pigs, which indicates that swine could serve as a reservoir for human NoV. In addition, the genetic similarity between human and swine NoV strains raises the possibility that porcine-human recombinants could emerge during co-infection of the same host (Wang *et al.*, 2005). Similarly, bovine NoVs can also produce recombinants as human NoVs. Thus, a cow co-infected with both bovine and human strains of NoV could conceivably produce a recombinant virus with altered virulence properties. It was also detected in 1.6% of bovine fecal samples from Canada (Mattison *et al.*, 2007). Partial genome sequence revealed GII.4 genotype. They also found one raw pork sample to be positive for NoV of the GII.4 cluster. The findings suggested that NoV may have a zoonotic route of transmission to humans (Wang *et al.*, 2005). However, infected humans may pass the virus to livestock as well, and some outbreaks of gastroenteritis in farm animals may be prevented by controlling the access of ill workers to livestock.

Prevalence in India

Since almost every child in India is infected with rotavirus, the deaths due to rotaviral diarrhoea represent 5% of all deaths occurring among children <5 years of age and 1 death among every 250 children born. The prevalence of rotavirus diarrhoea in India has been found to vary from 5-71% in hospitalized children less than 5 yr of age with acute gastroenteritis. The prevalence of childhood rotavirus in the north Indian cities of

Delhi, Chandigarh and Aligarh has been reported to vary from 6-45% (Jain *et al.*, 2001, Singh *et al.*, 1990). It was detected from acute gastroenteritis cases of children <5 yrs of age from Chandigarh (16-19%) (Sharma *et al.*, 1994) and Aligarh (19%)(Malik *et al.*,1987). The samples from children of Deharadun and Bareilly revealed the prevalence rate of 36.5% by Reverse Transcription-Polymerase Chain Reaction (RT-PCR) (Rawat, 2009). In the western states of India, in Pune, rotavirus was detected in 28-30% of children <5 yr of age with acute diarrhoea (Kelkar *et al.*, 1999, Ghosh *et al.*, 1991). In eastern India, in Kolkata the incidence of rotavirus associated diarrhoea varied from 5-22%. On the other hand, in Manipur the incidence was as high as 41% (Jain *et al.*, 2001). In southern India, rotavirus was detected in 17.8% of children with acute gastroenteritis with the peak prevalence in December to February and June to August in Vellore, 20.8% in Chennai and 16-22% in Bangalore (Brown *et al.*, 1988, Ananthan and Sarvanan, 2000). In 1985, an outbreak of asymptomatic rotavirus infections was observed in the new-borne unit of All India Institute of Medical Sciences (AIIMS) in New Delhi, India. The infections were clearly nosocomial (Jayashree *et al.*, 1988). In 1997 and 1998, group B rotaviruses were identified as the cause of sporadic cases of diarrhoeal disease in adults in Kolkata, India, representing the first description of cases of human group B rotavirus disease outside China (Krishnan *et al.*,1999).

Very limited work has been carried out about animal rotaviruses in India leading to the overall prevalence rate of 10-75%. In Hisar, 20-60% prevalence of rotaviruses was reported in bovine calves (Mittal *et al.*, 1986, Singh and Pandey, 1990, Gulati *et al.*, 1995). However, in Pantnagar and Bareilly, the overall 11-35% prevalence has been reported for bovine calves (Kumar, 2006). The prevalence of 17.1% and 25.0% of rotavirus reported in cattle farm located in Ambala (Haryana) and Meerat (U.P.), respectively (Grover *et al.*, 1988). Though the prevalence of rotavirus in diarrhoeic cattle and children is well documented in India, asymptomatic, carrier and atypical cases are still not well investigated. Prevalence of 8.08% from healthy calves, 18.8% in diarrhoeic calves, 2.4-12.3% in asymptomatic children and 4.0-29.3% in symptomatic cases of children are reported in India. Recently, bovine rotavirus genotypes have also been reported from Kashmir (Wani *et al.*, 2004). In case of piglets, marginal work carried out in India has shown prevalence of 10 and 10.26% by SDS-PAGE in Banglore and Ranchi, respectively (Sarkar and Soman, 1989; Jhala and Raghavan, 1996), whereas in NEH region, it was 30.0% by SDS-PAGE and/or RT-PCR (Dubal, Z.B, 2009).

In India, studies have been carried out on human norovirus at AIIMS New Delhi, CMC Vellore, NICED Kolkata and NIV Pune and the prevalence is 8-15% (Girish *et al.*, 2008, Chabra and Chitambar, 2008). A serological and molecular study from southern India described the presence of NoVs in 8% of sporadic cases of acute gastroenteritis (Kang *et al.*, 2000). A study conducted in Vellore, South India showed 68 (19.4%) samples were positive for human Caliciviruses (HuCVs), 18 (5.1%) for Sapoviruses (SaV) and 53 (15.1%) for NoV (Monica *et al.*, 2007) from 350 children hospitalized with diarrhoea. A recent study at AIIMS, New Delhi demonstrated HuCVs in 54 (24%) of 226 sporadic cases of acute gastroenteritis by RT-PCR of the RdRp gene (Girish *et al.*, 2008). In Pune, GII infection was detected in 11.9% (28/236) specimens. These included 24 of 192 (12.5%) specimens from hospitalized and 4 of 44 (9.0%) specimens from OPD case (Chabra and Chitambar, 2008). No report to date is available on animal norovirus infection in India.

GENOTYPIC DIVERSITY OF ROTAVIRUS AND NOROVIRUS IN HUMANS AND ANIMALS

Humans

In mixed infections with rotavirus, gene reassortment could theoretically lead to 110 different G and P combinations, but fortunately, this level of reassortment does not happen and only five strains are commonly detected (P[8]G1; P[4]G2; P[8]G3; P[8]G4; and P[8]G9) in humans all over the world. In most of the studies from India, the most prevalent strains are G1, G2, G3, G4 and G9 and P[8], P[6] and P[4], however, some other G types such as G6, G8, G10 and G12 have also been recently identified as cause of diarrhoea. The common worldwide strains G1P[8], G2P[4], G3P[8], and G4P[8] were underrepresented among Indian children (33%), whereas strains of P type [6] G1P[6], G2P[6], G3P[6], G4P[6], and G9P[6], which primarily infect asymptomatic newborns but are rare in children with diarrhoea were common in India (43%). A number of uncommon genotypes, G1P[4] (4%), G2P[8] (2.5%), G2P[6] (0.6%), G4P[4] (2.5%), and G4P[6] (1.25%), were also observed. Twenty two per cent of specimens showed mixed infections, and 24 per cent of the total samples remained untypeable. In very recent study at IVRI, Bareilly revealed the identifications of G11P[6] and G11P[8] genotypic combinations which are rarely observed in humans all over the world and were not yet reported from India (Dubal Z.B, 2009). Characterization of rotaviral isolates in another study indicated the predominance of P[6] type in combination with G1, G2 and G12 types in human (Rawat, 2009). The genotypic diversity of rotaviral strains from world verses India are depicted in Fig. 27.3 (Gulati *et al.*,1998).

Full genomic analysis of a human group A rotavirus G9P[6] strain from Eastern India provides evidence for porcine-to-human interspecies transmission. On sequencing of fourth gene segment of rotavirus strain 116E, isolated from asymptomatically infected neonates in Delhi revealed that, this gene is closely related to VP4 gene of bovine B223 strain (P[11]) at both nucleotide (90.8% identity) and amino acid (92.2% identity) levels. Similarly, another strain isolated from asymptomatic neonates from Bangalore (strain I321) belongs to G10, where both VP4 and VP7 genes were highly homologues to the respective genes of serotype 10 of bovine rotavirus B223 (G10P[11]) strain (Das *et al.*, 1993). Another two strains *i.e.* G9P[11] from North India and G10P[11] from South India had high incidence in asymptomatic neonates showed that the gene encoding VP7 of G10 strain was closely related to neonatal asymptomatic strain I321 and also with the sequence derived from bovine strains isolated in India. Whereas, the P[11] sequences are highly conserved and were 90% homologues at nucleotide level to strain I321 and to bovine rotavirus isolate from Japan (Das *et al.*, 1993, Itturizza *et al.*, 2004).

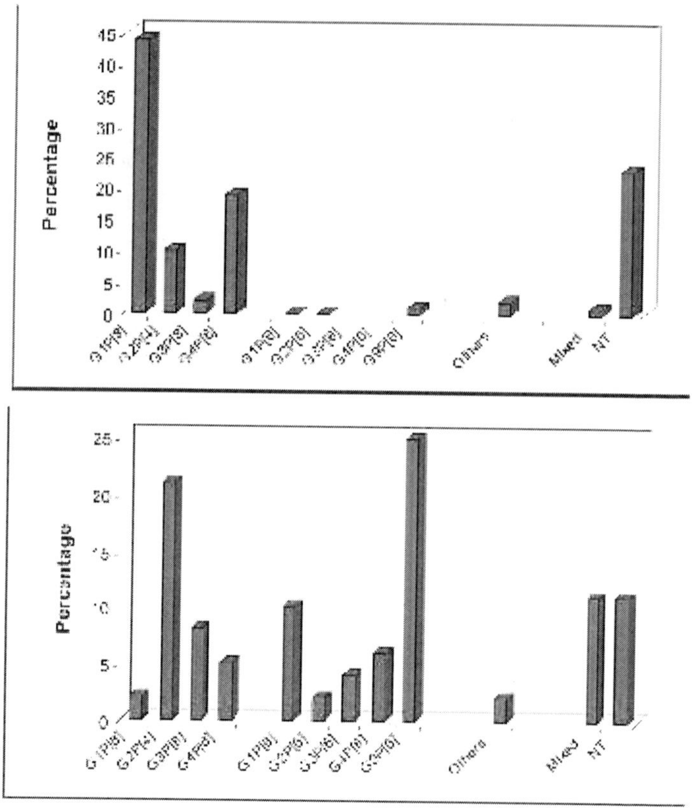

Fig. 27.9 : Human G and P genotypes of rotaviruses : World verses India

In a study from Vellore, South India, 7 genotypes of norovirus were found, all but one within genogroup II. The only genogroup I strain found was a GI-3 in a co-infection with a GII-2 strain. GII-4 was the most frequently identified genotype, followed by GII-2, while in the hospital GII3 was the most frequently identified genotype followed by GII-1 and GII-4 in equal.

A recent study at AIIMS, New Delhi demonstrated HuCVs in 24% sporadic cases of acute gastroenteritis by RT-PCR of the HuCVs identified, GGII of NoVs were the most predominant strains 34/59 (58%), followed by GI of SaVs 22/59 (37%), GI of NoVs 2/59 (3.3%), and GGII of SaV 1/59 (1.7%). Five samples had mixed infections with GII of NoVs and GI of SaVs (Girish *et al.*, 2008). In Pune, nucleotide sequence based analysis of GII strains indicated circulation of GIIb strains at a significant level in hospitalized (12.5%) and OPD (75%) children (Chabra and Chitambar, 2008). Recently, a new variant of Norovirus GII.4/2007 and inter-genotype recombinant strains of NVGII causing acute watery diarrhoea among children was detected from Kolkata, India (Nayak *et al.*, 2009, Mukharjee *et al.*, 2009)

Animals

In bovines, G6 and G10 among the G types and P[1] and P[11] among the P types are recognized as most common types circulated rotaviruses all over the world (Gouvea *et al.*, 1994, Minakshi *et al.*, 2005, Fukai *et al.*, 1999). In porcines, G5, G11, P[6] and P[7] constitute as the major rotavirus genotypes, distributed all over the world. Some of the human and other animal strains also been isolated and reported from bovines and porcines *viz.* G1, G2, G3, G6, G7, G8, G9, G10 and G11 (Minakshi *et al.*, 2005) and P[6], P[8], P[13], P[14], P[19], P[23] and P[26] (Maneekarn *et al.*, 2006). In case of animals, limited genotyping of bovine rotaviruses leads to the identification of G6P[14], G10P[14]; G10P[11], G6P[1] and G10(Ghosh *et al.*, 2007, Gulati *et al.* 1999). None to marginal work on porcine rotaviruses leads to the identification of P[25] from Kolkata (NICED, Annual report 2004-05). In another study, G4P[6] genotype was identified from piglet which is more commonly found in human beings. Genetic analysis of *VP7* and *VP4* genes of this G4P[6] isolate revealed very close association with human rotavirus strains which provides evidence for human-to-porcine interspecies transmission (Dubal, Z.B, 2009).

NoVs also cause diarrhoea in animals with genogroup GII reported in pigs and GIII in cattle. The porcine strains are very closely related to the human strains and there are reports of reassortants. However, no reports are available for animal NoVs in India.

REFERENCES

Ananthan, S. and Saravanan, P., *Indian J. Med. Res.*, 2000, **111**, 50-56.

Brown, D.W.G., Mathan, M.M., Mathew, M., Martin, R., Beards, G.M. and. Mathan, V.I., *J. Clin. Microbiol.*, 1988, **26**, 2410-2414.

Broor, S., Ghosh, D. and Mathur, P. *Indian J. Med. Res.*, 2003, **118**, 59-67.

Bull, R.A., Tu, E.T. and McIver, C.J., *J. Clin. Microbiol.*, 2006, **44**, 327-333.

Cook N., Bridger, J., Kendall, K., Gomara, M.I., El-Attar, L. and Gray, J., *J. Infect.*, 2004, **48**, 289-302.

Chhabra, P. and Chitambar, S., *J. Clin. Virol.*, 2008, **42**, 429-432.

Das, S., Sen, A., Uma, G., Varghese, V., Chaudhuri, S., Bhattacharya, S.K. Krishnan, T., Dutta, P., Dutta, D., Bhattacharya, M.K., Mitra, U., Kobayashi, N. and Naik, T.N., *J. Clin. Microbiol.*, 2002, 40, 146-149.

Das, M., Dunn, S.J., Woode, G.N., Greenberg, H.B. and Rao, C.D., *Virol.*, 1993, **194**, 374-379.

Dubal, Z.B., 2009, Ph.D. Thesis submitted to Indian Veterinary Research Institute (IVRI), Izatnagar, Bareilly, U.P.

Fukai, K., Sakai, T. Hirose, M. and Itou, T., *Vety. Microbiol.*, 1999, 66, 301-311.

Glass, P.J., White, L.J., Ball, J.M., Leparc-Goffart, I., Hardy, M.E. and Estes, M.K., *J. Virol.*, 2000, **74**, 6581-6591.

Ghosh, A.R., Nair, G.B., Dutta, P., Pal, S.C. and Sen, D., *Trans R Soc Trop Med Hyg.*, 1991, **85**, 796-782

Ghosh, S., Varghese, V., Samajdar, S., Sinha, M. and Naik, T.N., *J. Clin. Microbiol.*, 2007, **45**, 2751–2753.

Girish, R., Choudekar, A., Broor, S., Bhatnagar, S., Parveen, S. and Patwari, A., *J. Clin. Virol.*, 2008, **43**, 42-48.

Gouvea, V., Santos, N. and Timenetsky, M.C., *J. Clin. Microbiol.*, 1994, **32**, 1333-1340.

Minakshi, Prasad, G., Malik, Y. and Pandey, R., Indian J. Biotech., 2005, 4, 93-99.

Grover, Y.P., Minakshi, Patnaik, D.P. and Pandey, R., *Indian J. Comp. Microbiol. Infect. Dis.*, 1998, **19**, 121-123.

Gulati, B. R., Maherchandani, S. and Pandey, R., *Indian J. Virol.*, 1995, 11, 7-12.

Gulati, B.R., Patnaik, D.P., Singh, R. and Pandey, R., *Indian J. Anim. Sci.*, 1998, **68**, 781-792.

Gulati, B.R., Nakagomi, O., Koshimura, Y., Nakagomi, T. and Pandey, R., *J. Clin. MIcrobiol.*, 1999, **37**, 2074-2076.

Hardy, M.E., *FEMS Microbiol. Lett.*, 2005, **253**, 1-8.

Hopkins, R.S., Gaspard, G.B., Williams, F.P., Karlin, R.J., Cukor, G. and Blacklow, N.R., *Am. J. Pub. Health*, 1984, **74**, 263–265.

Hung, T., Chen, G.M., Wang, C.G., Yao H.L., Fang Z.Y., Chao T.X., Chou Z.Y., Ye W., Chang X.J., Den, S.S., *Lancet*, 1984, **1**, 1139-1142.

Iturriza Gomara, M., Kang, G., Mammen, A., Jana, A.K., Abraham, M., Desselberger, U., Brown, D. and Grayi, J., *J. Clin. Microbiol.*, 2004, **42**, 2541-2547.

Jain, V., Parashar, U.D., Glass, R.I. and Bhan, M.K. *Indian J. Pediatr.*, 2001, **68**, 855-862.

Jayashree, S., Bhan, M.K. and Raj, P., *Scand. J. Infect. Dis.*, 1988, **20**, 249-253.

Jhala, M.K. and Raghavan, R. *In Proc. XVII Annual Conference of IAVMI.*, Bhubaneshwar, 1996, pp. 16-18.

Kang, G., Hale, A.D., Richards, A.F., Jesudason, M.V., Estes, M.K. and Brown, D.W.G. *Trans. R. Soc. Trop. Med. Hyg.*, 2000, **94**, 681–683.

Kelkar, S.D., Purohit, S.G. and Sinha, K.V., *Indian J. Med. Res.*, 1999, **109**, 131-135.

Kim, J.S., Kang, J.O., Cho, S.C., Jang, Y.T. Min, S.A., Park, T.H., Nyambat,B., Gentsch, D.S. Bresee, J.S., Christopher Mast, T. and Kilgore P.E., *J. Infect. Dis.*, 2005, **192**, 549-552.

Khamrin, P., Maneekarn, N., Peerakome, S., Okitsu, S., Mizuguchi, M., and Ushijima, H. *Emerg. Infect. Dis.*, 2008, **14**, 985-986.

Kirkwood, C.D., Clark, R., Bogdanovic-Sakran, N. and Bishop, R.F., *J. Med. Virol.*, 2005, **77**, 96-101.

Ko, G., Garcia, C. and Jiang, Z.D., *J. Clin. Microbiol.*, 2005, **43**, 6126-6129.

Krishanan, T., Sen, A., Chaudhury, J.S., Das, S., Naik, T.N and Bhattacharya, S.K., *Lancet*, 1999, **353**, 380-381.

Kumar, M., 2006, M.V.Sc. Thesis submitted to Indian Veterinary Research Institute (IVRI), Izatnagar, Bareilly, U.P.

Linhares, A.C., Pinheiro, F.P., Freitas, R.B., Gabbay, Y.B., Shirley, J.A. and Beards, G.M., *Am. J. Epidemiol.*, 1981, **113**, 703–710.

Malik, A., Rattan, A. Malik, M.S. and Shukla, I., *J. Trop. Pediatr.*, 1987, **33**, 243-245.

Maneekarn, N., Khamrin, P., Chan-it, W., Peerakome, S., Sukchai, S. and Pringprao, K., *J. Clin. Microbiol.*, 2006, 44, 4113–4119.

Mattison, K., Shukla, A., Cook, A., Pollari, F., Friendship, R., Kelton, D., Bidawid., S. and Farber, J.M., *Emer. Infect. Dis.*, 2007, **13**, 1184-1188.

Mittal, S.K., Srivastava, R.N. and Prasad, S., *Indian J. Ani. Sci.*, 1986, **56** : 1127-1131.

Monica, B., Ramani, S., Banerjee, I., Primrose, B., Iturriza-Gomara, M. And Gallimore, C.I., *J. Med. Virol.*, 2007, **79**, 544-551.

Mukherjee, A., Singh, Ng. B. and Chawla-Sarkar, M., *In Proceedings of 97th Indian Science Congress*, Jan. 3-7, 2010. pp 105.

Muller, H. and Johne, R., Berl. Munch. Tierarztl. Wochenschr., 2007, **120**, 108–112.

CDC, *MMWR*, 2001, **50**, 1-17.

Mukherjee, A., Dutta, D., Ghosh, S., Bagchi, P., Chattopadhyay, S., Nagashima, S., Kobayashi, N., Dutta, P., Krishnan, T., Naik, T.N. and Chawla-Sarkar, M., *Arch. Virol.*, 2009, **154**, 733-46.

Maunula, L., Miettinen, I.T. and von Bonsdorff, C.H., *J. Infect. Dis.*, **11**, 1716-1721.

Nayak, M.K., Chatterjee, D., Nataraju, S.M., Pativada, M., Mitra, U., Chatterjee, M.K., Saha, T.K., Sarkar, U. and Krishnan, T., *J. Clin. Virol.*, 2009, **45**, 223-229.

Parashar, U.D., Hummelman, E.G. and Bresee, J.S., *Emerg. Infect. Dis.*, 2003, **9**, 565-572.

Park, S.I., Jeong, C., Park, S.H., Kim, S.K., Park, S.J., Kim, H.H., Hyun, B.H., Cho, K.O., Kang, M.I. and Yang, D.K., *Vet. Microbiol.*, 2007, **124**, 125-133.

Phan, T.G., Kaneshi, K., Ueda, Y., Nakaya, S., Nishimura, S. and Yamamoto, A.J. *Med. Virol.*, 2007, **79**, 1388-1400.

Ramani, S. and Kang, G., *Indian J. Med. Res.*, 2007, **125**, 619-632.

Rawat, S., 2009. M.V.Sc. Thesis submitted to Indian Veterinary Research Institute (IVRI), Izatnagar, Bareilly, U.P.

Sarkar, J.K. and Soman, J.B., *Virus Information Exchange Newsletter*, 1989, **6**, 157.

Sharma, P., Sehgal, R., Ganguly, N.K., Vaidyanathan, U. and Walia, B.N., *J. Trop. Pediatr.*, 1994, **40**, 58-59.

Singh, V., Broor, S., Mehta, S. and Mehta, S.K., *Indian J. Med. Res.*, 1990, **91**, 9-14.

Singh, A. and Pandey, R. *Indian J. Microbiol.*, 1990, **30**, 233-236.

Vinje, J., Hamidjaja, R.A. and Sobsey, M.D., *J. Virol. Meth.*, 2004, **116**, 109-117.

van der Poel, W.H., van der Heide, R., Verschoor, F., Gelderblom, H., Vinje, J. and Koopmans, M.P., *Vet. Microbiol.*, 2003, **92**, 297-309.

Wani, S.A., Bhat, M.A., Ishaq, S.M. and Ashrafi, M.A., *Rev. Off. Int. Epizoot.*, 2004, **23**, 931–936.

Wang, X.Y., Xu, Z.Y., Seidlein, L., Zhang, Y.L., Zhao, S.J., Hao, Z.Y., Han, O.P., Kilgore, P., Xing, Z.C., Han, C.Q., Ma, J.C., Chen, J.C. and Clemens, J., *J. Infect. Dis.*, 2005, **192**, S100-S105.

WHO, *World Health Report* 2004, Report of the Director General, WHO.